HERBS THAT HEAL

PRESCRIPTION FOR HERBAL HEALING

HERBS THAT HEAL

PRESCRIPTION FOR HERBAL HEALING

By

MICHAEL A. WEINER, Ph.D.
and JANET WEINER

A
QUANTUM
BOOK

HERBS THAT HEAL

PRESCRIPTION FOR HERBAL HEALING

BOTANICAL ILLUSTRATIONS COURTESY
OF NATURE'S HERBS, A TWINLAB AFFILIATED COMPANY

PUBLISHER:
QUANTUM BOOKS
6 KNOLL LANE
MILL VALLEY, CA 94941

Typesetting: WORDSWORTH, San Geronimo, CA

Library of Congress Cataloging in Publication Data
Card Number 93-086281

Weiner, Michael A.   ISBN 0-912845-11-2
Herbs That Heal: Prescription for Herbal Healing
448 pages, 135 illustrations, including references and indices
1. HERBS - Therapeutic use;
2. BOTANY - Medical

The purpose of this book is to provide an interesting and historical document to the general public concerning herbal remedies that have been used for centuries. In presenting this information, we neither suggest or recommend its use. Nor is this volume intended as a substitute for personal medical care. *Only a physician familiar with herbal medicine may prescribe the use of these remedies, and he or she should be consulted as to which remedies, and in what dosage, should be used.*

*For Becky & Russell
who gave us both the
faith, love & trust to
complete our beings.*

HERBS THAT HEAL
PRESCRIPTION FOR HERBAL HEALING

TABLE OF CONTENTS

INTRODUCTION

Herbs are everywhere! From India to Indiana, from the field to the consumers, herbs are now mainstream. From earliest recorded history, we know that herbal medicines helped to sustain Earth's peoples. Healing plants gathered from wet jungles to dry deserts still do serve as medicine for 90 percent of the world's population. Now we have seen the coming of the second "herbal revolution."

With the mass introduction of herbal capsules, people everywhere, even in hi-tech societies, are now enjoying the benefits of Earth's medicines. Industry sales tell the story. With growth of herb sales running about 30% more than each succeeding year for the past four or five years, we have hard evidence of the entry of herbs into almost every home, whether they be for cooking or for healing.

In the coming years as we enter the second millennium, we may expect even greater usage. With the entry of herbal preparations into supermarkets, drug stores, even convenience stores, people everywhere are seeking herbal relief for all the ills that plague them.

For aches and pains, Willow bark is a natural product that competes with aspirin and other analgesics. Why do people want this "old fashioned" remedy? Because Willow blocks pain without causing stomach bleeding.

Echinacea is sought and utilized by large groups of people now that they have learned that the root of this plant, the panacea of the Plains, may be our immune system's most powerful ally. Extracts have been shown to stimulate the human immune system directly while also destroying the germs of infection.

Ginkgo, which is now the leading prescription drug in Germany, will soon be taken by most Western elders as this ancient tree has been by Asians for nearly 3,000 years. The mounting body of research evidence points to outstanding effects of Ginkgo on many age-related disorders. By improving circulation, Ginkgo is a powerful treatment for restoring and boosting memory. A recent study published in a major scientific journal shows that an extract of this ancient botanical successfully restored erections to impotent men.

Instead of valium™ people will discover the calming effects of Passionflower and Valerian. These thousand-year-old tranquilizers are better because they calm without causing cellular damage. They are medicines that evolved with humankind.

Even conventional doctors are beginning to acknowledge that many of today's important pharmaceuticals have a rich ethnobotanical history. There is growing recognition that plants have contributed to medical therapy since the beginning of the world's civilizations. And, as people tire of the cost and damaging side-effects of prescription drugs, we will see the entry of herbal medicines into prescription drugs, again. Modified slightly they will be patented by pharmaceutical giants and marketed for their safety and efficacy. These phytopharmaceuticals, once our only drugs, will soon reappear in drug stores.

Herbs That Heal: Prescription for Herbal Healing is dedicated to this "second coming" of phytotherapy to educate the interested and serve as a backbone reference to the best plants intended for our use.

Mill Valley, California
June 1993

CHAPTER 1

THERAPEUTIC INDEX

BACTERIAL AND/OR FUNGAL INFECTIONS

BOILS

BREAKBONE FEVER (a tropical, "malaria-like" affliction)

SKIN PROBLEMS

CHAPTER 2

THE HISTORY OF HERBAL MEDICINE

L ong before the beginning of society, before the dawn of history, herbal medicine was man's first line of defense against the many ills and accidents that plagued us. Ancient humans learned from instinct, from the observation of animals, from birds, using leaves, earth, mud, and water. These were the first soothing applications. By trial, early humans learned which served them best. Eventually this knowledge was applied to helping others. Though the methods were basic and crude, several of today's medicines still spring from sources as simple as those which were within reach of ancient man.

In the earliest times, the application of these herbs and other healing substances, such as minerals, animal products, and extracts, were often accompanied by magical rites. While such spiritual rites still accompany the application of herbal medicine in the few primitive societies which remain, for most of mankind herbal medicine is today the only medicine available to treat their many ills. In the technological world in which we dwell, many of our most useful drugs are still connected to the early medical folklore of plants. Examples of these are reserpine from *Rauvolfia serpentina* (Indian snakeroot); digitoxin from *Digitalis purpurea* (Foxglove); quinine from *Cinchona* species (Peruvian bark); morphine from *Papaver somniferum* (opium poppy); cocaine from *Erythroxylon coca* (coca leaves); atropine from *Atropa belladonna* (deadly nightshade); and d-tubocurarine from *Strychnos* and other species (arrow poisons). These are but some of the useful drugs of today which have their roots in folk medicine and new experimental drugs, such as taxol from the Pacific Yew (*Taxus brevifolia*), which are showing enormous promise against certain forms of cancer. Others, of course, exist. And even in an age of synthetic pharmaceuticals approximately 25% of all prescription drugs sold in the United States are derived from a higher plant.

Mesopotamia, China, and Egypt

Ancient Mesopotamia, often called the cradle of civilization, provides us with the earliest known record of the practice of the art of medicine as we know it today. In those days medicine was largely herbal medicine. In this era, about 2600 B.C., the Babylonians already had a primitive form of medicine. The practitioners of healing in this era were priest, physician, and pharmacist all in one. Clay tablets describe early medical treatments and the first symptomology for illnesses as well as the prescription and the directions for compounding various remedies. Being the cradle of Western civilization as we know it, this early medicine in ancient Babylonia is thought to have spread to the neighboring countries along the caravan routes to and from India, Arabia, and Egypt.

Correspondingly during this same early period, in China people of the Hsia and Shang Dynasties employed similar methods to combat various diseases. In this early time the records we have show 36 names of diseases, but mention only prayers for healing with no reference to herbal treatments. While many other medical classics were thought to have been written in China, only the *Shan Hai Ching* survived. It dates from about 250 B.C. Another document is the *Hai Ching*, dating from 120 B.C. These records describe approximately 250 plants and animals in which only 68 are used as medicinals, 21 of which are from plants and 47 are from animals. Included in these early descriptions of herbal remedies are cinnamon, angelica, gambeer, peony, juju, dragon bone, and talc. Tracing the development of herbal medicine in China through contemporary times, we note a dictionary of Chinese herb drugs that was recently published by the People's Republic of China, which covers 5,767 various kinds of medicinal substances. In clinical practice, however, approximately 200 herbs including ginseng are most commonly used. In Japan, about 250 herbs are commonly used. Chinese herbology is a part of Chinese medicine and is a comprehensive system of health which teaches that health and disease are owing to the balance and imbalance of living forces acting alike on man and animals. Consequently, Chinese herbs are rarely utilized individually, but are always compounded in a carefully balanced mixture, aiming always to reestablish the inner harmony of the human organism.

Egyptian medicine dates from the Royal Courts of King Zoser in about 2900 B.C., but truly accurate records of medical practices have not been uncovered which date earlier than 1900 B.C. The best known and most important record of early drug making is the *Papyrus Ebers,* a sort of formulary or collection of various prescriptions, which contains about 800 different prescriptions and mentions 700 drugs of vegetable, mineral, and animal origin. In addition to formulas for inhalation, suppositories, gargles, snuffs, enemas, poultices, decoctions, infusions, pills, lotions, ointments, plastids, fumigations, we find that beer, milk, wine, and honey were common vehicles for most of the drugs that were mixed together. The Egyptian herbologist was very aware of beauty as well, for we find approximately 74 prescriptions pertaining to hair washes, dyes, oils, and depilatories. In ancient Egypt there were several echelons in the preparation of drugs. They were the gatherers and preparers of drugs and "chiefs of fabrication," or the equivalent of chief herbalists. They are thought to have worked in the "house of life."

Ancient Greece and Rome

Moving to ancient Europe, we focus on Theophrastus of Eresus, who was an early Greek philosopher, a natural scientist, and known as the father of botany. Theophrastus is still recognized today for his intensely accurate observations on all types of subjects including the botanical. He is credited as being one of the earliest scientific observers. It is in his *The History of Plants,* the ninth book, that we find him dealing with the medical qualities and peculiarities of herbs. Not only does he accurately describe herbs, but he also very aptly describes the preparation and uses of drugs obtained from plants.

In the first century A.D., Dioscorides was born at Anazarbos in a part of Asia Minor which was then a part of the Roman Empire. In order to study the herbs then known, he accompanied Roman armies throughout Asia Minor and traveled in Spain, Greece, Italy, and Gaul. Recording what he observed as he observed it, he finally wrote a book from his travels that made him famous. Galen, the Roman scientist who lived a century later, stated, "In his book, Dioscorides has written in a useful way on the entire materia medica because he not only deals with the herbs but includes the trees, fruits, seeds, the natural and artificial juices, and furthermore the metals and animals substances. In my opinion, he is the one among the various authors who has presented the most perfect discussion of the drugs." For fifteen centuries, Galen's words maintained the supremacy of Dioscorides in the world of plant drugs, his texts considered basic science in the field as late as the 16th century. Mentioned previously, Galen, who lived between 130 to 200 A.D., was not only a historian of sorts, but practiced and taught medicine and early pharmacy in Rome. He created principles for the preparation and compounding of medicines which were maintained for over 1500 years. Galen went beyond his predecessors by attempting to find a scientific basis for the dispensing of drugs and in his introduction of cautious dosage. He developed many methods for mixing, extracting, refining, and combining plant and other drugs.

The Middle Ages

During the Middle Ages, known also as the Dark Ages, much of the cultural and scientific knowledge of earlier civilizations in the Western world was destroyed. Fortunately, however, the more ancient knowledge of herbalism and medicine was preserved and utilized mainly in the monasteries. During this period it was the monks who did much to take care of the evolving science. Thus, for example, Latin writings on medicine were early on preserved in the libraries of monasteries. The early knowledge of herbal medicine was taught in the cloisters as early as the 7th century.

Manuscripts from many ancient writers and many ancient lands were translated and copied for monastic libraries. Gathering herbs in the field, the monks raised them in their own herb gardens. They prepared and used these for the benefit of the sick and injured amongst themselves and the surrounding areas. In many countries today, herb gardens may still be found in monasteries.

Before turning to the modern era, or post-Medieval times, we should make note of several scientists who were writing in Arabic. The findings of al-Razi, also known as Rhazes, who worked in about the year 923, was of scientific importance in the history of herbalism. Another important figure from this part of the world is the Spanish born Ibn-al-Baitar who lived between 1197 until 1248. He compiled a methodical and critical compendium of more than 2,000 herbal drugs. Yet when discussing the Arabian era in the history of herbal medicine one genius stands above all the others, the Persian Ibn Sina, also known as Avicenna in the English language. Sometimes known as the "Persian Galen," Avicenna lived from about 980 until 1037 A.D. He has been called an intellectual giant who was herbalist, physician, poet, philosopher, and diplomat. His works were accepted as authoritative in the Western world until as late as the 17th century, and are still considered influential in parts of the Orient. So here we have an early herbal scientist whose work dominated through the long Middle Ages and even into the Renaissance. It should be noted that Avicenna first adopted and then elaborated on Galen's ideas.

At this point in the history of herbal medicine, we see the development of the first official pharmacopoeia. (A Pharmacopoeia is a book of standards used by pharmacists in preparing and dispensing medicines as dictated by physicians.) In the year 1498, there was published the *Nuovo Receptario* and it was based almost solely on the Greek and Arabic drug therapy that preceded it. This pharmacopoeia, the first of its kind, was written in Italian and it was later translated into Latin in 1518 and soon became available throughout the Western world. Soon thereafter, official pharmacopoeias began to appear in other regions of Europe.

Herbal Medicine in the New World

In the beginning of the 1600s, early settlements began to appear in North America. This period marks the beginning of the first new age in herbalism because it was the interaction between the Europeans and the Native Americans that brought forth a pollination in the science of herbs. Many Europeans brought with them their knowledge of healing plants. They cultivated their own herb gardens upon arriving in the New World. These early American herbalists often learned about new drug plants from Native Americans. The earliest records demonstrate that many Native American plants were soon adopted by the European settlers. These included boneset, mullein, goldenseal, and jack-in-the-pulpit.

We now enter the first truly modern period of herbal medicine. The German chemist Serturner began experimenting with opium in 1803 and soon delineated opium's chief narcotic principle, morphine. He also recognized and proved the critical importance of an entire new class of organic substances, the alkaloids. This was based upon the fact that morphine, which was then a new substance, was alkaline in nature, and he saw it as the first of a new class of organic bases which formed salts with organic as well as with inorganic acids. It's interesting to note that this young man was only 23 years of age at the time of his discovery.

Late in the 18th century there was reported in Europe the value of "Peruvian barks," which were used to alleviate the symptoms of malaria and other strong intermittent fevers. Many scientists then tried to isolate the secret of cinchona bark. It was two young French chemists, Pelletier and Caventou, who first discovered quinine and cinchonine in cinchona bark. Soon after this discovery, the large scale manufacture of quinine was begun, but Pelletier because of his love for humanity refused to patent or create a monopoly for the manufacture of this important fever-lowering drug.

Earlier we described herb gardens in monasteries. The concept of obtaining God's healing powers from the earth achieved a renaissance among the Shakers, who are Protestant sectarians who settled in North American colonies. While they began their first cultivation and study of medicinal herbs in the early 1700s, their most important community was at New Lebanon, New York. The Shakers gathered and cultivated approximately 200 varieties of medicinal herbs. They dried, ground, and pressed them into solid bricks which were then sold to pharmacists and physicians around the world. They later made solid and fluid extracts. By 1850, the herb gardens of New Lebanon, then known as "physics gardens," occupied about 50 acres and were largely cultivated with hyoscyamus, belladonna, taraxacum, aconite, poppy, lettuce, sage, summer savory, marjoram, dock, burdock, valerian, and horehound. There were approximately another 50 minor plants raised by these people.

The 18th and 19th Centuries

Focusing on the English speaking world, the 18th and 19th centuries saw the proliferation of numerous healers whose repertoire consisted largely of herbal remedies. Then as now there were many healers but few who documented their techniques and remedies in any recognizable or lasting form. Therefore, we can best summarize the history of herbal medicine in these centuries by listing some of the chief books of medicinal plants which survive from this period. These include the beautifully illustrated volumes by Stephenson and Churchill, *Medical Botany* (1836), or by Bentley and Trimen, *Medicinal Plants* (1880). Both sets were published in England. The United States saw the publication of Charles F. Millspaugh's *Medicinal Plants* (1892), which treated 1,000 species. There were several other herbals published but none of equal quality.

In the 20th century few truly comprehensive American herbals have been published. Most notably *Weiner's Herbal,* published in 1980 and republished in a revised edition in 1990, is perhaps the best known and most well documented.

The Age of Technology

We now enter the age where technological progress permits the manufacture of highly reliable preparations of herbal medicines. Before glancing at some of the processing methods, it may be useful to look at the various ways in which herbs are still prepared in China, and compare these with the dominant forms in the United States. Traditional Chinese drugs are often found in the following forms: slices, powder, pills, plasters, medicated liquors, herb distillates, pellets, and medicinal teas. New dosage forms also appear in the Orient. These include: tablets, capsules, tinctures, fluid extracts, ointments, instant granules, and others which are the same as those found in Western medicine, including syrups, suppositories, aerosols, injections, and ampules. In today's bustling industrial world, people are too busy to prepare their own herbal remedies and generally do not like the traditional preparations because they are usually odorous, bitter, pungent, and difficult to consume. So even in Asia, scientifically prepared herbal preparations have become very popular and have gained a fine reputation and wide acceptance.

Why Herbs Are Processed

In addition to saving time in their preparation, that is, for convenience, there are other goals of drug processing. These include the reduction of toxicity and adverse affects. For example, in their raw states certain herbs may cause irritation of the throat, which is true for pinellia, a Chinese herb. Processing will reduce or eliminate this side effect. Another example is the Chinese herb Genkwa, which generally causes abdominal aching in the raw state but after fermentation it does not cause this process. In addition, herbs may be processed to promote their therapeutic effects. The alkaloids of certain herbs are hardly soluble in water, but after vinegar processing they are readily soluble and this enhances their potency. By processing licorice with honey, the effects are increased. Crude drugs are also processed to remove contaminants and unpleasant odors. In the raw state, the contaminants may include mold, rot of other forms, and animal waste. Processing renders the herbal product perfectly safe for human consumption. After processing herbs may be screened, cut, and extracted. These processes have been developed over thousands of years. Currently in America, we have certified potency herbal products as well as magnified dosages of various components of specific herbs which give them a more powerful therapeutic effect.

The Question of "Standardized Herbs"

There's a potency war brewing. The bottom-line, however, may prove that the 1970s aphorism "small is beautiful" or "less is more," is the answer. Simply upping the percentage content of an active constituent in an herbal preparation may yet prove harmful.

For now, the answer is to welcome standardization and to proceed with caution—making standardized herbal extracts *only* from plants which have been subjected to safety and efficacy studies. Examples includes herbs such as ginseng, ginkgo, ginger, milk thistle, echinacea, turmeric, essential oil or orange (d-limonene), valerian, St. John's Wort, horsetail, bilberry, and others with good efficacy and safety data.

Standardization was introduced to counter the negative effects of poor quality control which plagued the herb industry in the 1970's. With standardized herbs we can reliably count on receiving the same quantity of one or more active constituents per unit taken. Thus, a one gram capsule of milk thistle said to contain 80% silymarin— the chief active principle— can be reliably assumed to contain this consistent quantity.

In nature, herbs vary in their content of active constituents. Soils, climates, harvesting methods, processing, packaging and storage circumstances all affect the relative potency of a finished herbal product. When an active principle in the finished product is so identified on the label, the miscellaneous subjective effects can be objectively controlled, and the consumer can rely upon receiving a stated quantity and balance of activity.

A reasonable course of action, at this stage of knowledge, would be to proceed cautiously, as stated above, standardizing active constituents of herbs with well-established safety and efficacy. By also including the whole plant in the final product, some measure of the inherent natural "checks and balances" or synergism will be retained. With this method, we see an *enhancement* of natural medicinal activity rather than an imbalanced drug-effect.

Increased control of active ingredients, and a general increase in sophistication throughout the industry, coupled with greatly rising demand for herbal products at the consumer level, leads to me conclude that being bullish on herbs is a very safe course, indeed.

Bullish on Herbs

The future of herbal medicine in America is very bright. People have rediscovered plant remedies and are once again looking to nature for solutions to the ills that flesh is heir to.

This is a natural progression when we consider that the ethno-medical folklore of preindustrial cultures (so called, "primitive") consists of prescriptions for treating most physical ailments. Taken together with the fact that the main active ingredient of approximately 25% of all prescription drugs sold in the U.S. was derived from plants, we can see why folklore has given life to the new scientific interest in herbs.

Ever since the two principle anti-cancer drugs, vincristine and vinblastine, were isolated from the "Madagascar Periwinkle" (*Catharanthus roseus*) in the 1960's we have seen interest in the promise of herbal medicine. These powerful plant-derived drugs arrest cell division so dramatically that one of them, vincristine, is used for the treatment of acute leukemia, especially in children. With other drugs these plant-derived compounds are used to treat other cancers including Hodgkin's disease. Currently, taxol, derived from the Pacific Yew tree, is being used to treat "incurable" cancers.

These great success stories stimulated a world-wide investigation of centuries old folk medicine and the consumer usage of herbal preparations, mainly teas, in the United States.

In the late 1970's, the interest in herbs seemed to have waned. A new decade was beginning, one that would lead mankind into the new century, a century of high technology, and herbs were assigned an archaic aura. The new President ushered in a glittering decade. Hippies were dead. "Natural" was passé and all that glittered was thought to be golden.

As the 1980's matured, and the romance with surface realities reevaluated, people once again wondered if nature, that most unfickle phenomenon, might not yet hold some answers for mankind's infirmities.

In the decade of the '90s, we see a new and wonderful outcry to preserve our natural environment. There is a realization that the rainforests are a repository of hundreds if not thousands of potential medicines. Herbal preparations are being tried, for the first time by some, again by many.

AIDS will not go away. The virus keeps changing form too adeptly for the chemists who create synthetic drugs. Yet here again nature may hold some answers in the form of remarkable compounds derived from plants (see *Echinacea, St. John's Wort, Shiitake Mushrooms, Goldenseal,* and other immune-enhancing herbs in Chapter 4).

Herbs in the 21st Century

While estimates of the percent of new prescriptions in the U.S. which contain an active ingredient originating in nature run between 25 and 40 percent, these compounds represent a very short list with very wide usage. Very few *new* compounds derived from nature have entered the American pharmaceutical marketplace in the past 20 years. The same few developed years ago reappear in new permutations and combinations.

The lack of patent protection, not the lack of efficacy, keeps the pharmaceutical giants in the United States from investing in the development of drugs from plants. Herb companies and smaller pharmaceutical firms have been and will continue to meet the growing consumer demand for nature's remedies, however. In Japan, France and some developing nations drugs from herbs will become big business.

This is not to create the mistaken idea that the United States will *not* take part in the coming herb-based revolution in medicine. Currently, pharmaceuticals derived from plants are a $10 billion business in the U.S. and this is just a baseline for medicine from botanicals. By the middle of this decade, we can expect vast new markets for this class of products, because over 200 research groups worldwide are engaged in creating new medicinals from nature. Surprisingly, the largest number of these research groups are based in the U.S. (97 out of a total of 209 world wide research groups are U.S. based).

Europeans have long been able to purchase herbal-based medicinal preparations on an OTC ("over-the-counter") basis. These remedies are utilized as a second-line treatment immediately following alterations in diet, a first-line approach. Such herbal preparations are tried before people turn to physicians for third-line treatments, the potent pharmaceuticals.

In America, our first and second-lines of treating common ailments have largely disappeared. People have been taught to "see a doctor" for the smallest ache, often coming home with a potent pharmaceutical "prescription" just as likely to cause harm as to effect a cure.

With the growth of the herbal industry Americans will join the Europeans in taking charge of their own first-symptom health-care. The wildly escalating costs of medical care and the legion of tragic iatrogenic effects of prescription drugs have given new meaning to the old saying, "Physician, heal thyself!"

When I was younger, an older, wiser man said to me, "If you don't know how to take care of your health by the time you're forty, you *deserve* the doctors!"

Herbal remedies are coming of age in America, *and none too soon.*

CHAPTER 3

INTRODUCTION TO HERBALISM

The Medicine Shelf

Your spice shelf probably contains several herbs with active medicinal properties. Thyme, for example, though used primarily for its savory flavor, has also been valued as a medicinal since ancient times. The leaves of this small, branched shrub contain the oil thymol, which has antiseptic, expectorant, and bronchodilator effects. Thymol also releases gas trapped in the stomach and relaxes the smooth muscle of this organ. This is why thyme is so effective in cases of colic and flatulence.

Ginger, another common spice, also has important medicinal values. As a tea, this widely used condiment is a popular remedy for encouraging menstruation when it has been suppressed by a cold. For headache and toothache, an infusion is rubbed directly on the affected part; the borneol in Ginger relieves pain.

Garlic, now a staple for most cooks because of its unique flavor, contains selenium, an important trace mineral with remarkable biological effects. Long reputed for its ability to lower blood pressure, this tangy rhizome has antibacterial and diuretic properties as well. The juice is very effective for treating insect stings; and dripped into the ear (on a piece of cotton), it is a remarkable treatment for earaches!

Other common herbs with medicinal activity include Pennyroyal, noted for stimulating the menses; Peppermint, a truly effective gas expeller; Dandelion, an ancient home remedy for mild constipation; Anise, which increases milk secretion in nursing mothers; Arrowroot (a valuable source of calcium), which was utilized by Central and South American Indians as an antidote for various poisons; and many others.

Herbs as Prescription Drugs

We have noted that common kitchen spices have strong medicinal properties. But did you know that you may already be getting herbal medicines in your prescriptions?

Over $3 billion is spent each year on pharmaceuticals derived from plants. To demonstrate the impact of plants as medicines, the twelve most commonly utilized pure compounds derived form drug plants and used in prescriptions are presented in Table 1.

TABLE 1

Most Commonly Encountered Pure Compounds
from Higher Plants Used as Drugs in the U.S.A.

Active Plant Principle	Total Number of Prescriptions	Percent of Total Prescriptions
Steroids (95% from diosgenin)	225,050,000	14.69
Codeine	31,099,000	2.03
Atropine	22,980,000	1.50
Reserpine	22,214,000	1.45
Pseudoephedrine	13,788,000	0.90
Ephedrine	11,796,000	0.77
Hyoscyamine	11,490,000	0.75
Digoxin	11,184,000	0.73
Scopolamine	10,111,000	0.66
Digitoxin	5,056,000	0.33
Pilocarpine	3,983,000	0.26
Quinidine	2,758,000	0.18

Even more remarkable is the fact that of the over 38 million prescriptions evaluated that contained crude plant drugs or extracts from plants.

TABLE 2

Most Commonly Encountered Higher Plant
Extracts Used in Prescriptions

Crude Botanical or Extract	Total Number of Prescriptions	Percent of Total Prescriptions
Belladonna (*Atropa belladonna*)	10,418,000	0.62
Ipecac (*Cephaelis ipecacuanha*)	7,047,000	0.46
Opium (*Papaver somniferum*)	6,894,000	0.45
Rauwolfia (*Rauvolfia serpentina*)	5,822,000	0.38
Cascara (*Rhamnus purshiana*)	2,451,000	0.16
Digitalis (*Digitalis purpurea*)	2,451,000	0.16
Citrus Bioflavonoids (*Citrus* spp.)	1,379,000	0.09
Veratrum (*Veratrum viride*)	1,072,000	0.07

(Total prescription volume was 1.532 billion prescriptions.)

Natural plant drugs have been used since antiquity, and are still the only form of medicine for a large majority of the world's population who do not have access to hospitals and pharmacies.

Herbal medicine is often based on rational principles, as we see in Table 3 on page 54. The left column contains the names of compounds derived from plants; in the middle columns are the type of chemicals they contain; and on the right we see the type of effects they produce in the body.

Using herbal medicine is not so far removed from our daily lives as we may think. Many prescription drugs contain herbal compounds not unlike the remedies listed in this book.

TABLE 3

*Typical Plant Principles Used to Illustrate Pharmacological
Principles in Standard Textbooks*

Name of Compound	Type of Compound	Type of Pharmacological Action
Bulbocapnine	Alkaloid	Centrally acting skeletal muscle relaxant
Morphine, Codeine	Alkaloid	Analgesic
Papaverine	Alkaloid	Smooth muscle relaxant
Colchicine	Alkaloid	Anti-gout
Camphor	Monoterpene	Analgesic
Picrotoxin	Sesquiterpene	Stimulates central nervous system
Strychnine, Caffeine	Alkaloid	Stimulates central nervous system
Cocaine	Alkaloid	Local anesthetic
Atropine, Scopolamine	Alkaloid	Parasympatholytic
Pilocarpine, Physostigmine	Alkaloid	Parasympathomimetic
d-Tubocuraine	Alkaloid	Peripherally acting skeletal muscle relaxant
Ephedrine	Alkaloid	Sympathomimetic
Nicotine, Lobeline	Alkaloid	Ganglionic blocker
Digitoxin, Digoxin	Cardiac glycoside	Cardiotonic
Quinidine	Alkaloid	Antiarrhythmic
Sparteine, Ergot Alkaloids	Alkaloid	Uterine stimulant
Reserpine, Veratrum	Alkaloid	Antihypertensive
Reserpine	Alkaloid	Psychotropic
Anthraquinone glycosides	Anthraquinone	Cathartic
Psyllium, Agar	Mucilages	Laxative
Castor Oil	Fixed Oil	Laxative
Quinine	Alkaloid	Antimalarial
Emetine	Alkaloid	Anti-amebic

CHAPTER 4

HERBS AND MEDICINAL PLANTS

A - Z Reference Guide to Over 220 Medicinally Active Herbs

How to Gather, Prepare, and Preserve Herbs

Gathering Herbs

If you wish to collect your own herbs from the countryside or the herb garden, be sure to gather them at the peak of their growth, usually during the spring and early summer. The best time of day is in the early morning after the dew has dried; herbs that are moist when collected are not suitable for drying. Leaves and flowers should be picked when young, just after opening. Discard discolored, withered, or insect-damaged plant parts, and snip off all stalks.

Seeds should be collected after sun-ripening on the plant.

Roots and barks should be gathered in the early spring, when the sap rises and the leaves are just budding, or after the plant has shed its leaves in the autumn.

Caution: Never collect any herbs that may have been contaminated with insecticides or other chemical sprays.

Drying Herbs

Herbs collected for drying must not be damp. Leaves and flowers should be hung in small bunches out of direct sun (except in Alpine climates) and where there is plenty of air circulation. they may also be spread on flat surfaces and turned frequently.

If you can, allow seeds to dry on the plant.

Handle fruits like leaves and flowers; larger fruits can be sun-dried in cooler climates, or they may be sliced, seeded, and dried slowly in an oven at low temperature with the door slightly open (turn them frequently).

Prepare roots and barks for drying by wiping them clean--do not wash them. In cold climates some artificial heat may be needed. They should be turned frequently during drying. They may also be cut up, strung with a needle, and hung in a well-ventilated room.

Storing Herbs

Dried herbs should be kept in a **dry** room that is not too hot. They can be stored in brown paper bags tied at the neck with a string, or they can be broken up and stored in jars or tins.

Herbal Preparations

Medicinal plants can be eaten raw, and ideally this is the way to use them. But since many medicinal herbs have an unpleasant taste, and since they are often used dried, they are usually taken in the form of decoctions or infusions. Dried herbs are twice as strong as fresh, so when using fresh plant products larger amounts are necessary.

DECOCTIONS are used for the tougher plant parts, such as roots, barks, seeds, and stems, to extract the active or useful principles. In a covered container, slowly boil the vegetable material in water for a certain length of time, usually 20 to 30 minutes. The liquid is then allowed to cool slowly in the *closed* container. Where proportions are not given, use about one teaspoon of the raw material to 1 1/2 pints of water.

INFUSIONS are used for the softer plant parts--the leaves, flowers, and entire herbs. They are made in the manner of tea: Place the herb in a pot that has a tight cover. Pour boiling water over the vegetable material; then cover the pot and allow the infusion to steep for 5 to 20 minutes. Strain and drink the infusion. Where the proportions are not given, use about 1/2 ounce of plant material to 1 pint of boiled water.

FLUIDEXTRACTCS contain alcohol as a solvent, where each milliliter represents 1 gram of the drug.

TINCTURES are *diluted* alcoholic solutions of herbs, the standard strength being 10 percent for powerful drugs and 20 percent for less powerful ones.

JUICES form tubers and fleshy leaves are mixed with water, fruit juices, other mild herb "teas," aromatics, or carminatives, and sipped directly.

As a final note it is important to remember that in the golden age of botanical medicine, the late nineteenth century, few people actually prepared herbal remedies themselves. The skills of the trained physicians/herbalist were called upon, and most herbal remedies were administered in the form of tinctures. Since few highly trained herbalists are in practice today, many people are learning to prepare herbs themselves.

ACACIA

SCIENTIFIC NAME: *Acacia vera,*
　　　　　　　　A. arabica,
　　　　　　　　A. senegal
PARTS USED: Bark, exudate (gum)

DOSAGE:

　　The gum is given either in powder or dissolved in almond milk or similar flavored beverages: $1/2$ ounce of the gum to a pint of liquid.

ACACIA: *"Gum arabic" swells and soothes membranes when it comes into contact with water, making it an effective throat lozenge.*

Traditional Usages

The gummy Acacia exudate, soluble in water, is used for its demulcent properties (soothing to mucous membrane surfaces). For shielding sore throat due to cough, a dried piece of Acacia gum is allowed to dissolve slowly in the mouth, maintaining a constant supply to the irritated area. Bronchial passages are similarly relieved by sucking on such a natural lozenge.

Externally an application of powdered gum has been employed to check hemorrhage from leech bites. Applied in a mucilaginous state, it has been used to soothe burns and scrapes, as well as the sore nipples of nursing mothers.

Probably the principal use of the gum has been as a vehicle for other medicines, as in the suspension of insoluble powders, in lozenges, and other uses.

Recent Scientific Findings

There is full justification for the use of Acacia (gum arabic) as a **demulcent**, since when the gum comes into contact with water it swells, develops a tenacious character, and **coats and soothes mucous membranes**. The gum consists of a mixture of high-molecular-weight carbohydrate substances. When taken internally they are broken down to simple sugars (i.e., glucose) which are well known to have nutrient value. Further, since gum arabic also swells to some extent when taken orally, it has been used as a mild laxative, although not extensively in recent years.

ADDER'S TONGUE

SCIENTIFIC NAME: *Erythronium americanum*

PARTS USED: All parts active; leaves preferred

DOSAGE:

Bulbs: 1.3 to 2.0 grams of the bulb will produce rapid vomiting.

Leaves: Since the leaves are stronger in action, very cautious doses are recommended by practitioners, starting with 0.25 gram one time per day, and observing the results. If tolerated, the dose is often increased to 0.50 gram per day, but not to exceed 0.75 gram. The fresher the plant material, the greater is the danger of toxicity due to higher alkaloid content.

ADDER'S TONGUE: *This colorfully named plant has long been used to treat wounds.*

Traditional Usages

The plant derives its name from the coloring and shape of the leaf, which resembles an adder's tongue. It is possible that the traditional use of the plant as an external application for the treatment of wounds derived from its appearance (the "doctrine of signatures"), which would suggest that it be used for snakebites and, by extension, for other wounds and ulcers. At any rate, various oil infusions and ointments made from the leaf and spike have been used to treat wounds, and poultices of the fresh leaves have been applied to soothe and heal bruises.

The bulbs of this plant have been recorded as emetic (producing vomiting) and as a substitute for Colchicium in the treatment of gout. In the fresh state it has been reported to be a remedy for scurvy.

Recent Scientific Findings

Experimentally, Adder's Tongue has been found to contain alkaloids. Since the plant is closely related to other plants that produce colchicine, it may be presumed that colchicine is present in Adder's Tongue. **Colchicine is a specific agent used for the diagnosis and treatment of gout.** However, it is extremely toxic, and caution must be exercised concerning the ingestion of even the smallest amount of any plant containing colchicine. (See *Meadow Saffron* for more information on colchicine.)

AGRIMONY

SCIENTIFIC NAME: *Agrimonia pilosa*
PARTS USED: Herb, root, fruit

DOSAGE:

Root: Boil 1 teaspoon of dried root bark per 1½ pints water in covered container for about ½ hour at a slow boil. Allow liquid to cool slowly in the *closed* container. Drink 1 cup at a time, twice daily.

AGRIMONY: *Long used in traditional Chinese medicine, modern research is also finding this herb possesses a number of possible medicinal applications.*

Traditional Usages

Agrimony's first recorded use dates from a Chinese herbal published nearly a thousand years ago. In traditional Chinese medicine, Agrimony is classified among the blood regulating drugs. It has a tendency to invigorate the functions of the stomach, liver, and bowels, eliminating foul matter from the system.

It is highly recommended in the treatment of stones of gravel in kidneys or bladder. It is also used to stop hemorrhages.

As a gargle, the decoction is considered very effective in relieving soreness and inflammation of the mouth and throat. It is also useful for diarrhea, though it needs to be used consistently for a period of time.

Recent Scientific Findings

A member of the rose family. Agrimony contains bitters, mucilage, and phytosterol. It is rich in tannins.

A study on Agrimony and several other plants effect on diabetes found that Agrimony retarded the development of streptozotocin diabetes in mice. An extract has been found to have **hypotensive action**. An extract also demonstrated anti-viral activity in mice.

In other studies, Agrimony exhibited a hemostasis effect, stimulating platelet formation and **hastening blood coagulation**. As an **anticancer agent**, a decoction has inhibited proliferation of certain cancer cells.

Agrimony has been found to have a **cardiotonic effect**. At lower doses it regulates heart rate; at high doses it slows the heart beat.

ALFALFA

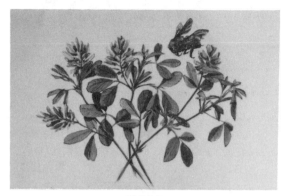

Alfalfa

SCIENTIFIC NAME: *Medicago sativa*
PARTS USED: Leaves

DOSAGE:

Leaves: Approximately 1 ounce of leaves to 1 pint of water. Boil water separately and pour over the plant material and steep for 5 to 20 minutes, depending on the desired effect. Drink hot or warm, 1 to 2 cups per day, at bedtime and upon awakening.

ALFALFA: *For centuries, this grain has been used for its nutritional value.*

Traditional Usages

Alfalfa seeds were ground between stones by Native Americans, who used this "flour" as bread or mush. Also, fresh branches were boiled and then eaten as greens.

Alfalfa has a reputation for treating both arthritis and diabetes.

Recent Scientific Findings

Alfalfa possesses extremely high nutritional value. **An excellent source of vitamins A and D,** Alfalfa leaf is used in the popular infants' cereal pablum. Also rich in vitamin K, Alfalfa leaf has been used in medicine **to encourage blood clotting.**

Alfalfa also **lowers blood cholesterol.** Additionally, the plant has been folklorically used as a "natural" cure for jaundice.

Other recommended uses for Alfalfa are for asthma and hayfever. Alfalfa has also been found to retard the development of streptozotocin **diabetes** in mice.

ALOE VERA

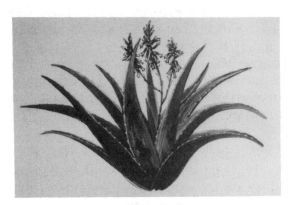

Aloe Vera

SCIENTIFIC NAME: *Aloe vera*
PARTS USED: Leaves

DOSAGE:

As a purgative, aloes were administered in the form of tincture or extract, the dose being 100 to 300 milligrams.

Caution: Do not use during the menstrual period, nor while pregnant. Do not use for hemorrhoids.

ALOE VERA: *Known to the ancient Egyptians as a beauty aid for the skin, this remarkable plant promotes healing from burns and wounds.*

Traditional Usages

Ever since the age of Cleopatra, when Aloe was used to **treat burns**, this remarkable plant has enjoyed popular acclaim and wide usage. The first known use of Aloe as a medicinal came in 333 B.C. when Alexander the Great heard of this plant and sent a commission to the island of Socotra to investigate and return with samples. During the 1800s and early 1900s much of the Aloes exported to Europe came from plants cultivated in the Dutch West Indies on the islands of Aruba and Barbados. These are variously identified as Curacao Aloe, *Aloe vera*, and Barbados Aloe. African Aloe varieties are Cape Aloe, Uganda Aloe, and Natal Aloe, collectively referred to in commerce as Zanzibar Aloe.

There are about 180 Aloe species, of different sizes and forms. The several Aloes are cultivated for ornamental purposes; with their stiffness and radial symmetry, they fit well into rock gardens and since their home is the African desert, they grow well in direct sunlight. The true Aloe (*Aloe barbadensis*; synonym *A. Vera*) yields "Barbados aloes."

Along with Aloe's use since ancient times as a beauty aid for the skin, externally the raw mucilage from the fresh plant has long been employed as an analgesic for burns, scrapes, sunburn, and insect bites, as well as to promote healing of such injuries. A fleshy stalk is broken off, the skin of the plant split to expose the interior, and the edges are spread apart for effective wrapping of the afflicted area. One stalk can be used piece by piece until gone since it forms its own natural container as the plant skin's surface dries and forms a seal which preserves the remainder of the stalk.

For the treatment of *chronic* constipation *only*, aloes were felt to be particularly effective, as their action is largely limited to the colon. However, they were not recommended as a general laxative. As the action produced by aloes often caused griping (painful muscle spasms of the bowels), it was common to include a carminative such as Fennel to soothe the side effects of this purgative action. Aloes were also often utilized to treat various forms of amenorrhea (absent or suppressed menses).

Recent Scientific Findings

I first learned of this plant's properties in 1968 when I read **it was being utilized to treat radiation burns** by a research group at the University of Pennsylvania. Very significantly, this university research team found the mucilaginous Aloe to be the most effective treatment for minor radiation burns. Subsequent trials of my own demonstrated what folklore had long told: **Aloe was an effective, safe, inexpensive treatment for burns and wounds.**

The leaf juice of *A. ferox* and *A. vera*, when incorporated into a water-soluble ointment base or used as the fresh juice, has well-established emollient effects on the skin. Such preparations are widely utilized to treat **minor sunburn** cases and also to **treat burns from X-ray treatment of cancer and related diseases.** The active principle has not been identified, but is probably a polysaccharide that forms a protective and soothing coating when applied to the skin. If the juice is dried and then applied to burns, it is not effective. This ancient healing plant should remain forever one of humankind's most important frontline remedies against wounds.

The authors of one study wrote that *A. vera* improves wound healing when administered either orally or topically. "It not only contributes to a decrease in wound diameter, but also leads to better vascularity and healthier granulation tissue. The fact that Aloe is effective orally suggests that it is not broken down by the gastrointestinal tract and is absorbed into the blood. **Aloe possibly improves wound healing by increasing the availability of oxygen and by increasing the synthesis and the strength of collagen.** Aloe Vera has become a subject of scientific study concerning inflammation and wound healing. As knowledge about Aloe increases, significant benefits of a practical nature in the management of healing wounds can be expected." (Davis, et al.)

Aloe's ability to accelerate wound healing was demonstrated in a study with patients with full-face dermabrasion (surgical removal of skin imperfections, such as scars, by abrasion). One side of the face was treated with the standard polyethylene oxide gel while the other side received the standard gel saturated with stabilized Aloe Vera. Overall, wound healing was approximately **72 hours faster** on the Aloe side. The authors concluded that "This acceleration of wound healing is important to reduce bacterial contamination."

One note of caution: Adverse reactions to Aloe have taken place following dermabrasion. It is recommended that patients refrain from using Aloe Vera topically in the first weeks after surgery. Aloe has also been found to aid in the **treatment of frostbite.**

In another study on *Aloe* by a group of researchers in the Netherlands, **immune-enhancing activity** was discovered. Beginning with the traditional medical usages for this plant, these workers purified an aqueous gel-extract. A highly active polysaccharide fraction was isolated from the *Aloe* gel. This component proved active in the production of antibodies and also stimulated another aspect of the immune response (i.e., complementary activity). The authors compared the effectiveness of this gel fraction of *Aloe* with *dextran sulphate*, a sulphated polysaccharide found principally in certain seaweeds. (For about 40 years Japanese researchers have been testing dextran sulphate and ably demonstrating its anti-tumor and anticlotting properties.)

The known healing effects of Aloe Vera on infected wounds are thought to be explained by the local activation of complement which is thought to lead to an influx of monocytes and PMN's to the injured area.

In one study, an Aloe extract prepared with 50% ethanol applied topically decreased inflammation by 29%. Another research team combined Aloe with hydrocortisone and tested against acute inflammation. The authors speculated that **Aloe Vera has significant potential as a biologically active vehicle for steroids.**

If the leaves of various *Aloe* species are extracted in a special way, and the resulting product is concentrated, a mixture of anthraquinones results. This mixture is known in the U.S. and Canada as "aloes" or "aloin," and it is well established to be an **effective laxative** in humans. The laxative effect is **much stronger than that produced by Senna or Cascara products.**

Another preparation from Aloe, **carrisyn**, is a polysaccharide. It has been claimed that **carrisyn** directly kills various types of viruses, including herpes and measles, and **possibly HIV.** However, research is still in the preliminary stages.

ANEMONE

SCIENTIFIC NAME: *Anemone* spp.
PARTS USED: Root and flower

DOSAGE:
Dried powder: The dose is 0.13-0.2 grams, although larger amounts may possibly have been taken safely.
Fluidextract: Made from the fresh herb, 4.6-7.8 milliliters, divided over 24 hours.

ANEMONE: *Ancient Chinese and Greek physicians extolled these beautiful plants, which contain the compound anemonin.*

Traditional Usages

In ancient texts of Greek and Chinese healers we find continual reference to the healing virtues of the lovely Anemones. Dioscorides revered Anemone in the form of **external plasters** or baths for **skin ulcers** and inflamed eyes. Pliny advocated its use for **toothache** and **swollen gums.** The Chinese employed *A. pulsatilla* for ailments ranging from dysentery to madness.

One type of Anemone, l verleaf (*A. hepatica*) is so named because its leaves resemble the shape of the liver; according to the "doctrine of signatures" a tonic of this particular Anemone consequently will aid liver disorders.

There are several other Anemones: *A. ludoviciana* (American Pulsatilla), *A. pratensis* (European Pulsatilla), *A. ranunculoides* (Yellow Wood Anemone), and *A. appennina* (Blue Anemone). These are also employed in folk medicines in various capacities. Some have been used as sedatives, demulcents, and vulneraries, and others were once employed as a primary treatment in early cases of tuberculosis.

Recent Scientific Findings

Many Anemone species have been studied in the laboratory, both for their chemical content and for the effects of their extracts in animals and in the test tube. They are all remarkably similar in their chemical and pharmacological properties, a majority of the effects explained by the presence of the simple chemical compound known as protanemonin, which is converted to the active substance anemonin. It also contains protoanemonin, the lactone of gamma-hydroxy-vinylacrylic acid.

Anemonin is highly active against a large number of different disease-producing microorganisms, has **sedative** properties, **lowers blood pressure**, **stimulates the gallbladder**, **relaxes smooth muscle of the gut**, **allays pain**, and in pure form will produce a blistering effect on the skin or mucous membranes. When a sufficiently dilute water extract of Anemone is used, this blistering effect has not been observed because the anemonin is diluted. There is enough of this substance present, however, to slightly irritate the mucous membranes, giving rise to an expectorant, as well as perhaps a diuretic effect. Anemone is considered one of the most effective of all drugs for **amoebic dysentery**.

A 1988 analysis determined that anemonin is the primary compound responsible for the **fever lowering** effects, while both anemonin and protanemonin produce a **sedating effect**. A 1990 study determined that protoanemonin has in vitro **activity against fungi**.

ANGELICA or DONG QUAI

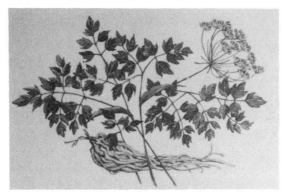

Angelica

SCIENTIFIC NAME: *Angelica sinensis, A. acutiloba*

PARTS USED: Root, herb, and seed

DOSAGE:

Seeds: The recommended medicinal dose was 1 teaspoon of seeds per cup boiling water, to be drunk at room temperature, 1 to 2 cups per day.

Root: 1 tablespoon, boiled in a covered container of 1½ pints water for about ½ hour, at a slow boil. Allow liquid to cool slowly in the *closed* container. Taken cold, 1 swallow or 1 tablespoon at a time, 1 to 2 cups per day.

Herb: Approximately ½ ounce of herb to 1 pint of water. Boil water separately and pour over the plant material and steep for 5 to 20 minutes, depending on the desired effect. Drink hot or warm, 1 to 2 cups per day.

ANGELICA: *Called "the women's herb" in China, modern research substantiates Angelica's effects in regulating uterine function.*

Traditional Usages

Long utilized as a folkloric remedy for "female complaints," in China Angelica is called "the woman's herb." The Chinese name for this herb means "missing the husband," or "returned to the husband's home." It is generally employed in traditional medicine as a food (in soup) or **as a "tea" for irregular, painful, or meek menstruation**, especially when associated with the **symptoms of PMS** (tension, cramps, weakness, etc.).

In addition Angelica has a long history as a remedy for diabetes, hypertension, cancer, angina pectoris, and nephritis. In Europe, Angelica was used for **infant flatulence** and **colic** and **heartburn** in adults. In the *British Flora Medica* we find the following report:

> The Laplanders considered this plant as one of the most important productions of their soil. During that part of the year which they pass in the woods, they are subject to a severe kind of colic, against which the root of Angelica is one of their chief remedies. They also frequently mix the unexpanded umbels with the leaves of the Sorrel and boiling them down in water to the consistence of syrup, mix it with reindeer's milk, and

thus form a stomachic and astringent medicine.

The essential oils distilled from Angelica fruit and roots are utilized in the perfumery, cosmetic, and distillery industries. The oil is found in Benedictine, chartreuse, and gin.

Recent Scientific Findings

Angelica contains essential oils (including ligustilide, safrol, carvacrol, and n-butylidenphthalide); fatty acids (palmitic, linolic, stearic, arachidonic); commarins (bergaptene); as well as a host of other compounds including Beta-sitosterol, and several B-vitamins. These constituents are responsible for the extremely dynamic activity exhibited by this pharmacologically active herb.

Interestingly, while this herb has been shown to have genuine effects in regulating uterine function, depending upon how it is prepared, **it both stimulates and inhibits uterine muscles.** Here is what the *Oriental Materia Medica* advises:

> Experiments indicate that its non-volatile water-soluble compounds stimulate uterine muscle, while its volatile oil inhibits uterine muscle, producing a relaxing action. Therefore, to cause the uterus to contract the herb should be decocted for a long period of time to get rid of the volatile oil. If the uterus is to be relaxed then the herb should be put into the decoction later (that is, the other herbs should be decocted first for some time before *tang-kuei* [Angelica] is added and it should be boiled over a low flame to prevent loss of the

volatile oil). Animal studies show that the uterus upon being pressed will exhibit irregular contractions, but after administration of *tang-kuei* the uterus will contract regularly. This means that *tang-kuei* can regulate the function of the uterus and that is most probably the mechanism of *tang-kuei's* ability to treat menorrhalgia. Mice given feed containing 5% *tang-kuei* have higher DNA (deoxyribonucleic acid) content in their uteri, have higher glucose metabolism, and thus have a higher multiplication rate of uterine tissue.

According to extensive clinical trials, Angelica has proven to be **antibacterial, antifungal, an immuno-stimulant** (inducing production of interferon), and has **exhibited anti-tumor activity.** A study from Japan, by Dr. Yamada in 1990, suggests anti-tumor activity in *in vitro* experiments utilizing polysaccharide fractions from Angelica. A 1991 Japanese study employed several different extracts of Angelica root to test their anti-tumor properties. The authors concluded that two of the extracts may be useful to develop the effective method of cancer prevention.

Two chalcones isolated from Angelica root showed antibacterial activity. A 1990 study involving two other extracts focused on anti-ulcer effects. The authors found that the derivatives "significantly inhibited acid secretion and the formation of stress-induced gastric lesions. These results suggest that the antisecretory effect is due to the inhibition of gastric H+."

Ferulic acid is a phenolic compound contained in Angelica. Researchers discovered that ferulic acid showed an inhibitory effect on uterine movement and contractions. A mixture of herbal components, TS, which included Angelica hoelen, peony, alisma, and cnidum significantly increased progesterone secretion, suggesting "an exquisitive blended effect of herbal components of TS on progesterone secretion by corpora lutea."

Two 1991 studies involved Angelica's effect on **arrhythmia** (irregular heartbeat). The results showed that the total **incidence of arrhythmia were greatly reduced by Angelica.**

ANISE

SCIENTIFIC NAME: *Pimpinella anisum*
PARTS USED: Seed

DOSAGE:

   Seeds: Steep 1 teaspoon of crushed seeds per cup boiling water, 3-5 minutes. Drink cold, 1 to 2 cups per day, 1 tablespoon at a time.

ANISE: *The aromatic seeds may also promote iron absorption.*

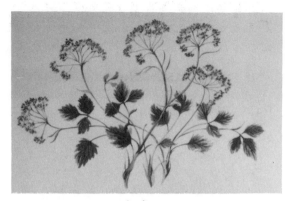

Anise

Traditional Usages

The 1918 *U.S. Dispensary* says, "It is one of the oldest aromatics, having been used by the ancient Egyptians; is spoken of by Theophrastus; and was cultivated in the imperial German farms of Charlemagne."

The seeds are abundant in Malta and Spain. The Spanish seeds are smaller than the German or French and are usually preferred. Anise seeds' fragrant odor is increased by friction. They taste warm, sweet, and aromatic. These properties, which depend on a volatile oil, are imparted sparingly to boiling water, freely to alcohol. The volatile oil extract is the envelope of the seeds, and is separated by distillation. Their internal substance contains a bland fixed oil. By expression, a greenish oil is obtained, which is a mixture of the two. The seeds are sometimes adulterated with small fragments of argillaceous earth. Their aromatic qualities are occasionally impaired due to a slight fermentation they undergo when collected before maturity. The seeds are the source of oil in Anise, utilized extensively in flavoring.

A decoction of Anise seed added to milk is used to **remedy infant colic and flatulence**. It also **increases milk secretion** for nursing mothers. Due to its pleasant aroma, it is often added to preparations to make them more palatable, mainly masking disagreeable odors. (These properties are known as **carminative** and **aromatic**.)

Recent Scientific Findings

Containing 80- to 90-percent anethol and methyl clavicol, Anise seeds have been shown to be an **effective expectorant** (promotes discharge of phlegm from lungs).

A 1990 study tested the effect of certain beverage extracts, including anise, on the absorption of iron. The results showed that anise was the most effective of the extracts tested in **promoting iron absorption**. The authors recommended offering beverages with anise, mint, caraway, cumin, tilia, and liquorice to children and adults as a preventive agent to iron deficiency anemia.

Along with its aromatic properties, anise seeds have been shown to possess **insecticidal** properties.

ARROWROOT

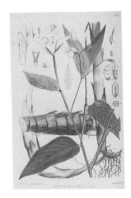

Arrowroot

SCIENTIFIC NAME: *Maranta arundinacea*

PARTS USED: Root

DOSAGE:

Root: 1 tablespoon, boiled in a covered container of 1½ pints water for about ½ hour, at a slow boil. Allow liquid to cool slowly in the *closed* container. Taken cold, 1 swallow or 1 tablespoon at a time, 1 to 2 cups per day.

ARROWROOT: *The natives of Central and South America used this root as an antidote to arrow poisoning; it is now recognized as a superior carbohydrate.*

Traditional Usages

The Arrowroot plant is a native of South America and of the West Indies, where it is predominantly cultivated. It also grows in Florida, and has been cultivated in the southern states.

It is probable that other plants contribute to furnish the Arrowroot of commerce. It is procured in the West Indies from *Maranta allouya* and *M. nobils,* beside *M. arundinacea.* Other species serve as sources of Arrowroot in the East Indies.

The mashed rhizome of Arrowroot were once used by Central and South American Indians as an **antidote for arrow poisoning**—hence the plant's name.

It is recorded that the Mayas utilized the root to make **poultices for smallpox** and, when drunk as a beverage, as a remedy for pus in the urine. This latter usage is due to the root's demulcent properties, which made it valuable in bowel complaints as well as urinary problems.

Recent Scientific Findings

Today Arrowroot is commonly used in baked products. It is a **superior carbohydrate** as well as a **source of digestible calcium,** which makes it a valuable element in the diet of children after weaning and of delicate persons during convalescence. It may be prepared as a jell, gruel, blancmange, and beverage, as well as in baking.

When mixed with hot water, the root starch of this herbaceous perennial becomes gelatinous and serves as an **effective demulcent** to soothe irritated mucous membranes.

ARTICHOKE

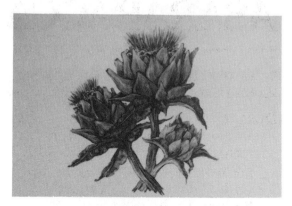

Artichoke

SCIENTIFIC NAME: *Cynara scolymus*
PARTS USED: Flowerhead bud and root

DOSAGE:

Leaves: 1 to 4 grams of the dried leaves or stem three times per day.

ARTICHOKE: *This tasty vegetable contains flavonoids that protect the liver.*

Traditional Usages

Artichokes have long been eaten as a vegetable. The leaves were used for their diuretic properties. The leaves and roots were employed to help prevent atherosclerosis and to treat diabetes. Other reputed uses include for jaundice, anemia, and dyspepsia.

Recent Scientific Findings

Silymarin is a flavonoid long recognized for its ability to benefit people with **liver disorders** and as a protective compound against liver-damaging agents. Wild artichoke contains silymarin. A group of researchers pretreated rats or mice with a single dose of silymarin isolated from Artichoke. After introducing a liver toxin, they found that the silymarin completely abolished the lethal effects, pathological changes, and significantly decreased the levels of serum enzymes normally induced by the toxin. These results, along with numerous other studies (see *Milk Thistle*), *confirm, once again, silymarin's ability to protect the liver.*

Recently, it has been found that Globe Artichoke contains the extract cymarin, which is similar to silymarin. Researchers discovered that this extract promotes liver regeneration and causes hyperaemia. It was also found that an Artichoke extract caused dyspeptic symptoms to disappear. The researchers interpreted the reduction in cholinesterase levels to mean that the extract effected fatty degeneration of the liver. In another study, Artichoke lowered lipids. Interestingly, in 1969 a team of French researchers patented an Artichoke extract as a treatment for kidney and liver ailments.

In the 1940s, a series of experiments by Japanese, Swiss, and American researchers discovered that **Artichokes lowered blood cholesterol.** The lead and cadmium content of 20 species of edible vegetables collected in Spain was investigated for their lead and mercury content. The researchers found that Artichoke, along with tomato, cucumber, and green beans, contained the lowest concentrations of lead and mercury, in comparison to "soft" vegetables such as lettuce, spinach, and parsley.

ASARABACCA

SCIENTIFIC NAME: *Asarum europaeum*

PARTS USED: Rhizome, root, and leaves

DOSAGE:

Caution: Do not use as a cathartic. As a snuff, 0.065-0.13 gram is snuffed up the nostrils. (This plant is an ingredient of the European Schneeberger snuff.)

ASARABACCA: Modern research supports the traditional use of the leaves as an expectorant.

Traditional Usages

This plant is known for its emetic, diuretic, and cathartic properties. It has been substituted for Ipecac to produce vomiting; the French use it for this purpose after drinking too much wine.

In powder form and taken as a snuff, it causes a profuse discharge of mucus from the nasal membranes, and hence has been used to remedy headache, drowsiness, giddiness, catarrhs, and other conditions caused by congestion. Asarabacca has been a component in many popular commercial medicinal snuffs. There are numerous reports of the folkloric anticancer use of this plant.

Recent Scientific Findings

Asarabacca has been extensively investigated, both chemically and pharmacologically. It is rich in flavonoids. The leaves contain a highly aromatic essential oil that contains constituents that verify the value of extracts as an errhine (for promotion of nasal secretion). Based on human experiments, the expectorant properties of both the roots and the leaves are quite good.

In Rumania, human experiments where infusions of Asarabacca were administered to people suffering pulmonary insufficiency, the preparations were said to have a **beneficial effect on the heart condition, including a diuretic effect.**

Human experiments have shown that the emetic effect of the leaves is not as pronounced as that of other, more effective drugs. There is no experimental evidence to support the use of any part of Asarabacca as a cathartic, although from the types of irritant chemical compounds known to be present in this plant, one would expect that catharsis would result from ingestion of extracts prepared from Asarabacca. However, **it is violent in its action and its use in home practice is discouraged.**

ASHWAGANDHA
("Indian Ginseng")

SCIENTIFIC NAME: *Withania somnifera*
PARTS USED: Root

DOSAGE:

Root: 1 teaspoon of dried root bark per 1½ pints water, boiled in covered container for about ½ hour, at a slow boil. Allow liquid to cool slowly in the *closed* container. Drink 1 cup at a time, twice daily.

ASHWAGANDHA: *In use for more than 2,500 years, this Indian shrub is proving adaptogenic properties described in ancient texts.*

Traditional Usages

"The notion of resistance to disease and the idea that such resistance can be modified by life experience and by emotional states, forms one of the basic tenets of Ayurveda, the ancient Indian system of medicine, thus avoiding the Cartesian dichotomization of mind and body," writes S. Ghosal concerning research on Ayurvedic medicines.

From antiquity to the present day, Ayurvedic medicine has employed a wholistic approach to physical and mental well-being. Preserved through the ages on delicate manuscripts and scrolls, Ayurveda retains a vital place in modern India. Used for more than 2,500 years, Ashwagandha, is among several plants the renowned

Ayurvedic text *Charaka Samhita* (1000 B.C.), terms **"vitalizers,"** describing properties that today fall under the category of "adaptogens."

Since antiquity, Ayurvedic physicians have used Ashwagandha as a rejuvenative tonic both alone and in combination with other products. The ancient Ayurvedic texts say Ashwagandha, when taken with milk, oil, or water for 15 days, "imparts strength for the emaciated body, as good as rain does to a crop."

Traditionally, the various preparations and forms of Ashwagandha, such as powder, decoction, oil, smoke, poultice, etc., have been utilized for a variety of conditions including **arthritis, asthma, bronchitis, cancer, candida, fever, inflammations, nausea,** and **rheumatism.** However, its most important use is as a tonic to promote vigor and stamina.

Recent Scientific Findings

Today's researchers continue to study and substantiate, through modern science, many traditional applications for Ayurvedic herbs. Over the last forty years, an increasing number of studies have been made of Ashwagandha's constituents by scientists interested in the **sedative and tranquilizing properties** of Ashwagandha roots and the traditional uses of the plant in the treatment of numerous maladies. The result has been that a large number of compounds have been isolated. At present, Ashwagandha is known to contain 11 alkaloids, 35 withanolides, and several sitoindosides, a new group of bioactive chemicals first isolated in late 1980s. Yet even with all the high technology tools of modern analysis, the complexity of the plant and it's constituents are not fully understood. Further studies are continuing to examine additional chemical constituents of this plant in an effort to explain and understand its unique actions.

An adaptogen is an agent that causes adaptive reactions. Adaptogenic drugs appear to increase SNIR (State of Non-specifically Increased Resistance) in the human body, protecting against diverse stresses. Pharmacological research has shown that Ashwagandha is effective for a variety of ailments, including leucoderma, bronchitis, asthma, and marasmus, and that it is also useful as a hypotensive, antispasmodic, antitumor, antiarthritic, antipyretic, analgesic, anti-inflammatory, and antidiabetic. Because of its usefulness in diverse pathological states, it is reasonable to conclude that the herb acts by inducing SNIR in the human body.

Much of the research has concerned Ashwagandha's **anti-stress** and **anti-cancer** properties. One study concluded that mice treated with Ashwagandha exhibited better swimming performance, a standard means for assessing stress. The duration of swimming increased significantly in treated mice. The researchers also found Ashwagandha reduced the incidence of gastric ulcers produced by high doses of aspirin and by physical stress. In a later study on albino mice, *Withania somnifera* was found to completely reverse the effects of urethane on total count, lymphocyte count, body weight and mortality. It also afforded significant protection to the extent of 75% in the incidence as well as in the number of lung adenomas.

In studying the effects of two new sitonindosides derived from *Withania somnifera*, Ghosal found the compounds produced significant anti-stress activity in albino mice and rats and augmented learning acquisition and memory retention in young and old rats. These findings are consistent with the use of *W. somnifera* in Ayurveda to attenuate cerebral function deficits in the geriatric population and to provide non-specific host defense. Ghosal concluded:

> Pharmacologists have long sought a drug for the treatment of **memory disorders**, a drug which could enhance the acquisition, storage and retrieval of learning and memory. Most of the synthetic drugs (e.g., the nootropic agents) in use are psycho-stimulants which cause improved performance mainly due to improvement in attention by way of arousal induced by these agents and they have no significant effect on memory storage and retrieval. The present study suggests an opportunity for the improved use of this Ayurvedic 'Rasayan' (*Ashwagandha*) for **immunomodulation** and for **learning** and **memory**.

Human studies have shown similar results. A 1965 study employed Withaferin A, a compound extracted from Ashwagandha leaves. Results demonstrated marked **tumor-inhibitory activity** when tested *in vivo* against cells derived from human carcinoma. In a double blind trial conducted with children between the ages of 8 and 10, it was found that milk fortified with Ashwagandha resulted in increased body weight and total protein.

In another double blind clinical trial to study the process of aging, 101 healthy male adults between the ages of 50-59 were surveyed. After treatment for one year, statistically significant differences were found between the Ashwagandha group and the placebo group in hemoglobin and serum cholesterol. The treated group exhibited significant increases in hemoglobin and red blood cell count. **Serum cholesterol levels were much lower** in the treated group. **No side effects** of the drug were observed.

This plant has also been shown to possess anti-inflammatory activity, making it useful in arthritis. In several animals studies *W. somnifera* was proven to have more activity than four other herbs which were tested. Interestingly, these "others" are all respected as folkloric treatments for arthritis.

Ashwagandha's antiarthritic activity was also demonstrated in a human clinical trial. A herbal formula consisting of Ashwagandha, Turmeric, and Boswellin was evaluated in a randomized, double-blind, placebo-controlled study. After a one-month evaluation period 12 patients with **osteoarthritis** were given the herbal formula or placebo for three months. The patients were evaluated every two weeks. Then after a 15 day wash-out period, the treatment was reversed with the placebo patients receiving the drug and vice versa. Again results were evaluated over a three month period. The patients treated with the herbal formula showed a significant drop in severity of pain and disability score.

As the concept of functional foods to reduce the incidence of various diseases becomes widespread in the United States, preventive herbal extracts such as Ashwagandha will find a vital place among the diets of many Americans.

ASTRAGALUS

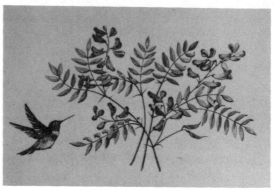

Astragalus

SCIENTIFIC NAME: *Astragalus membranaceus*

PARTS USED: Root

DOSAGE:

Root: One teaspoon of root to 1½ pints water. In a covered container, slowly boil for 20 to 30 minutes. Allow the liquid to cool slowly in the *closed* container. Drink 1 cup at a time, twice daily.

ASTRAGALUS: *This traditional Chinese medicinal has yielded striking results in stimulating the immune system.*

Traditional Usages

Astragalus is a commonly used traditional herb in Chinese medicine, where this potent plant is known as Radix Astragali, or as part of a Chinese herbal mixture called *Qiang gan ruan jian tang*. "Yellow leader," as it is known, is recognized for its importance as a tonic herb, and for centuries the Chinese have utilized Astragalus to enhance natural defense mechanisms. Its use was first recorded in a herbal over 2,000 years ago. Astragalus is a tonic used to increase *ch'i* or "wind energy," overcome fatigue, control diabetes, lower blood pressure, and to treat coronary heart disease and anemia.

Recent Scientific Findings

Certain species of Astragalus are the source of the widely used food additive, tragacanth gum. *Astragalus membranaceus* has been screened for its **immunomodulating activity**, and found to augment the proliferation of mononuclear (MNC) white blood cells (macrophages and lymphocytes) in vitro. Recent studies originating out of the M.D. Anderson Hospital and Tumor Institute in Houston, Texas have yielded a stronger focus on the immunomodulating scope of *Astragalus membranaceous.*

As with many plant extracts, certain fractions may possess biological activities that are in direct contrast with those of other fractions. Chu and his colleagues performed several extraction procedures and manipulations on air-dried roots of Astragalus, ultimately producing 8 different fractions, fraction 7 being the original crude extract. The authors used a testing model developed in their laboratory, designed to evaluate the competence of human T-lymphocytes in attacking foreign cells (rat skins). The animals were rendered immuno suppressed, due to the administration of cyclophosphamide, a potent immunosuppressive agent routinely used in human organ transplantation procedures. This minimized the influence of the animal's immune system upon the actions of the implanted human cells.

Individuals with various types of cancer, and "normal" controls served as blood donors for the MNC's. MNC's were treated with one of the eight fractions derived from the original roots of Astragalus. Fractions 2, 3, 7, and 8 displayed significant immunomodulating activity in cells from controls in this system. Fractions 3, 7, (the original crude extract) and 8 all produced a significant increase in the immunocompetence of the animals. However, fraction 2 led to a further reduction of immune function, indicating this fraction to have **immunorestorative** effects.

The treatment of MNC's from cancer patients revealed additional striking results. Only fractions 3, 7, and 8 were used in this part of the study. Five of the 13 cancer patients' MNC's experienced immune restoration in their T-cell activity. The MNC's from the remaining 8 patients had intact T-cell function before incubation with the fractions; following incubation T-cell function was actually increased.

The authors pointed out that **the immune responsivity seen in most of the Astragalus-treated cells from cancer patients was greater than that observed in the cells from untreated normal donors.** Cancer patients' cells treated with fractions 3 and 8 displayed the greatest degree of immune restoration, being significantly greater than that of untreated normal control values. Treatment with fraction 7 did not produce a significantly greater response.

Comparison of the stimulating effects of fractions 3, 7, and 8 on MNC's from both cancer and normal donors revealed fraction 3 to possess a higher stimulating activity in cancer patients than in normals. No difference existed between the two groups for the other two fractions. Fraction 3 also proved to have superior immunorestorative actions in cancer patients alone, relative to the crude extract (7), and the extract derivative (8).

A companion study evaluated the ability of immunosupressed animals treated with fraction 3 to generate an immune response against untreated human MNC's. This is similar to a reversal of the previous experiments, where the animals T-cells are tested in their capacity to attack human T-cells. They found fraction 3 to completely reverse the effects of cyclophosphamide-induced immuno suppression upon their test system. Although fraction 3 was administered intravenously, it is very likely that oral administration of a carefully fractioned Astragalus preparation would also exert significant immunorestorative activity in such conditions as cancer and AIDS.

A third subfractionation was performed, using AR-4E as the parent fraction. This step produced four more subfractions (AR-4E1 - AR-4E4), with AR-4E2 having the greatest anti-tumor potential. This third generation fraction was composed of 87% hexose-type sugars e.g. galactose, arabinose, and rhamnose. The authors performed extensive analysis of the chemical properties of this latter fraction, leading them to conclude that the structure of the side chain of the polysaccharide fraction determines its anti-tumor activity, but not its anti-complementary activity.

These structure-activity relationship studies are crucial to the understanding of the specific component(s) responsible for the biological effects of a given plant extract, and in the development of powerful plant drug extracts with a high degree of specificity. Reducing a plant extract to a single molecule or compound does indeed lead one into the world of conventional medicine, as many drugs currently used were once derived from plant sources. However, this process also provides a marker, or series of markers, whereby crude plant extracts can be objectively assessed for their content of active principles.

The structure-activity relationship studies reviewed here are crucial to the understanding of the specific component(s) responsible for the biological effects of a given plant extract, and in the development of powerful plant drug extracts with a high degree of specificity.

Several new studies focusing on the *whole* plant also demonstrate the immune-enhancing properties of this remarkable plant. Extracts of Astragalus injected into mice were seen to increase the Th cell activity in *both* normal and immunodepressed mice. Even an *oral* dose of an ethanol extract of the root of this herb was shown to alleviate liver injury that had been experimentally induced in mice, and also to protect liver cells from pathological changes.

In a study of **chronic cervicitis** it was found that this disorder was associated with *three* types of virus; **papillomavirus type 16, herpes simplex virus type 2, and cytomegalovirus (CMV)**. Treatment with recombinant interferon alpha 1 improved clinical symptoms in 93.8% of cases. The study authors then added *A. membranaceus* to the therapy and concluded it was "synergistic to interferon therapy." Perhaps the future of medicine will show that a **combination of ancient and modern therapies** will offer the best hope for medical treatment.

Within the last 10 or 20 years interest in AM, for immune-enhancement, has moved from its home (in China) to the U.S. and Japan. An Italian study found that **Astragalus extracts were immunostimulatory** on mononuclear cells from normal healthy donors and cancer patients. The authors believe that the observed enhancement of Th cell activity results from increased induction of these Th cells, both in normal mice or immunodepressed mice. Perhaps most interestingly, the biological activity of Astragalus extracts were found to depend on the *carbohydrate* content, lending support to the continued use of the whole plant in herbal medicine.

BARBERRY

SCIENTIFIC NAME: *Berberis vulgaris*
PARTS USED: Root bark and berries

DOSAGE:

Root: When used in medicine the dosage was 1 teaspoon of dried root bark per 1½ pints water, boiled in covered container for about ½ hour, at a slow boil. Allow liquid to cool slowly in the *closed* container. Drink 1 cup at a time, twice daily. If the more potent *powdered* root bark was prepared as above, just 1 cup daily was considered sufficient.

BARBERRY: *Used by the ancient Egyptians, this plant is rich in the astringent berberine.*

Traditional Usages

Barberry is noted throughout herb literature for its important economic and medicinal properties. The ripe fruit is eaten as a preserve; the roots yield a yellow dye which at one time was utilized in the dyeing of wool, cotton, and flax.

In ancient Egyptian medicine, syrup of Barberry combined with Fennel seeds was reputedly of value in warding off the plague. This possibility is not to be laughed off, since the ancient Hebrews relied on Hops for the same purpose. Hops contain effective **antibacterial** principles, and were in fact **valuable against the infectious agent *Yersinia pestis*, the plague bacillus.** In exploring the possible validity of Barberry and Fennel seed for the same purpose we would have to evaluate **potential antibacterial properties.**

Soon after Barberry's introduction to North America, several tribes employed it for medicinal purposes. The Penobscots of Maine pulverized the roots or bark in water and applied them to **mouth ulcers** or to relieve **sore throat.** The Catawbas drank a tea of the boiled roots and stems for **stomach ulcers.** Since Barberry was employed in Europe for similar purposes, it is safe to assume that the Native Americans borrowed these uses from the early settlers.

The fruits of this shrub were formerly used in England to **reduce fevers,** while the bark was employed as a purgative and as a diarrhea treatment. During the early part of the nineteenth century, the acidic berries were also used in Egypt to reduce fevers. Throughout other traditional herbal literature we find patterns of usage surrounding the following ills: **high fevers, jaundice, and chronic dysentery.**

Recent Scientific Findings

The most credible medicinal uses are centered in the herb's strong **purging** effects, and as a **gargle** for sore throats. While the root bark, rich in berberine, is used for the former effect, the Barberry fruit itself is crushed for that latter; it also finds application as a mouthwash.

Barberry owes virtually all of its effects to its high content of the alkaloid berberine, which is present in all parts of the plant. Berberine, when applied externally, causes an astringent effect, and if placed in the eye will reduce the "bloodshot" appearance, since the blood

vessels are constricted by the alkaloid. Due to the berberine, Barberry berries would be useful as a **mouthwash** and **gargle** for their astringent effect, and some **local anesthetic effect.**

If the correct amount is used, Barberry roots will act as a **purgative.** Barberry root preparations are even more useful, however, to halt diarrhea. Such preparations are well established as effective in stopping diarrhea in cases of **bacterial dysentery.** Since berberine is not very well absorbed if taken by mouth, the risk of any possible toxic effects is reduced.

BAYBERRY

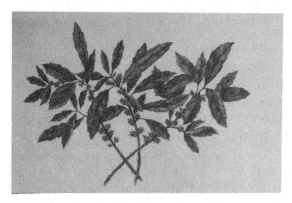

Bayberry

SCIENTIFIC NAME: *Myrica cerifera*
PARTS USED: Bark

DOSAGE:

Bark: 1 teaspoon of dried root bark per 1½ pints water, boiled in covered container for about ½ hour, at a slow boil. Allow liquid to cool slowly in the *closed* container. Drink 1 cup at a time, twice daily.

BAYBERRY: *At one time the bark was a popular drug in domestic American medicine.*

Traditional Usages

Bayberry bark was popular in domestic American medicine for its **astringent** and **tonic** properties. A decoction was used in cases of **diarrhea, dysentery, dropsy, uterine hemorrhage**, and as a **gargle** for **sore throat**. A poultice was applied to sores and ulcers. The root bark was official in the *National Formulary* for only twenty years, from 1916 to 1936.

The wax which forms around the berries was also used medicinally. It was boiled "to an extract [as] a certain cure for the most violent cases of dysentery." Some physicians of the eighteenth century even considered this wax a narcotic!

Native American use of the plant was quite limited. Only one tribe, the Louisiana Choctaws, employed it as a fever remedy. They boiled the leaves and stems and drank the resulting tea.

Recent Scientific Findings

Bayberry's use in modern medicine continues to be limited, as there are other more effective astringent and tonic herbs.

Interestingly, the extract has proven to be useful as an insect attractant, particularly for male Mediterranean fruit flies. Thus it may become of importance as a natural means of controlling fruit fly infestations.

BEARBERRY
(UVA URSI)

SCIENTIFIC NAME: *Arctostaphylos uva-ursi*

PARTS USED: Leaves

DOSAGE:

    Leaves: When made up by herbalists, the leaves were often soaked in brandy or alcohol for a few hours, then added to boiling water, using 1 teaspoon of the soaked leaves per cup of water. Two to three cups were taken per day, cold. An alternative preparation consisted of the dried leaves powdered and boiled in water without the alcohol soak.

BEARBERRY: *The leaves of this evergreen shrub have a long history of use as a diuretic.*

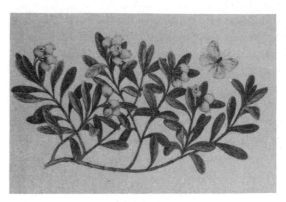

Bearberry

Traditional Usages

It appears that the medicinal properties of Bearberry were discovered independently by Native Americans and white settlers. The Thompson tribe of British Columbia drank a tea of steeped Bearberry leaves to **promote the flow of urine** and to strengthen the bladder and kidneys. The Menominees added the leaves to their **menstrual remedies.** The Cheyenne and Sioux used Bearberry to **promote labor contractions.** The early fur traders of the Scottish Northwest Company reported that many tribes used the leaves with honey, pollen, and other herbs as a **longevity elixir.**

Although this evergreen shrub was used in ancient medicine, it was not popularly employed for kidney disorders until the mid-eighteenth century. From that time on, Bearberry leaf was a recognized diuretic. The *London Pharmacopoeia* admitted it in 1763 and it was included in the *U.S. Pharmacopoeia* from 1820 until 1936.

The strong astringent properties of the leaves have led to usage as diuretics and tonics. Inflammations of the urinary tract, especially in acute cystitis, were formerly treated with a decoction of these leaves. (Patients were forewarned to expect a sharp greenish color of their urine during treatment.) Bearberry leaves, prior to the discovery of synthetic diuretic and urinary antiseptic drugs, were the major medicine available to physicians for these purposes.

Recent Scientific Findings

We have known for a number of years that the diuretic, astringent, and urinary antiseptic value of Bearberry leaves can be accounted for by the fact that they contain the active principles hydroquinone and arbutin. In the body, arbutin is rapidly converted to hydroquinone, which is what causes the harmless effect of changing the color of the urine.

A study examined the combined effect of arbutin isolated from Bearberry leaves and indomethacin on immuno-inflammation, edema, and arthritis. When arbutin and indomethacin were administered simultaneously, the inhibitory effect was more potent than indomethacin alone. The authors stated that these results suggest that arbutin may increase the inhibitory action of indomethacin on **edema** and **arthritis**.

A similar 1990 series of studies by a Japanese research group employed a 50% methanolic extract from Bearberry leaf with prednisolone to determine its effect on immuno-inflammation. Like the indomethacin research, the authors found that when simultaneously administered, the inhibitory effect was more potent than that of prednisolone alone. They also isolated arbutin from the methanolic extract and found similar results.

Additionally, Bearberry leaves contain **allantoin,** a substance that is known to **soothe and accelerate the repair of irritated tissues.**

A liquid extract of Bearberry given in the form of a chamomile tea was reported to be useful in the treatment of **cystitis** in paraplegics. Unlike nitroguantoin, Bearberry did not cause gastric irritation.

Experiments conducted by Rumanian scientists in 1980 have proven Bearberry exhibits **anti-trichomonal activity** in "in vitro" tests. Current pharmacology indicates Bearberry demonstrates **antiviral (particularly strong against herpes and flu)** and antibacterial action, enhances **cytotoxic** activity, and also exhibits **antifungal** and **anti-plaque** action.

A dietary study involving a herbal mixture containing Bearberry, Goldenseal, Mistletoe, and Tarragon found significant effects on the symptoms of **diabetes** without affecting glycemic control.

BEE POLLEN

SCIENTIFIC NAME: *Entomophilous,* var. spp.
PARTS USED: Plant pollen collected by bees, mixed with honey and nectar, and then fermented in the hive.

DOSAGE:

Caution: It is advised that readers use only commercial products and follow the label directions.

BEE POLLEN: *Pollen extracts have been shown to increase stamina.*

Traditional Usages

Pollen extracts are a highly concentrated energy source for protein and carbohydrates. They are often taken as a **food supplement**. Among athletes, pollen has a reputation for **increasing stamina** and, in general, **improving athletic ability.**

More recently, in Eastern Europe and Russia pollen has been used to treat a variety of ailments, including **anemia, diarrhea, mental illness, obesity, rickets**, and **skin problems.**

Royal Jelly is the larval bee food produced from saliva of the Honey Bee (*Apis mellifera*). It is the sole food of bee larvae for first 3 days of life. It is also the continued food for the queen bee(s). This food is what causes queen bees to differentiate and develop. In folk medicine, Royal Jelly has been used as a **youth enhancer, hair restorer,** and **fertility aid.**

Recent Scientific Findings

Animal studies of pollen extract have demonstrated **remarkable lipid-lowering effects.** Researchers found that rats fed an atherogenic (i.e., causes atherosclerosis) diet consisting of a high saturated fat content and concurrently fed pollen extract attained a lowered total cholesterol content and a rise in serum HDH cholesterol.

At Pratt Institute in New York, bee pollen was shown to **improve endurance and speed.** This finding was substantiated by a study in which four groups of rabbits were fed differing diets. (The rabbit was chosen by this group of Polish scientists owing to its susceptibility to atherosclerosis and its similarity to man in bile acid metabolism. While I strongly *oppose* most animal experimentation, I feel it would be a double tragedy to *not* report on valuable work already completed.)

> The study showed that the pollen extracts not only significantly lowered blood lipid levels, but they also suppressed the development of atherosclerotic plaque formation.

These effects are thought to be due to the known constituents of pollen extract, such as polyunsaturated fatty acids (23% Linolenic acid) and sterols, 21 amino acids, all known vitamins, enzymes, and coenzymes, minerals, and trace elements.

The researchers utilized a pollen extract that is a trademarked product derived from six plant species: rye grass, maize, timothy grass, pine, alder flower, and orchard grass. These extracts (Cernitin T60 and Cernitin GBX—also known in the industry by the names AB Cernelle, Vegeholm, Sweden) are uniquely treated. Pollen grains have their membranes removed with a solvent and are then flushed out through the hila. The solvent is later removed and the pollen extract digested microbiologically. This process, transforms the difficult to absorb high-molecular weight material to low-molecular weight substances which are easily absorbed in the G.I. tract. Because the final product is free of antigens and other high-molecular weight substances, it ought not produce allergic reactions in humans.

There has been no evidence to support the folkloric uses of Royal Jelly. However, it has exhibited anti-inflammatory action and analgesic activity in mouse and rat experiments.

In regards to allergy, an interesting 1991 paper proposed that mammals evolved allergic reactions "as a last line of defense against the extensive array of toxic substances that exist in the environment in the form of secondary plant compounds and venoms." The authors stated that allergic responses, such as sneezing, coughing, diarrhea, and scratching, help the body expel the toxic substance that triggered the response. Since toxic substances also bind to the DNA of target cells, they are potentially mutagenic and carcinogenic as well. "Thus, by protecting against acute toxicity, allergy may also defend against mutagens and carcinogens." This fascinating hypothesis explains why allergies occur to many foods, pollens, etc,; why allergic cross-reactions occur to allergens from unrelated botanical families; why allergy appears to be so capricious and variable; and why allergy is more prevalent in industrial societies.

Caution: Persons with pollen-sensitive allergies may find bee pollen aggravating.

BELLADONNA

SCIENTIFIC NAME: *Atropa belladonna*
PARTS USED: Leaves

DOSAGE:

Leaves: Tincture of Belladonna is occasionally employed by traditional physicians, in a dosage of 0.5 milliliter by mouth every 4 hours or as needed. When the plant itself is used, 1 teaspoonful of the leaves is steeped in 1 pint of boiling water for 3-5 minutes. The infusion is drunk cold, 1-2 teaspoonfuls 2 to 3 times daily.

Caution: Contains potent alkaloids. Heavy overdose can have very serious effects. Blindness, as noted, can occur if taken by people using drugs for glaucoma.

BELLADONNA: *This toxic plant contains atropine, an alkaloid with a variety of medical uses.*

Traditional Usages

This plant's name is the combination of the two Italian words, *bella* (beautiful) and *donna* (lady). Some writers contend that Belladonna berries were used by Italian ladies as a cosmetic dye and to dilate the pupils of the eyes to give them a captivating look. In the Middle Ages, it was believed the devil watched over Belladonna, his favorite plant.

Externally applied as a plaster or in ointment form, this plant has had long use as an effective **painkiller.** The highly toxic nature of Belladonna urges extreme caution in employing it internally.

Belladonna and **Black Nightshade have often been confused.** Unscrupulous or ignorant drug collectors regularly substituted Black Nightshade leaves for Belladonna leaves. Because of this, earlier publications on medicinal plants featured photographs of both species in microscopic detail to alert wholesale drug dealers.

Recent Scientific Findings

The alkaloid atropine obtained from Belladonna is used in medicine for five purposes: to check mucus secretion, to stimulate circulation, to overcome spasm of the involuntary muscles, locally to dilate the pupil of the eye and paralyze the muscles of visual accommodation, and externally as a local anodyne.

As a circulatory stimulant, atropine is highly useful in such applications as countering the depressant effects of various compounds, including Opium. Increasing heart rate by vagal inhibition, atropine is valuable in severe emergencies such as surgical shock.

Belladonna contains the potent alkaloids atropine (as already noted), hyoscyamine, and scopolamine, in all parts of the plant. These alkaloids are known to have an anodyne effect when applied to the skin. For example, Belladonna platers have been utilized for decades, especially to alleviate back pain. When taken internally, the alkaloids are absorbed and produce a strong antispasmodic effect on the smooth muscle of the gut. These alkaloids block the nerve supply to the stomach and cause a relaxation that results in less pain, due to reduced stress on the organ. Both atropine and hyoscyamine have a depressing effect on higher nerve centers, which accounts for the energetic narcotic effect of Belladonna preparations. However, the scopolamine is most probably responsible for most of this effect, since it has a greater depressant action on the higher nerve centers than atropine or hyoscyamine.

A word of warning should be interjected here: **Belladonna preparations are very potent and the greatest caution should attend their use.** Even light overdosing will result in dilation of the pupils of the eyes, which results in a "blurry" vision and inability to see things clearly. An additional, very characteristic effect of Belladonna derivatives is a "drying up" of the mouth, which can be uncomfortable. Persons being treated for glaucoma should never take Belladonna preparations, or any of the alkaloids contained in this plant, since the usual treatment for glaucoma is with drugs that have an effect opposite to Belladonna's. Should both drugs be used at the same time in a glaucoma patient, the effects of each would be nullified and the patient would most likely suffer irreversible blindness, unless this self-negating treatment was discovered early and discontinued.

BETEL NUT PALM

SCIENTIFIC NAME: *Areca catechu*
PARTS USED: Nuts

DOSAGE:
    Nuts: The nuts are chewed as desired.

BETEL NUT PALM: *In Southeast Asia, these nuts have long been chewed and habitual use may lead to cancer.*

Traditional Usages

This tall, elegant plant bears betel nuts, which are used by millions in Southeast Asia (Malaysia, New Guinea). The inside of the nut is powdered and chewed with lime enclosed in a fresh leaf from the *Piper betel* tree, while the red juice is spat out. There is a **relief of tension**, with a **definite sedative effect**. Normandy Islanders utilize these sedative nuts to "soothe a mad person."

Medicinally, the betel nuts were used for various digestive ailments including intestinal worms and irregularity.

Recent Scientific Findings

The nuts contain the alkaloids arecoline and arecaidine. Arecoline has known **anthelmintic** and **tranquilizing properties**. While habitual chewers of the nut have a high incidence of buccal cancer, attributed by some to the condensed tannins the nut contains (11-26 percent tannins), it is likely that other components of the nut or nutritional factors may also be involved. In fact, the very young unfolded leaves are even eaten as a vegetable. **A 1991 case control study in Thailand confirmed the cancer-promoting dangers of chewing this stimulant nut.**

In addition to their sedative effects, the nuts are also used to increase perspiration (in the common cold), to **kill worms, and in veterinary medicine as a laxative and worm remedy.**

In Europe, ground nuts are used in some **tooth powders.**

BILBERRY

SCIENTIFIC NAME: *Vaccinium myrtillus*
PARTS USED: Fruit

DOSAGE:

Berries: 1 teaspoon dried berries with 1 cup of water, 1 cup per day.

BILBERRY: *Modern research is finding that a variety of promising applications, including for atherosclerosis and ulcers.*

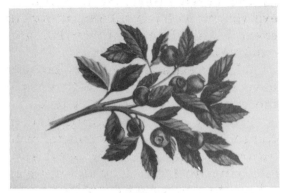

Bilberry

Traditional Usages

Traditionally, both the leaves and berries of this shrub has been used as an **astringent**. A decoction of the berries was employed for **fevers**. The juice of the berries was used as a **gargle** and **mouthwash** for catarrh.

Recent Scientific Findings

Extracts of Bilberry have been found to be **antiviral** in cell culture for **herpes simplex virus II**, **influenza**, and **vaccinia viruses**. In vitro testing of Bilberry extracts for antimicrobial activity is encouraging. Extracts have been found to kill or inhibit growth of **funguses**, **yeasts**, and **bacteria**. They have also been shown to **kill protozoans** such as *Trichomonas vaginalis*.

Anthocyanins in Bilberry act to prevent capillary fragility and inhibit platelet aggregation. Bilberry is therefore demonstrated to be an anti-inflammatory herb. Anthocyanins stimulate the release of vasodilator prostaglandin *in vitro*. These compounds, therefore, have potential for the prevention of thrombosis. They also causes coronary vasodilation in animals which would reverse attacks of angina. Moreover, they prevent atherosclerosis in cholesterol-loaded animals.

Since Bilberry extracts reduce capillary permeability, there is antihistamine activity, too. Many clinical tests have shown that Bilberry anthocyanosides given orally to humans **improve vision** in healthy people and also help treat people with eye diseases such as **pigmentary retinitis**.

Toxicology reports are especially promising regarding the anthocyanins. Tests in rats, mice and rabbits showed no abnormalities or toxicity. Even pregnant women who were given extracts of Bilberry (and vitamin E) were seen to have **fewer varices and various blood problems**. The study author concluded that the extract "was well tolerated and no side effects were found in either the mother or the infant."

A 1988 research project indicated that one Bilberry extract possesses a promising **anti-ulcer** activity. The researchers speculated this was probably due to the extract potentiating the defensive barriers of the gastrointestinal mucosa. In experiments with rats, **Bilberry proved to exert a significant preventive and curative anti-ulcer activity.**

Bilberry extracts have been found to have **anticancer** activity with certain cancer cell strains in laboratory tests.

Bilberry extracts administered in controlled experiments, conducted with persons suffering from **diabetes**, exhibited resulting normalization of capillary collagen thickness and reduced blood sugar levels in humans and animals.

BIRCH

SCIENTIFIC NAME: *Betula* spp.
PARTS USED: Leaves and bark

DOSAGE:

Leaves: Approximately 1 ounce of leaves to 1 pint of water. Boil water separately, pour over the plant material, and steep for 5 to 20 minutes, depending on the desired effect. Drink hot or warm, 1 to 2 cups per day.

BIRCH: *This tree's marvelous bark was once a common remedy.*

Traditional Usages

This tree's beautiful distinctive bark was also a common remedy. The boiled bark was used as a poultice for minor wounds. The leaves and bark, both separately and together, were steeped to make a tea drunk for a variety of ailments including **fevers, rheumatism,** and abdominal complaints. A tea from the boiled fruit was used during **menstruation.** The smoke from the burning fruit was inhaled to treat respiratory problems. White settlers also used Birch as a mouthwash and to treat intestinal worms. Indeed, in some regions of the U.S. the twigs are still chewed as a dentrifice.

Recent Scientific Findings

Unfortunately, there is little research to confirm or deny Birch's folkloric claims. Birch contains methyl salicylate, which is often used in ointments and liniments for conditions such as **rheumatism.**

BITTER-SWEET

SCIENTIFIC NAME: *Solanum dulcamara*
PARTS USED: Twigs, root, leaves

DOSAGE:

Root: When used in medicine the dose was 2 teaspoons of the root per pint of boiling water, drunk cold, 2 to 3 tablespoons, 6 times per day. A fluidextract was once official in the National Formulary in doses of 2 to 3.9 grams.

BITTERSWEET: *At one time this was employed extensively for skin irritations.*

Traditional Usages

Bittersweet, or Woody Nightshade, was used extensively in treating a variety of diseases. Internally, for example, it was reported to be beneficial in **chronic rheumatism**. However, its most usual application was **external**, for **treating skin eruptions and irritations.** A poultice of the leaves was applied for this purpose, especially in injuries of the knee joint, and in hard and painful swellings of the female breast. Bittersweet was also reportedly helpful for **bruises**, promoting the absorption of blood from the swollen tissues.

Recent Scientific Findings

Bittersweet is one of 27 herbs included in the March 1977 issue of the U.S. Food and Drug Administration Bulletin of Unsafe Herbs, "being a poisonous plant containing the toxic glycoalkaloid solanine, as well as solanidine and dulcamarin." However, some authorities report both the toxic and the medicinal properties of the plant to be rather insignificant; various investigators have administered considerable quantities without any noticeable medicinal of toxic effect.

We have been unable to document the rationale for the use of the root bark of Bittersweet in relieving skin irritation. **The fruits of this plant, however, are commonly implicated in cases where children ingesting them are often poisoned.** The severity of poisoning seems to depend on the stage of ripeness of the fruit.

Caution: **See above.**

BLESSED THISTLE

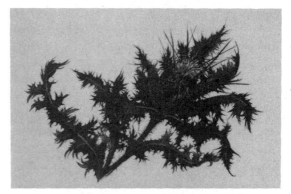

Blessed Thistle

SCIENTIFIC NAME: *Cnicus benedictus*
PARTS USED: Herb

DOSAGE:

Root bark: 1 teaspoon of dried root bark per 1½ pints water, boiled in covered container for about ½ hour, at a slow boil. Allow liquid to cool slowly in the *closed* container. Drink 1 cup at a time, twice daily.

BLESSED THISTLE: *Human experiments have confirmed this herb's folkloric use as a gastrointestinal.*

Traditional Usages

Blessed Thistle has been recorded as a medicinal since the first century A.D. Credited with the medical virtues of a **diuretic, diaphoretic, febrifuge,** and cholagogue, it has been used to treat a variety of ailments. It is a bitter tonic and a good appetite stimulant, and is still utilized today to treat **indigestion.** At one time this herb was ascribed the nearly supernatural qualities of a "cure all." The Zuni used Blessed Thistle to treat venereal disease, and to lower fever.

Blessed Thistle was considered an excellent **appetite stimulant.** It was also taken to relieve flatulence and indigestion, as well as to treat **liver** and **gallbladder** disorders.

Recent Scientific Findings

At one time this herb was ascribed the nearly supernatural qualities of a "cure all," but current knowledge yields no evidence to support such a belief. On the other hand, the use of leaf decoctions as a bitter tonic is well founded. The bitter principle in this plant is known to be cnicin, and human experiments have shown that extracts of Blessed Thistle stimulate the production of gastric juices, confirming its folkloric use as a gastrointestinal.

Cell cultures have shown cytotoxicity against cancer cells using extract of blessed thistle and **antitumor activity** in mouse cancer (sarcoma) as well.

In vitro studies with extracts of Blessed Thistle have shown considerable **antibacterial activity** against a wide variety of organisms, including *Nycobacterium phlei*. **Anti-yeast activity** against *Candida albicans* has been found in vitro using extract of Blessed Thistle.

BLOODROOT

SCIENTIFIC NAME: *Sanguinaria canadensis*

PARTS USED: Root

DOSAGE:

Root: For medicinal use, 1 level teaspoon of the ground root is steeped for ½ hour in 1½ pints of boiling water, then strained. Of the liquid thus produced, 1 teaspoon was taken 3 to 6 times per day. Avoid prolonged internal use.

BLOODROOT: *Once a common Native American medicine for rheumatism, this root's alkaloid extract prevents cavities and plaque.*

Traditional Usages

The Bloodroot owes its name to the red juice in the roots and stems, which was used as a facial dye by North American tribes. Among Native Americans of the Mississippi region, Bloodroot was a favorite remedy for **rheumatism**. The Rappahannocks of Virginia also made a tea from the root which they drank for rheumatism.

The Iroquois used Bloodroot to treat **ringworm**. The Pillager Ojibwas squeezed the root juices on a piece of maple sugar and held the astringent lump in their mouths to cure **sore throat**.

Bloodroot became popular in domestic American medicine for its ability to remove mucus from the respiratory mucous membranes, and was official in the *U.S. Pharmacopoeia* from 1820 to 1926. A powder was also applied externally to skin eruptions, nose polyps, ulcers, and badly healing sores.

Recent Scientific Findings

An **acro-narcotic poison on overdose, the plant has been reported to cause death.** It is one of the 27 plants included in the USFDA unsafe herb list, published in March 1977.

Bloodroot contains tormentil, which contains high amounts of tannic acid, explaining the plant's astringent properties. The root is emetic and purgative in large doses; in smaller doses it is stimulant, diaphoretic, and expectorant.

Experimentally Bloodroot preparations are known to induce emesis, have expectorant properties, and be irritant. These activities are all due to the presence of the toxic alkaloid sanguinarine. Topically, sanguinarine and/or Bloodroot preparations have been helpful in the treatment of **eczema** and most probably would give a **mild local anesthetic** effect. Mausert recommends an external application of the powder for **nose polyps, ulcers,** and **bad sores,** stating that it encourages new and healthy tissues.

> Several recent studies, including a long-term clinical evaluation, found that an extract of Bloodroot, sanguinaria, in toothpaste and mouth rinses helped prevent cavities and destroy plaque.

BONESET

SCIENTIFIC NAME: *Eupatorium perfoliatum*

PARTS USED: Tops and leaves

DOSAGE:

Leaves: Moderate dose (for fever): A mild infusion is brewed, 1 teaspoon of leaves per cup of boiling water, steeped 3-5 minutes. Drunk warm will produce perspiration and gentle vomiting. Drunk cold, effect is that of a simple tonic.

Strong dose: To be drunk as hot as the patient can tolerate, a strong decoction is brewed, using one ounce of plant material boiled with 3½ pints of water, boiled down to 1 pint and administered in doses of 4 ounces to ½ pint. This will produce vomiting rather rapidly.

BONESET: *In the late 19th century, this plant was extensively used in American medical practice.*

Traditional Usages

Boneset was a favorite remedy of North American tribes. The Menominees used it to **reduce fever**; the Iroquois and Mohegans for fever and colds; the Alabamas for upset stomachs; and the Creeks for **body pain.** Among settlers Boneset soon became a very popular remedy for fever and colds; it was in use at least 100 years before it was listed in any American medical text. In 1887, Dr.

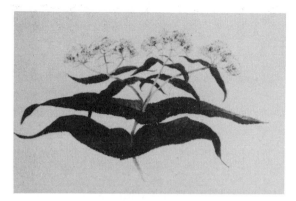

Boneset

Millspaugh wrote that "There is probably no plant in American domestic practice that has more extensive or frequent use than this [boneset]."

The plant derives its common name from its usefulness in treating a kind of influenza prevalent in the United States in the 19th century known as "break-bone fever," which was characterized by pains that felt as if all the bones of the body were broken. The plant has also been used in the treatment of intermittent fevers, although its action was acknowledged to be inferior to that of Quinine. As a mild tonic, it was given in cases of dyspepsia and as an aid to indigestion in the elderly.

Boneset is said to act as a mild tonic and diaphoretic in moderate doses and as an emetic and purgative in larger doses. Drunk as hot as possible, it was given to induce vomiting and the evacuation of the bowels; when drunk at warm temperature, the action was somewhat milder, producing increased perspiration and somewhat later a mild evacuation of the bowels. Boneset's ability to produce perspiration made it useful in catarrhal conditions, especially influenza; the administration of a warm infusion would produce perspiration and sometimes vomiting, often arresting the complaint.

Of this numerous genus, comprising not less than 30 species within the limits of the United States, most of which probably possess analogous medical properties, three have found a place in the *Pharmacopoeia* of the United States—*E. perfoliatum, E. teucrifolim,* and *E. purpureum*—the first in the primary, the last two in the secondary list. *E. connabinum* of Europe, the root of which was formerly used as a purgative, and *E. Aya-pana* of Brazil, the leaves of which at one time enjoyed a very high reputation as remedy in numerous diseases, have fallen into neglect.

Recent Scientific Findings

The leaves contain several sesquiterpene lactones that stimulate the appetite. In sufficient amounts they would have anthelmintic effects. Toxic relatives of Boneset, such as White Snakeroot (*E. rugosum*) have been responsible for numerous cases of agricultural animal poisonings, as well as human poisonings.

Researchers experiment with a sesquiterpene lactone from Boneset, EVP, concluded that EVP may possess antitumor activity in vivo.

BORAGE

SCIENTIFIC NAME: *Borago officinalis*
PARTS USED: Whole plant

DOSAGE:
> *Not recommended.*

BORAGE: *The seed oil of this popular salad green is producing promising results in arthritis patients.*

Traditional Usages

Popular in salads and as a pot herb, Borage has also been credited with mild medicinal properties as a demulcent, refrigerant, gentle diaphoretic, cordial, and aperient. An infusion was drunk as a general tonic when one was feeling out of sorts. In 1611, Mattioli wrote, "It strengthens the heart and vital spirit, takes away anxiety, depression and grief." The plant has also been used to make other less palatable medicinals more agreeable.

Recent Scientific Findings

Even though Borage is a widely used and popular herbal preparation and salad green, it should never be taken internally for any reasons. Borage contains substances known as pyrrolizidine alkaloids (i.e., lasiocarpine) of the type that are known to cause liver damage (hepatotoxicity), and to induce cancer in laboratory animals when fed to them over a long period of time.

Whether the amount of these liver poisons in Borage is sufficient to cause liver damage or cancer in humans has not yet been established. However, until this has been determined, we recommend that Borage not be taken orally by humans in any amount.

However, experimental evidence indicates that Borage oil is an excellent dietary fatty acid. Experiments have found that certain dietary oils, including Borage oil, may have therapeutic potential. One study determined that Borage oil augments arterial control of vascular resistance. Both a 1988 and a 1990 study found dietary oils may exert beneficial effects on inflammatory skin disorders.

More significant is Borage's **anti-arthritic** and **anti-rheumatic** properties. Diets enriched with Borage seed oil have **suppressed inflammation** in a variety of models. In one study, Borage seed oil was administered for a 12 week period to patients with **rheumatoid arthritis** as well as a normal control group. Of the seven rheumatoid arthritis patients given Borage seed oil, six experienced clinical improvement.

BOSWELLIN

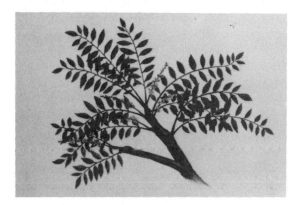

Boswellin

SCIENTIFIC NAME: *Boswellia serrata*
PARTS USED: Gum resin

DOSAGE:
　　Follow label directions of commercial preparations.

BOSWELLIN: *Known as "Indian frankincense," a purified compound from its gum resin has been found to have beneficial effects on rheumatic disorders.*

Traditional Usages

There are many medicinal plants of great therapeutic value referred to in the ancient treatment systems of **Ayurveda.** The two important Ayurveda treatises, *Sushrita Samhita* and *Charak Samhita,* describe the **anti-rheumatic** activity of guggals (gum resins of certain trees), especially those of the tree *Boswellia serrata,* whose extract the ancients claimed to have potent **anti-inflammatory** and **anti-arthritic** properties.

Boswellia serrata is a moderate to large branching tree generally found in dry hilly areas of India. The tree exudes a gummy oleo-resin when it is tapped by scraping away a portion of the bark. The chemical constituents of the gum resin include essential oils, terpenoids, and gum. Also known as Indian frankincense, *Boswellia serrata's* essential oil is an ingredient in many Oriental perfumes and is closely related to the incense of Biblical renown. Along with its aromatic properties, the gummy exudate is lauded by the Ayurvedic texts as a remedy for **diarrhea, dysentery, pulmonary diseases, boils, ringworm** and other afflictions, as well as **rheumatoid arthritis.**

Recent Scientific Findings

To verify the Ayurvedic claims, the Regional Research Laboratories in India undertook a series of studies. The researchers hoped "to discover herbal-based **anti-inflammatory products** having beneficial effects on rheumatic diseases without any adverse and undesirable side-effects." **Rheumatic disorders** affect people throughout the world and are a major cause of disability. It is not usually possible to cure the disease. However, through proper treatment it is possible to alleviate pain, prevent further tissue injury, and increase mobility.

By means of a chemical process of defattening and extracting, the Indian researchers derived a purified compound from the gum resin exudate of *Boswellia serrata*. The researchers found this extract to be more beneficial, less toxic, and more potent than the standard "drug of choice," Ketoprofen (benzoyl hydrotropic acid). In turn, Ketoprofen is preferred

over other anti-inflammatories such as indomethacin, phenylbutazone or acetylsalicylic acid.

Researchers concluded that boswellic acids (BA), as non-steroidal, anti-inflammatory agents, are beneficial because they suppress the proliferating tissue found in inflamed areas and also prevent the breakdown of connective tissue. "It appears from the experimental studies done so far that it acts by a mechanism similar to non-steroidal groups of anti-arthritic drugs with the added advantages of its being free from side effects and gastric irritation and ulcerogenic activity."

Because of the success of these studies, Indian authorities approved the marketing of a product made from the purified compound under the trade name **Sallaki.** Since then, in several other acute and chronic experimental test models of inflammation, *Boswellia serrata* has shown potent anti-inflammatory and anti-arthritic activity. In animal studies, Boswellin was also seen to promote a reduced rate of body weight loss associated with inflammatory disorders, reduced secondary lesions, and to be free from any effect on the CNS and cardiovascular system.

In human studies, Boswellin has been found to **improve blood supply to the joints and restore integrity of vessels weakened by spasm.** In one clinical trial conducted for four weeks on early cases of **osteoarthritis** of the knee, 26 patients showed a good response. The researchers concluded, "If the drug had been continued for a longer period, they would have shown excellent results." In another clinical trial at the orthopedic department of Government Medical College, Jammu, India, 122 out of 175 rheumatoid arthritis patients who were either bedridden or incapacitated from doing normal work and suffered from morning stiffness showed an abatement of symptoms two to four weeks after the initiation of therapy. None of these patients complained of any undesirable side effect. The authors concluded, "All these patients were happier with this therapy than with any other drugs given previously."

Boswellin's **antiarthritic** properties were demonstrated in a human clinical trial. **A herbal formula consisting of Boswellin, Ashwagandha, and Turmeric was evaluated in a randomized, double-blind, placebo-controlled study.** After a one-month evaluation period 12 patients with osteoarthritis were given the herbal formula or placebo for three months. The patients were evaluated every two weeks. Then after a 15 day wash-out period, the treatment was reversed with the placebo patients receiving the drug and vice versa. Again results were evaluated over a three month period. **The patients treated with the herbal formula showed a significant drop in severity of pain and disability score.**

Boswellia serrata is proving to be a potent addition to the drugs physicians may use to deal with **rheumatoid arthritis.** And, as the Regional Research Laboratory researchers concluded, physicians "may in due course be convinced of its superiority over the conventional drugs as it is a plant product being used since the ages and is absolutely free from any toxic and side effects."

BROOM

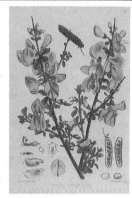
Broom

SCIENTIFIC NAME: *Sarothamnus scoparius*
PARTS USED: Tops and seeds

DOSAGE:

Leaves: A decoction is made from the leaves, 1 teaspoon of plant material per 1 cup of boiling water, drink cold, 1 to 2 cups per day.

Seeds: The dose of the seeds, crushed and powdered, is $\frac{1}{2}$gram to 1 gram.

BROOM: *This beautiful shrub contains an alkaloid that appears to regulate the heart.*

Traditional Usages

This familiar and beautiful shrub is a plant of many uses. The seeds, dried and roasted, have been used as a coffee substitute, and the twigs have been employed as a fiber, to make brooms, and as a substitute for jute.

Medicinally, Broom was used for **urinary tract disorders**, especially in cases where the urination is scanty or painful. It was also employed to increase the flow of urine in dropsical conditions and relieve bladder spasms. It was believed to have a tonic effect on the heart.

Recent Scientific Findings

Collected before blooming, the flowering tops are a source of sparteine sulfate. The medicinal action of the plant, which has a most disagreeable taste in decoction, is **diuretic** and **cathartic**, while it is emetic in large doses. It has been especially valued in treating dropsical conditions, particularly those associated with heart diseases, as it is efficacious in acting on the kidneys to produce urine flow. **Because of its action on the kidneys, it is contraindicated in acute renal disease.**

Recent research has uncovered possible effects on **heart arrhythmia**. Since Broom contains no glycosides, it is not one of the plants with digitalis properties (such as Foxglove). Instead, Broom contains sparteine, an alkaloid which appears to **regulate the action of the heart.**

BUCHU

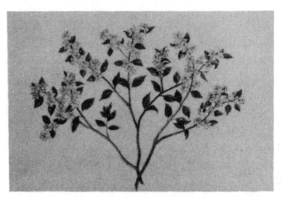

Buchu

SCIENTIFIC NAME: *Agathosma betulina,*
A. crenulata
PLANT FAMILY: Rue
PARTS USED: Leaf

DOSAGE:

BUCHU: *Used for centuries in South Africa, the leaves are rich in volatile oils.*

Traditional Usages

Buchu has been used in South Africa since long before colonization. Its name is a Hottentot word. These native South Africans used the dried leaves for various urinary disorders. Early in the 1800s, the leaves' medicinal qualities were introduced in Europe. In South Africa, Buchu is still commonly employed as a tincture for a variety of ailments, especially **urinary, kidney,** and **prostate** problems.

Buchu was used to relieve catarrhal

conditions and inflammation in the kidneys and cramps in the bladder. It has also been recommended for gravel and stones in kidneys and bladder. Its soothing and strengthening effect on the urinary organs has been highly praised.

Recent Scientific Findings

Buchu is one of the best and most useful herbs in urinary tract diseases that are attended with increased uric acid. Its effect is due to its volatile oils, including limonene and diosphenol (a phenolic ketone), as well as glycosides and flavonoids.

Buchu is not as strong as some diuretics, but is sometimes blended in conjunction with stronger agents due to Buchu's overall effects and restorative properties. Several proprietary drugs commonly used in South Africa for urinary disorders still contain Buchu leaves as a major ingredient.

BUCKBEAN

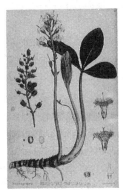

Buckbean

SCIENTIFIC NAME: *Menyanthes trifoliata*
PARTS USED: Leaves, root, and rhizome

DOSAGE:

Root, Rhizome, Leaves: The medicinal dosage is one teaspoon of root/rhizome/leaves, chopped fine, per cup of boiling water; drink cold one mouthful at a time, during the course of the day.

BUCKBEAN: *At one time, this plant was considered a panacea.*

Traditional Usages

The Buckbean, or Marsh Trefoil, was formerly considered a medicinal of great value in Europe, and in some countries it was regarded practically as a panacea. According to strength and dosage, its action ranges from that of a bitter tonic and cathartic all the way to purgative and emetic effects. In earlier times,

Buckbean was employed in the treatment of **dropsy, catarrh, scabies,** and **fever**. Early modern physicians used the plant for rheumatic complaints, skin diseases, and also to reduce fever. Buckbean is also reportedly excellent for relieving gas and excess stomach acid.

In domestic American medicine, a tonic was prepared consisting of 1.3 to 2.0 grams of the powdered leaves or root. While all parts of the plant are medicinally active, only the leaves were officially listed in the *U.S. Pharmacopoeia* from 1820 and 1842 and in the *National Formulary* from 1916 to 1926.

Recent Scientific Findings

This perennial herb contains a bitter glucoside, menyanthin. Due to its tart taste it is an ingredient in beer (Scandinavia) and also a substitute for tea.

Buckbean leaves contain a number of alkaloids, especially gentianne and gentianadine. In animals, gentianine shows **analgesic** and **tranquilizing** effects; gentianadine **lowers blood pressure** and has **significant anti-inflammatory activity**.

BUCKTHORN

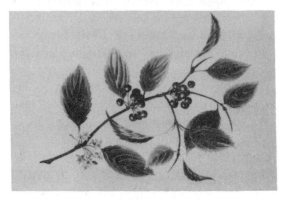

Buckthorn

SCIENTIFIC NAME: *Rhamnus cathartica, R. frangula*

PARTS USED: Bark and berries

DOSAGE:

Bark: 1 teaspoon of *dried* bark per 1 1/2 pints of water, boiled in a covered container for about 1/2 hour, at a slow boil. Allow liquid to cool slowly in the *closed* container. Administer cold, 1 tablespoon at a time, very carefully. (Note: bark must be at least two years old; fresh bark may cause vomiting.)

BUCKTHORN: *Used since the Middle Ages, research reveals that extracts of Buckthorn may have antiviral properties.*

Traditional Usages

Esteemed for its purgative powers, the freshly powdered bark of Buckthorn is highly irritating to the gastrointestinal mucous membrane, causing violent catharsis coupled with **vomiting** and **pain.** The *dried* bark is much milder, resembling Rhubarb in its action. Buckthorn has been utilized as a medicinal since the Middle Ages, when it was called Waythorn or Hartsthorn. It appeared in the London Pharmacopoeia in 1650.

The tribes of southern Vancouver Island prepared a decoction from the bark to treat digestive tract ailments. A European variety (*R. bulbosus*) was official in the *U.S. Pharmacopoeia* from 1820 to 1882. It was used as a counter-irritant, to promote blistering of pimples, etc. In 1887, a report stated that "violent attacks of epilepsy are recorded as having been induced by this plant, a sailor who inhaled the fumes of the burning plant was attacked with this disease for the first time in his life, it returned again in two weeks, passed into cachexia, nodous gout, headache, and terminated in death." Interestingly, a related species (*R. acris*) was crushed and the vapor inhaled as a cure for headaches by the Montgagnais of Newfoundland and Nova Scotia.

Recent Scientific Findings

The berries of *Rhamnus cathartica* are known to contain anthraquinone glycosides that are responsible for the cathartic effect attributed to them. Similarly, Buckthorn bark (*R. frangula*) is used widely in Europe as a cathartic in the same way that *R. purshiana* (Cascara Sagrada) is utilized in North America. The active principles in Buckthorn bark and Cascara Sagrada bark are similar, with Buckthorn the mildest anthraquinone herb and Cascara next

mildest. For additional information see *Cascara Sagrada.*

Buckthorn extract has been found to **kill several species of fungi,** including *Aspergillus, Trichophytum, and Fusarium.* Applied externally, Buckthorn extract has been found to be active **against herpes simples virus I and II in adult humans.** In cell culture, Buckthorn extract has been found to be an **antiviral agent** against **influenza virus A$_2$** and vaccinia virus. Moreover, it was found to have **cytotoxic activity** toward HELA cancer cells.

In a 1991 study, the authors found that aqueous extracts from Buckthorn showed **significant activity against staphylococcus and candida.** Antitumor activity of Buckthorn extract was found in mice with sarcoma 37 and leukemia P388. Another study found that an extract of Buckthorn **lowered arterial blood pressure in rats.**

BUPLEURUM OR CHAI HU

SCIENTIFIC NAME: *Bupleurum falcatum, Bupleurum chinense, Bupleurum longiradiatum*

PARTS USED: Root

DOSAGE:

Root: 1 teaspoon of dried root bark per 1 1/2 pints water, boiled in covered container for about 1/2 hour, at a slow boil. Allow liquid to cool slowly in the *closed* container. Drink 1 cup at a time, twice daily.

BUPLEURUM: *Long an integral part of Oriental medicine, a mixture containing the root shows promise as an adaptogen and in treating Alzheimer's.*

Traditional Usages

Also known as Hare's Ear, *Chai Hu* is the dried root of certain members of the Umbelliferae family. Traditionally, the species used have been *B. chinense* in China, *B. falcatum* in Japan, and *B. longiradiatum* in Korea.

In Oriental traditional medicine, certain herbal mixtures containing the plant have long been used for the treatment of chronic inflammatory and autoimmune diseases, as well as the management of certain neurological disorders. Bupleurum is classified as sudorific, meaning it was used to dispel and disperse "surface" problems.

Bupleurum was given for malaria, as well as blackwater fever and as a liver sedative.

Recent Scientific Findings

Stress can be of a non-specific origin, or can involve specific physical or psychological factors capable of producing a disease state. The ability of stress to cause disease may be related to its suppression of the immune system. Numerous plant extracts have been described as having **powerful anti-stress activity** (adaptogenic).

Shosaikoto is an extract containing *Bupleurum falcatum* (Bupf) by weight). The extract also includes *Piniella ternata* (21%), *Scutellaria baicalensis, Zizyphus vulgaris,* Korean ginseng (12.5% each), licorice root (8%), and ginger root (4%). Experiments have found that Shosaikoto possesses immunomodulating activity, stimulating immune cell activity in immune suppressed or normal mice, and suppressing immune responsivity in hyperimmune rats.

Recent studies have evaluated the effect of Shosaikoto on stress-induced immuno-suppression in mice. It was found that Shosaikoto stimulated the pituitary-adrenal cortex axis, leading to elevations in blood corticosterone levels and increases in adrenal gland weight, in normal mice.

Adrenal gland enlargement is one of the hallmarks of continuous exposure to a significant stressor. Indeed, adrenal glands from stressed rats in this study increased in weight by approximately 13%. However, two different Shosaikoto oral dosing schedules (equivalent to two and ten times the normal human dose) had no effect upon adrenal gland weight.

Shosaikoto was able to restore the immunosuppression resultant to the physical stress, although only at the lower dosage. These animals showed a significantly enhanced immune response to foreign red blood cells, relative to the untreated or high dose Shosaikato groups. Conversely, only the higher dosage of the plant extract combination was able to restore rectal temperature to normal following the final exposure to the stress. The authors concluded that Shosaikoto may act as an **immuno-restorative agent** via its direct **immunomodulating and/or anti-stress activities**. Additionally, they suggested that **Shosaikoto also acts upon the central nervous system in a manner similar to that of Valium.**

A companion paper by the same authors tested the effects of Shosaikoto upon age-induced amnesia in rats. Shosaikoto-treated animals displayed learning response times significantly lower than those of the control group of old animals, and equal to those of the young animals. Additionally, Shosaikoto appeared to **reduce age-related memory loss**, preserving memory function virtually identical to that seen in the young animals.

Analyses of neurochemicals from the brains of the various groups indicated that Shosaikato-treated animals had higher levels of dopamine, found to be low within the brains of Alzheimer's disease patients. **The authors suggested that the reputed beneficial effects of Shosaikoto in Alzheimer's may be due to its ability to elevate brain dopamine levels, possibly leading to improved memory and cognitive processing.**

A detail meriting attention is the amount of Shosaikoto fed to the animals in this study. These animals received only half of the low dose, and one-tenth of the high dose of Shosaikoto given to the animals in the stress study described above. The effects of higher doses upon neurological function/chemistry warrants further investigation.

These results show that the components of Shosaikoto act as biological response modifiers in the immune and central nervous systems. Their promise as **immunomodulating** and **neuroactivating** agents awaits further studies.

BURDOCK

SCIENTIFIC NAME: *Arcticum lappa*
PARTS USED: Root

DOSAGE:

    Root: One teaspoon of root (only 1-year-old root should be used) to 1½ pints of boiling water, steeped ½ hour. Drink at room temperature, 1 to 2 cups daily. (Mausert recommends that Burdock oil be rubbed into the scalp to prevent hair from falling out.)

BURDOCK: *Long used as vegetable and medicinal, the root of this weed has shown antibacterial and antifungal properties.*

Traditional Usages

    This common weed is a native of Europe and is abundant in the United States. The root, which should be collected in spring, loses four-fifths of its weight by drying. The root's odor is weak and unpleasant, the taste mucilaginous and sweetish with a slight tinge of bitterness and astringency.

    Widely eaten as a vegetable, Burdock has also been praised for its medicinal virtues since antiquity. A root decoction has been reported useful in the treatment of **gout, rheumatism,** and **dropsy.** In Japan, the tender leaf stalks and roots are boiled in two changes of water to remove the tough fibers, and then eaten. The Iroquois and other tribes learned how to prepare Burdock from Colonial settlers. The dried roots of young plants were

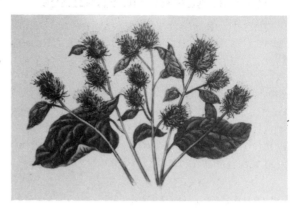

Burdock

added to soups, while the leaves were cooked and included in their diet as greens.

    In his *Travels in North America* the Swedish naturalist Peter Kalm wrote about Burdock in a 1772 visit to Ticonderoga, New York: "And the governor told me that its tender shoots are eaten in spring as radishes, after the exterior part is taken off." According to Woodville, an eighteenth-century writer on medical botany, the plant was very useful as **a diuretic,** and it effects cure without increased irritation and nausea as side effects.

    Externally the leaves have been applied to **benign skin tumors** as well as in the treatment of **knee joint swellings** unresponsive to other medicines. A poultice was made by boiling the leaves until most of the liquid was boiled off, then applying the hot, wet mass to the affected area. In tandem with the drinking of the root decoction, this same poultice was applied in the treatment of gout. Burdock poultices were also used to treat severe bloody bruises and burns.

Recent Scientific Findings

Burdock root extracts have been shown experimentally to produce **diuresis** and to **inhibit tumors** in animals. Extracts also **lower blood sugar** and have **estrogenic activity**. In test tube experiments, extracts show **antibacterial** and **antifungal** properties. The active antibacterial principle was isolated and partially characterized as a lactone.

These experiments indicate potential use of Burdock in **female complaints**, in **diabetes**, and for **bacterial** or **fungal infection**.

BUTCHER'S BROOM

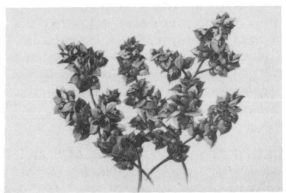

Butcher's Broom

SCIENTIFIC NAME: *Ruscus aculeatus*
PARTS USED: Rhizome

DOSAGE:

Root: When used in medicine, the usual dose is 2 teaspoons of powdered root per 1½ pints of boiling water, boiled in a covered container for about ½ hour, at a slow boil. Allow the liquid to cool slowly in the *closed* container. Drink cold, 2 to 3 tablespoons 6 times a day.

BUTCHER'S BROOM: *Modern research is confirming ancient Mediterranean healers' use of this plant as an anti-inflammatory agent.*

Traditional Usages

This member of the Lily family has very active chemical constituents, saponins, similar to those found in Licorice and Sarsaparilla. That this evergreen shrub, native to the Mediterranean region, has been found to contain highly active chemical constituents would not come as a surprise to ancient peoples. While the stiff, leaf-like twigs were once used by butchers to whisk scraps from their cutting blocks, ancient Mediterranean healers utilized the rhizome for a wide variety of **circulatory** and **inflammatory disorders. Varicose veins** were cured with this species according to the Roman scholar Pliny (c. 60 A.D.), while in more ancient years Greek doctors reported curing "swelling" with "the miracle herb."

Recent Scientific Findings

Beneath the stiff twigs of this plant long employed for mundane purposes courses chemical constituents with profound effects. Oral contraceptives are made from steroids derived in large part from the plant kingdom. So too are other important steroids, such as cortisone, testosterone and estradiol. Thanks to the pioneering efforts of many scientists who investigated the plant world for starter compounds these synthetic drugs are now available at very low prices.

The saponin glycosides found in some plants are the basis for the production of many useful steroid pharmaceuticals. During the course of investigations into finding new saponins, two new sapogenins were discovered in the rhizomes of Butcher's Broom. These were named Ruscogenin and Neo-ruscogenin and are chemically similar to diosgenin, the principle steroid starter compound found in Mexican yams (various species of *Dioscorea*).

Relatively recent pharmacological findings indicate **vasoconstrictive** and **anti-inflammatory** properties. Tests conducted on animals by Capra showed that the Ruscogenins have good **anti-inflammatory** activity. As for toxicity, tests in the mouse and rat showed that when administered orally, these compounds from Butcher's Broom were well tolerated.

The saponins it contains constricts the veins and decreases the permeability of capillaries. Consequently several writers state that this so-called "phlebotherapeutic agent" is utilized to treat disorders of circulation, such as **varicose veins** and **hemorrhoids.**

A **venotropic drug (RAES)** composed of an extract of Butcher's Broom along with hesperidin and ascorbic acid, was examined in a 1988 clinical trial. Four patients between the ages of 28 and 74 suffering from chronic phlebopathy of the lower limbs were evaluated in the double-blind, cross-over trial. The authors undertook two periods of treatment of two months with RAES or a placebo. They concluded that symptoms **"immediately changed significantly in correspondence with the administration of RAES. The biological and clinical tolerability were excellent."**

Another randomized double-blind study of 50 patients suffering from varicose veins employed a commercial preparation of Butcher's Broom extract. **The research indicated improvement in those treated with the extract.**

BUTTERCUP

SCIENTIFIC NAME: *Ranunculus* spp.
PARTS USED: Herb

DOSAGE:
Not recommended.

BUTTERCUP: *Employed by the ancient Greeks, an extract has recently been found to inhibit RNA and DNA synthesis in leukemia cells.*

Traditional Usages

Ancient physicians, including Hippocrates and Dioscorides, used various *Ranunculus* species as an external application to remove psora, leprous nails, steatomatous, and other tumors as well as fomentations to chilblains, and toothache. Arabic physicians found it to be a **powerful treatment for skin diseases** and the Bedouins used them as rubefacients.

In Europe, Buttercups were applied to the wrists and fingers to cure intermittent fevers. Early English practitioners utilized the bulb to produce vesication when a "lasting blister" was believed necessary, but they did not use it internally because of negative reactions such as violent attacks of epilepsy

Recent Scientific Findings

Buttercup contains anemonol and anemoninic acid. Among the components is protoanemonin, which has been found to be an **effective antifungal** agent.

An extract of Buttercup (BE) has been found to inhibit RNA and DNA synthesis by HL-50 promyelocytic leukemia cells. When the cells were exposed to BE for 18 hours, RNA synthesis was dramatically inhibited without loss of cell viability. After a period of 12 to 24 hours the researchers found the RNA level returned. This research warrants further study.

CASCARA SAGRADA

SCIENTIFIC NAME: *Rhamnus purshiana*
PARTS USED: Bark

DOSAGE:

   Bark: Boil 1 teaspoon of bark in a covered container of 1½ pints of water for about ½ hour, at a slow boil. Allow liquid to cool slowly in the *closed* container. Drink cold, 1 swallow or 1 tablespoon at a time, 1 to 2 cups per day.

CASCARA SAGRADA: *The bark of this tree remains the world's most popular laxative.*

Traditional Usages

   The bark of Cascara Sagrada has been called **the most widely used cathartic on earth.** Traditionally employed as a remedy by Native Americans, the bark became known to the settlers and eventually passed into use by the medical profession. The pharmaceutical house of Parke, Davis and Co. first marketed Cascara Sagrada in 1877, although the plant did not become official in the *U.S. Pharmacopoeia* until 1890.

   This tree is native to the northwest Pacific Coast, ranging from British Columbia to California. Various tribes throughout this range utilized Cascara Sagrada for its laxative effects. The Thompson tribe of British Columbia

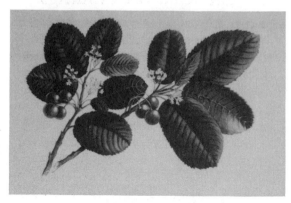

Cacara Sagrada

boiled a small amount of the bark or wood in water. This was a standard method of preparing plant medicines and consistently reappears throughout the literature on Native American remedies.

   The early Spanish priests of California most probably learned of this "sacred bark" from the natives of Mendocino County. In 1877, Dr. J.H. Bundy "rediscovered" this plant, probably through Native Americans, and introduced Cascara into medicine. It quickly became a **favorite laxative throughout the world.**

   Indiscriminate cutting destroyed great stands of these trees. As early as 1909 Alice Henkel wrote:

   Many trees are annually destroyed in the collection of cascara sagrada, as they are usually peeled to such an extent that no new bark is formed. It has been estimated that one tree furnishes approximately 10 pounds of bark, and granting a crop of 1,000,000 pounds a year, 100,000 trees are thus annually destroyed. . . .

Recent Scientific Findings

No synthetic substance can equal the mild and speedy action of the "holy bark"; it is marketed in pills, powders, and fluidextracts by many pharmaceutical companies. The basis of Cascara's laxative effect is the presence of a mixture of anthraquinones, either free (i.e., aloe-emodin) or as sugar derivatives (glycosides). The free anthraquinones remain in the intestines and cause catharsis by irritating the intestinal wall. Those anthraquinones present in the plant as sugar derivatives are largely absorbed from the intestine, circulate through the bloodstream, and eventually stimulate a nerve center in the lower part of the intestine, which causes a laxative effect.

Though its effectiveness has been proven, research continues. A 1991 study involving 271 human patients compared a Cascara-Salax laxative with two other regiments, a Senna and saline laxative as well as a polyethylene glycol electrolyte lavage solution (Golytel). The researchers found no differences between the regimens, either in the patient's impressions or for the convenience of the preparation.

Cascara bark should always be aged for at least one year before being employed as a laxative. During this period of time certain chemical changes occur in the bark that reduce the "griping" effect that often accompanies the use of a laxative preparation of this type.

Aqueous extracts of Cascara have been found to be antiviral against herpes simplex virus II and vaccinia virus in cell culture.

CASTOR BEAN

SCIENTIFIC NAME: *Ricinus communis*
PARTS USED: Seeds

DOSAGE:
> *Caution:* Highly poisonous.
> Use only manufactured products.

CASTOR BEAN: *Castor oil has a long history of success as a cathartic and purgative.*

Traditional Usages

Expressed from the Castor bean (seed), castor oil has an unpleasant, acrid taste. It has long been highly valued as a **safe and reliable cathartic and purgative** to be used in irritable conditions of the gastrointestinal tract and the genito-urinary system. Most commonly, it has been given to infants and young children. Often attempts are made to mask the unpleasant taste with the addition of aromatic and essential oils, but the dominant Castor taste is difficult to subdue.

Recent Scientific Findings

All parts of the plant, especially the seeds, or beans, are poisonous to humans and animals. The toxic action is due to ricin, a severe irritant that produces nausea, vomiting, gastric pain, diarrhea, thirst, and dimness of vision. Recently scientists found that ricin is not a single substance, but a complex mixture of toxic materials that are very difficult to separate and purify. Ricin causes red blood cells to hemolyze (dissolve), as well as disturbing the body's immune system.

In the preparation of castor oil, the seeds are usually pressed and the oil that exudes is collected and purified. **The toxic components of the seeds are completely insoluble in oil and therefore are not found in castor oil.** However, one should never eat the seed by itself; there are documented cases in which a single bean has been lethal when eaten.

However, if castor oil is to be used as a cathartic, one should be confident that it will not be poisonous. **Only the seeds are poisonous if ingested.**

CATNIP

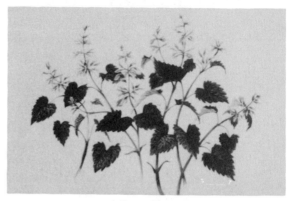

Catnip

SCIENTIFIC NAME: *Nepeta cataria*
PARTS USED: Leaves and flowering tops

DOSAGE:

Leaves: Approximately ½ ounce of leaves to 1 pint of water. Boil water separately and pour over the plant material and steep 5-10 minutes, depending on the desired effect. Drink hot or warm, 1 to 2 cups per day, at bedtime and upon awakening.

CATNIP: *This feline favorite also has a long history of use as a domestic remedy.*

Traditional Usages

The plant was originally distributed in Europe, Siberia, western Asia to the Himalayas. Introduced in North America, the weed now grows in dry soil from Canada to Minnesota and south to Virginia and Arkansas. It flowers June to

September, and when utilized medicinally the leaves and flowering tops were collected and then dried.

The Mohegans made a tea of catnip leaves for **infantile colic**. This became a popular domestic remedy and is still used today in some regions of the United States. Catnip was also used to **induce sweating to cure colds**. At the beginning of this century, the leaves and flowering tops were widely utilized in medicine as a **stimulant** or **to promote suppressed menstruation**. The plants was also thought to have a **sedative** effect. It was official in the *U.S. Pharmacopoeia* from 1842 through 1882 and in the *National Formulary* from 1916 to 1950.

Recent Scientific Findings

Surely a plant that has such a powerful impact on our feline friends, causing them to "roll upon, chew, and tear to bits any withered leaf till nothing remains," could not be destitute of medicinal value in humans. Catnip has been reported efficacious in the treatment of **iron-deficiency anemia, menstrual and uterine disorders,** and **dyspepsia,** and as a **gentle calmative**. It has been administered in a variety of forms, including infusion, injection, lavement, and in the bath. It has been drunk as a treatment for chronic cough, and chewed for relief of **toothache**. Containing a bitter principle, this perennial herb has also been useful for infantile colic. Extract of Catnip has been found to be **cytotoxic** to HELA-S$_3$ cancer cells in cell culture.

CAYENNE

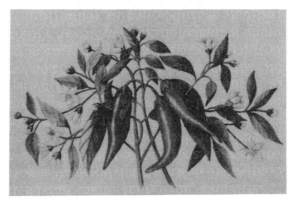

Cayenne

SCIENTIFIC NAME: *Capsicum frutescens*
PARTS USED: Fruit

DOSAGE:
　　Fruit: 1/4 to 1 whole teaspoon per cup of hot water.

CAYENNE: *This condiment is producing surprising results as a short-term anti-inflammatory agent.*

Traditional Usages

The stimulant effect of the common chili pepper is reflected in its use as a condiment in foods, with a resulting promotion of digestion. As a medicine, cayenne pepper is a **general stimulant,** and has been reported of value in the treatment of **dyspepsia, diarrhea,** and **prostration.** It has been used as a **remedy for nausea from seasickness.**

As a gargle, the seeds are valued as a treatment for **sore throat and hoarseness.**

In the treatment of ague (painful swelling of the face due to decayed or ulcerated teeth or a cold), inhalation of the steam of Cayenne and vinegar, coupled with a small mouth poultice containing one teaspoon of cayenne pepper, will reportedly afford relief by producing a free discharge of saliva.

Recent Scientific Findings

Cayenne pepper acts as a rubefacient when applied externally, and as a stimulant internally, due to the presence of *capsaicin,* which is the "hot principle" in the fruits of this plant.

Oleoresin of *Capsicum* is still used in the preparation of a number of popular proprietary products to be applied locally for **the relief of sore muscles,** and produces the desired effect by mildly irritating the surface of the skin, which causes an increased blood flow to the area of application. The increased blood flow reduces inflammation of the affected area. **Capsaicin,** a phenol present in Cayenne pepper, has shown a variety of medicinal benefits. **In a recent letter to *The Lancet,* it was reported that topical applications of *capsaicin* cream completely alleviated the severe stump pain experienced by a middle-aged female diabetic.** This double-amputee patient subsequently underwent a placebo trial, where it was proved that while this cream completely relieved the pain, the placebo having no effect. Given the successful outcome of this extreme example, it would be reasonable to expect capsaicin creams to yield beneficial topical results when applied to various painful neuropathies.

Further information regarding the **anti-inflammatory** property of capsaicin is revealed in the paper, "Direct Evidence for Neurogenic Inflammation and its Prevention by Denervation and by Pretreatment with Capsaicin," as quoted in Dr. Garcia-Leme's book, *Hormones and Inflammation,* 1989. In studies with rats given capsaicin systemically, the results proved, "sensory nerve endings became insensitive to chemical pain stimuli for a long time. Neurogenic inflammation cannot be elicited in animals pretreated with capsaicin."

Additionally, two Indian scientists recently reported that long-term treatment with capsaicin "desensitizes" the membrane against various gaseous irritant-induced free radical damage. They found that this compound protects lung tissue (in experiments with rats) by increasing superoxide dismutase (SOD), catalase (CAT) and peroxidase (POD) activities. In as yet unpublished studies by the same authors, pretreatment with capsaicin also protected the lung of rats from nitrogen dioxide and formaldehyde induced free radical damage.

Two double-blind studies with human patients investigated a capsaicin-based pharmaceutical's effect on the daily activities of patients suffering from the **nerve pain associated with diabetes.** Such neuropathy usually interferes with the ability to work, sleep, walk, eat, use shoes and socks, and enjoy recreational activities. This complication of diabetes often upsets and reduces the overall quality of a patient's life, the pain usually lasting for many years.

The failure of drugs such as tricyclic antidepressants, anticonvulsants, narcotic analgesics, and phenothiazines for this condition has led to the search for safer, more effective alternatives. The medical world has found that nature has succeeded where synthesis has failed.

Researchers at the prestigious Scripps Clinic and Research Foundation in La Jolla, California, enrolled 277 men and women with this painful condition and followed them for 8 weeks in this double-blind study. The capcaicin cream was tried against a neutral cream and applied to the painful areas four times daily. Statistically significant differences were observed, with improvement in favor of the capsaicin cream. Such a natural-based medicine is now being utilized to improve the lives of thousands.

The marvelous benefits of capsaicin were reported earlier by a group from Henry Ford Hospital in Detroit, Michigan. This double-blind study tested 15 patients with diabetes mellitus suffering from neuropathy. The authors concluded that this plant-derived compound is "potentially effective when burning pain is a major symptom of PDN. The side effects of capsaicin were limited and minimal. **This agent should be considered by clinicians for treatment of PDN.**"

Also human studies have been done on **Capsaicin's effectiveness in treating rhinitis.** The drug was given to patients three times daily for three days. The patients' symptoms were recorded over a one month period. The results indicated that the Capsaicin treatment markedly reduced nasal obstruction and nasal secretion.

Interestingly, both cayenne pepper preparations and the active principle *capsaicin* have been shown in humans and in animals to stimulate the production of gastric juices, **resulting in improved digestion.**

CEDAR BERRY OR SAVIN

SCIENTIFIC NAME: *Juniperus sabina*
PARTS USED: Oil from leaves and flowering tops, tops & branches with attached leaflets

DOSAGE:
Leaves and Flowering Tops: Approximately 1/2 ounce of leaves and flowering tops to 1 pint of water. Boil water separately, pour over the plant material, and steep for 5 to 20 minutes, depending on the desired effect. Drink hot or warm, 1 to 2 cups per day, at bedtime and upon awakening.

CEDAR BERRY: *Once a popular abortifacient, Savin may possess strong antibacterial properties.*

Traditional Usages

Savin is the essential oil from the leaves and flowering tops of *J. sabina*. The ends of the branches, and the leaves by which they are invested, are collected for medical use in the spring. When dried the color of the leaves fades.

The tops and leaves of the Savin have a strong, heavy, disagreeable odor, and a bitter, acrid taste. These properties are owing to a volatile oil which is obtained by distillation with water. They impart their virtues to alcohol and water.

There is reason to believe that *Juniperus virginiana*, the common red cedar, is sometimes substituted in the shops for the Savin, to which it bears so close a resemblance it is difficult to distinguish between them. The two species, however, differ in their taste and smell. In the red cedar, the leaves are sometimes terminate.

Savin has many recorded uses, but it must always be employed with caution. Although it is used internally relatively rarely, Savin was given in powdered form to stimulate the **menses** and for the seemingly opposite effect of **checking uterine hemorrhages.** Other uses range from a remedy for **worms** to a cure to **chronic rheumatism** as well as **chronic gout.**

Externally, powdered or infused Savin was applied to **warts, ulcers,** and **psoriasis**; some people used the juice from fresh leaves for these purposes. Since Savin is highly irritant, these applications seemed to help such skin afflictions by aggravating them, thereby speeding up the disease's natural progression to effect a quicker recovery.

Recent Scientific Findings

Savin has been used in the United States and in Europe as a **popular abortifacient,** but gained a reputation for toxicity during the 1930s, when a number of deaths were attributed to the use of Savin as an abortifacient. However, it was subsequently shown that the toxic material was a synthetic phthalate derivative that was added to the Savin. Thus, it is not clear from literature reports, most of which were published during that period of time, whether Savin itself is really toxic.

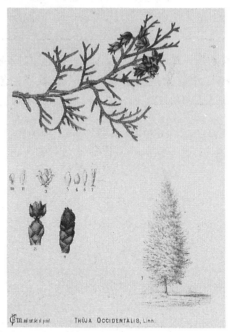

Cedar Berry or Savin

It is clear that Savin will contract uterine tissue in test tube experiments, and thus could possibly be beneficial in alleviating amenorrhea and atonic menorrhagia, as indicated by its folkloric uses. However, the employment of Savin itself cannot be recommended as a safe aid to alleviate these conditions, since it is a highly concentrated and complex mixture. But a tea prepared from the tops of *J. sabina* could exert a much milder and probably more beneficial effect.

In vitro **antimicrobial activity** of the essential oil of the Cedar Berry includes activity against a number of bacteria (e.g., *E. coli, Pseudonomas aurginosa* and *staphylococcus aureus*) and the pathogenic yeast, *Candida albicans.* **Antitumor activity** was found in the mouse against sarcoma 37 and spontaneous mammary cancer.

CHAMOMILE

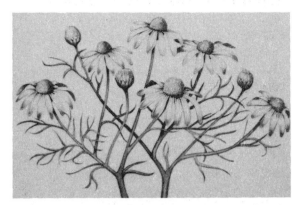

Chamomile

SCIENTIFIC NAME: *Matricaria chamomilla* (German) *Anthemis nobilis* (Roman)

PARTS USED: Flowers

DOSAGE:

Flowers: Approximately ½ ounce of flowers to 1 pint of water. Boil water separately and pour over the plant material and steep for 5 to 20 minutes, depending on the desired effect. Drink hot or warm, 1 to 2 cups or more per day. (Used as a hair wash, it will brighten the hair.)

CHAMOMILE: *This is one of nature's safest and most effective sedatives.*

Traditional Usages

There are two major types of Chamomile; they should not be confused. Roman Chamomile is derived from the flowers of *Anthemis noblis,* whereas German, or Hungarian Chamomile makes use of the flowers of *Matricaria chamomilla.*

The Greek name for German Chamomile signifies "ground-apple" and is appropriate. The whole plant when bruised affords a pleasant aromatic smell very similar to that of apples. German Chamomile is an annual herb.

German Chamomile, a showy annual cultivated in Europe, has long been taken in home remedies for anthelmintic and antispasmodic effects. The dried flower heads are known to stimulate the digestive process and are equally well established for their mild relaxing properties. It was a popular remedy for gas and cramps of the stomach.

Externally, an infusion was applied in compresses to relieve pain and swelling. The flowers have been used extensively as a rinse to keep the hair golden. This Chamomile species is also used for flavoring liqueurs and in perfumes, shampoos, and special tobaccos.

Also known as English Chamomile, Roman Chamomile flowers are an excellent stomachic in indigestion, flatulent colic, gout, and headaches in moderate doses. A strong infusion acts as an efficient emetic (try it combined with ginger!). The oil has stimulant and antispasmodic properties; it is useful in treating flatulence, and is added to purgatives to prevent griping pain in the bowels.

A related species, *A. cotula*, Stinking Chamomile or May Weed, was once widely used in the United States to promote sweating in chronic rheumatism, and was recommended by

Tragus, a 16th-century herbalist, in the form of decoction as a remedy for hysteria.

Recent Scientific Findings

Chamomile's **mild sedative effects** have been well documented. In 1973 a study was carried out in the United States in which 12 hospitalized patients having various types of heart disease were administered Chamomile tea in order to determines its effect. Each patients was given a 6 ounce cup of hot tea prepared form 2 commercial Chamomile tea bags. Approximately 10 minutes after the ingestion of the tea, ten of the patients fell into a deep sleep. They could be aroused, but immediately fell again into a deep sleep. The sleep lasted approximately 90 minutes. The only other effect seen in the patients was a small but significant increase in arterial blood pressure.

Experimentally in animals, the volatile oil from Chamomile flowers was given orally to rabbits with impaired kidney function, so that the amount of urea in the blood was increased. In all cases, the uremic condition in the rabbits normalized. This indicates a possible usefulness in regard to impaired kidney functions.

Another study in animals, using a flavonoid found in Chamomile flowers (apigenin), showed that this substance had **antihistaminimic** effects. When administered orally to arthritic rats, Chamomile's essential oil reduced the inflammation markedly. It was further shown that the constituents in the oil responsible for most of this effect was a substance known as alpha-bisabodol. In test-tube experiments Chamomile oil has also been shown to **relax smooth muscle of the intestine.**

Chamomile has also been a popular **eye wash** for treating **conjunctivitis** and other reactions. It has also been found to **promote wound healing.** A double-blind study with 11 patients found that Chamomile's effect was statistically significant in decreasing the wound area as well as the drying tendency.

With the exception of an occasional allergic response, there have been no adverse effects reported in the literature in humans for Chamomile. Thus, here is another safe sedative from nature's garden.

CHASTE BERRY

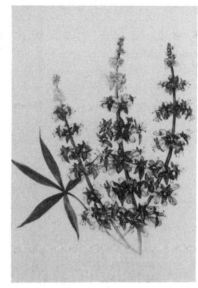

Chasteberry

SCIENTIFIC NAME: *Vitex agnus castus*

PARTS USED: Dried fruit

DOSAGE:

CHASTEBERRY: *Called "monk's pepper" during the Middle Ages, modern research has found that Chasteberry reduces or eliminates premenstrual symptoms.*

Traditional Usages

Chasteberry has been used since ancient times as a female remedy. One of its properties was to reduce sexual desire, and it is recorded that Roman wives whose husbands were abroad with the legions spread the aromatic leaves on their couches for this purpose. It became known as the chasteberry tree.

During the Middle Ages, Chasteberry's supposed effect on sexual desire led to it becoming a food spice at monasteries, where it was called "Monk's pepper" or "Cloister pepper."

In tradition, it was also known as an important European remedy for controlling and regulating the female reproductive system. Long used to regularize monthly periods and treat amenorrhea and dysmenorrhea, it also helped ease menopausal problems and aided the birth process.

The fruit's peppermint-like odor comes from its volatile oils.

Recent Scientific Findings

Chasteberry has not been significantly investigated for its therapeutic effects. However, preliminary investigations do indeed show the presence of compounds which are able to adjust the **production of female hormones**. It is thought to contain a progesterone-like compound and is now thought to be useful in the following conditions: **Amenorrhea, Dysmenorrhea, PMS, Endometriosis.**

The chemical constituents are the monoterpenes agnuside, eurostoside, and aucubin. Chasteberry also contains the flavonoids casticin, chryso-splenol and vitexin. While it is not known which constituent is responsible for its beneficial effects, it has been shown in laboratory animals in German experiments that extracts of *Agnus castus* can stimulate the release of Leutenizing Hormone (LH) and inhibit the release of Follicle Stimulating Hormone (FSH). An early German study with laboratory animals found that extracts of Chasteberry can stimulate the release of Leutenizing Hormone (LH) and inhibit the release of Follicle Stimulating Hormone (FSH). This hormonal effect has been confirmed in another laboratory report which suggests that the volatile oil has a progesterone-like effect.

Interest in this plant as an aid in Premenstrual Tension has arisen as a result of a clinical study carried out by Dr. Alan Stewart, who heads a clinic in a London hospital specializing in the treatment of premenstrual problems. Dr. Stewart's study indicated a 60% group reduction or elimination of PMS symptoms such as anxiety, nervous tension, insomnia, or mood changes, from subjects who were taking dried *agnus castus* capsules.

This trial, which is not yet published, studies the premenstrual symptoms reported by 30 women who took 1.5 gm/day dried agnus castus tablets, and 80 women who took placebo. The symptoms were classified into groups and assessed by a daily symptomatology diary and by questionnaire. Nearly 60% of the women reported that the symptoms were all or practically all gone, a much higher score than the placebo. **Symptoms such as anxiety, nervous tension, insomnia, or mood changes were most reduced.**

Employing an aqueous extract from the fruit, Agnolyt, a 1979 study reported good results on premenstrual water retention. Another study of Agnolyt discovered that women were able to sustain a good level of milk production for breast feeding. While it took some time for the drug to take effect, the women were able to continue use of the drug for months without harmful side effects.

CHERRY LAUREL

SCIENTIFIC NAME: *Prunus laurocerasus*
PARTS USED: Leaves

DOSAGE:

Leaves: "The proportion of HCN in he leaves varies according to the season, the age of the plant and the character of the soil and of the weather . . . [the] consequence of this variability . . . has prevented the general introduction of so variable a remedy." (U.S.D.) *Not recommended for home usage.*

CHERRY LAUREL: *The leaves contain hydrocyanic acid, a potent medicine.*

Traditional Usages

Water distilled from Cherry Laurel leaves was often employed in Europe for the same illnesses in which hydrocyanic acid was applied; dilute HCN was used in **respiratory ailments** and to **calm coughs**, as a **sedative**, as a **tonic** for **stomach upset** of nervous origins, and externally as a cure for **severe itching.**

Recent Scientific Findings

The leaves contain hydrocyanic acid (HCN), which gives a somewhat astringent and strongly bitter taste, with a flavor of peach kernel.

Hydrocyanic acid is an extremely fast-acting poison; overdoses can kill within minutes. Extreme caution should therefore be employed when using the distillate of Cherry Laurel leaves, since HCN content varies widely and **too high a content can prove fatal**. The Bitter Almond is preferred as a source of HCN when more uniform HCN content is desired in order to avoid accidental overdose.

Most *Prunus* species are much alike in chemical composition. Therefore, all remarks indicated for Wild Cherry (*P. virginiana:* see article) apply to Cherry Laurel as well.

CHERRY, WILD

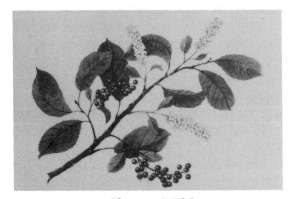

Cherry, Wild

SCIENTIFIC NAME: *Prunus virginiana*
PARTS USED: Stem bark

DOSAGE:
    Bark: Decoction interferes with the action of the bark. Never boil. For medicinal purposes, prepare an infusion (steeping in just-boiled water), using one teaspoon of the bark per cup of water.

CHERRY, WILD: *A Cherokee tea of the inner bark has remained in the U.S. Pharmacopoeia since 1820.*

Traditional Usages

The Mohegans allowed the ripe wild black cherry to ferment naturally in a jar for about one year and then drank the juice to cure dysentery. The Meskwakis made a sedative tea of the root bark, and this drink has long been popular in domestic American medicine. Cherokee women were given a tea of the inner bark to **relieve pain in the early stages of labor**. This preparation was soon adopted by the early settlers and in 1820 it became official in the *U.S. Pharmacopoeia*, where the bark is still listed for its **sedative** properties.

The most widespread popular use of Wild Cherry bark is as a **cough sedative**. It acts as a **tonic** and **calms irritation, diminishing nervous excitability**. It has been employed in the treatment of bronchitis, and because it **slows heart action**, has been used in heart disease characterized by **frequent, irregular**, or **feeble pulse**. It has also been considered a good remedy for weakness of the stomach or of the system coupled with general or local irritation.

When used in medicine the bark is collected in autumn when it contains the greatest concentration of precursors to hydrocyanic acid. Alice Henkel, an early expert on medicinal plants, cautioned against storing the bark for longer than one year, stating that it deteriorates with time. She added that young, thin bark was preferred and that bark from small or old branches was discarded.

Recent Scientific Findings

The *Prunus* genus includes the plums, almonds, peaches, apricots, and cherries. All these possess to some degree the glycoside amygdalin, which when combined with water reacts to form hydrocyanic acid. **The cancer treatment *laetrile*, currently employed with repeated reported success** in Mexico and Germany and seeking acceptance today in the U.S., contains amygdalin.

Both hydrocyanic acid and benzaldehyde, formed during the water extraction of the bark, contribute to the pleasant characteristic odor of Wild Cherry preparations. It should be pointed out that heat should be avoided during the preparation of Wild Cherry extracts, since both hydrocyanic acid and benzaldehyde are very volatile, and would be lost if heat is applied.

Hydrocyanic acid is toxic in sufficient dose, and there are many reports of animals being poisoned fatally by eating the leaves or fruits of many *Prunus* species. The degree of toxicity depends on a number of factors, and it is generally agreed that **the wilted leaves are the most toxic**.

CHESTNUT, SPANISH

SCIENTIFIC NAME: *Castasnea sativa* and other *Castanea* species

PARTS USED: Leaves and bark

DOSAGE:

Leaves and Bark: 1 teaspoon of leaves and bark, chopped fine, boiled in a covered container with 1 pint of water for about 1/2 hour, at a slow boil. Allow liquid to cool slowly in the *closed* container. Drink cold, 1 swallow or 1 tablespoon at a time, 1 to 2 cups per day.

CHESTNUT: *These tasty nuts were at one time a common remedy for whooping cough.*

Traditional Usages

Chestnuts are, of course, better known for their edibility. As well as being eaten roasted or boiled, they have traditionally been ground into flour in order to make breads and cakes, and to thicken soups. Eating too many can result in constipation.

Being astringent, the bark and leaves were used to make a tonic which was also reportedly useful in the treatment of upper respiratory ailments such as **coughs,** and particularly **whooping cough.**

The American Chestnut was utilized as a **remedy for whooping** cough by the Mohegans. They learned to use a tea of the leaves from whites, who derived the remedy from an unknown source. Dr. Millspaugh wrote that chestnut leaves were used for whooping cough. However, the 1942 *Dispensatory of the United States* characterized this belief as a superstition, declaring "there is . . . no sufficient reason to believe them to possess any therapeutic value except that of a mild astringent." As an astringent, the leaves were official in the *U.S. Pharmacopoeia* from 1873 to 1905.

Recent Scientific Findings

The bark of Spanish Chestnut is known to contain high concentrations of tannins, which explains the **astringent** effect claimed when water extracts of this plant are applied externally.

Although there is no direct experimental evidence to corroborate claims that the leaves of this plant have value in treating whooping coughs, they are rich in polysaccharides. If taken orally in a water infusion, polysaccharides would **produce a demulcent and soothing effect on the irritated mucous membranes,** and hence have a tendency to lessen the symptoms of whooping cough.

CHINESE CUCUMBER

SCIENTIFIC NAME: *Trichosanthes kirilowii*

PARTS USED: Root tubers

DOSAGE:

> *Not for home use; medical supervision required.*

CHINESE CUCUMBER: *Used for centuries in traditional Chinese medicine, this is the source of the drug Compound Q.*

Traditional Usages

In Oriental medicine, root preparations have been utilized for centuries to induce abortion and treat certain cancers. **Trichosanthin is used to bring about mid-trimester abortion** (*abortifacient*). It achieves this by selectively killing specialized cells found in the uterus. This drug is also employed (again in China) as a treatment for choriocarcinoma, a cancer of these cells found in the uterus. Apparently, trichosanthin is either selectively absorbed by these cancer cells or it has selective antiviral activity.

In traditional Chinese medicine, each part of the plant has been employed for various other ailments. The roots were also utilized to treat **jaundice, diabetes, hemorrhoids,** and **sore throats.** The seeds first recorded use dates from the 5th century A.D. Along with the same ailments as the roots, the seeds also were used as a **laxative** and to **reduce phlegm.**

Recent Scientific Findings

Chinese Cucumber has become the hottest herb of the past 40 years because it is the source of the **drug GLQ223, or "Compound Q." Early findings suggest this drug may work on the HIV virus.** Not since *Rauwolfia* (Indian snakeroot) was introduced from Ayurvedic medicine as an antihypertensive in the 1950's under the name reserpine has a herbal remedy generated so much hope and hype.

The plant itself is not being tested for anti-AIDS activity. **GLQ223 is a highly purified version of trichosanthin,** which is a protein isolated from root tubers of *T. Kirilowii* from southern China.

T. kirilowii contains compounds with **antibacterial** activity, **antiyeast** activity, **gallstone inhibitory activity, oestrogenic activity, uterine relaxant activity,** and **white blood stimulant activity** (from sitosterol). The plant also contains alpha spinasterol, which is **anti-inflammatory** and **antipyretic.** Other of its compounds induce **abortion, kill tumor cells,** and increase prostaglandin levels (PG72A), to mention only a few of the documented actions.

Exciting preliminary results show that **GLQ223 selectively destroys macrophages infected with the human immuno-deficiency virus type 1 (HIV-1).** Such infected T cells are thought to be the major sites of the virus in the human body. In addition, the $CD4^+T$ cells have been found to be a reservoir for latent HIV-1 viruses.

When Michael McGrath, M.D., of San Francisco General Hospital, first tested the drug, he thought it might destroy all macrophages in the body. Nevertheless, he deemed this radical treatment worth the risk. Dr. McGrath discovered that this plant-derived drug killed *only* infected T-cells! Here we had a *selective* agent to try against AIDS.

Along with GLQ223, another protein isolated from *T. kirilowii*, TAP 29, also has shown anti-HIV properties. Preliminary research reported to National Academy of Sciences in 1991 indicated that the therapeutic index of TAP 29 is at least two orders of magnitude higher than that of Compound Q. The researchers concluded, "Thus TAP 29 may offer a broader safe dose range in the treatment of AIDS."

As testing of this promising drug continues, people want to know if they can take the plant itself, is a hot-water infusion of the root safe and effective, will this plant work against other viral infections, and does Chinese Cucumber somehow stimulate the immune system.

First, it is important to emphasize here that **Compound Q, which is presently only available from China, is very dangerous!** It must *not* be utilized without strict and expert medical supervision owing to potential side-effects and toxicity. Some doctors have observed severe anaphylactic reactions in their patients. Other effects include flu-like symptoms such as fevers, as well as seizures, stupors, and even coma.

Trichosanthin is chemically similar to ricin toxin, from Castor Beans (*Ricinus communis*). Ricin is one of the most potent naturally-occurring toxins. Both trichosanthin and ricin belong to a family of proteins known as single-chain ribosome-inactivating agents. In simpler terms, these highly active compounds stop all division. They therefore have the capacity of stopping the division of *healthy* cells—and they can bring about death.

It is easy to kill infected monocytes with many different compounds. Chloroquine, an anti-malarial, for example, is an effective agent. St. John's Wort (*Hypericum perforatum*) has also been shown to be active against the AIDS virus in *test-tube experiments*. To be effective against the virus, *in a human*, relatively high concentrations of hypericin, the active ingredient, would be required—perhaps at a toxic level. At this time, we do not know if GLQ223 is any more effective than chloroquine or hypericin. Further, "Compound Q" may prove to be too large to reach the infected cells, its potency has not been established, and it may also kill healthy cells.

To develop an immunotoxin for an HIV infected cell, highly specialized procedures are required. The envelope glycoproteins, GP160, for example, are found on the surface of HIV cells and are the target receptors for immunotoxins. We do not know, however, if GLQ223 reaches these receptors.

Moreover, it has not yet been determined if trichosanthin is even extracted when Chinese Cucumber roots are boiled. So we do not yet know if a "tea" of this interesting species would have any medicinal properties, let alone be capable of killing viruses or stimulating immunity.

Further, assuming that small quantities of trichosanthin were found to occur in a hot-water extract, as an herbal tea, we do not know if this agent would be *absorbed* from the gastrointestinal tract. (It may prove to work only via the injectable route.)

For these reasons, we *cannot* recommend the self-administration of extracts of this species. Only careful human trials of the drug will answer the many questions which remain outstanding.

Unfortunately, though a number of other studies have taken place since the initial discovery, most have not been published in peer-review journals. To date, there is continuing controversy over both the results and the efficacy of the researchers. Martin Delaney, Executive Director of Project Inform, declared that Compound Q had produced "dramatic effects." Arnold Relman of the *New England Journal of Medicine* said Delaney was "irresponsible" for making such claims. Another article accused Delaney and another researcher, Dr. Larry Waites, of reporting fragmentary data and being over-optimistic in their assessments. AIDS researcher Marcus Conant said that the researchers' enthusiasm sometimes leads to over-optimistic interpretations.

One peer review study involved 18 patients receiving various doses of tricosanthin. Those patients who received the highest doses exhibited *in vitro* antiviral effects. However, the researchers felt these effects did not have therapeutic value, though they did declare the drug safe for further study.

A subsequent study involving 51 patients relied on higher doses. The researchers reported significant decreases in p24 antigen levels with an overall reduction of 67%. Those patients who received the full course of three infusions of the drug showed the best results. The researchers stated that "A picture is forming of a drug which seems to have at least some benefit for some patients, and on which a handful of patients have done extremely well while others appear to have shown little or no benefit and a few have suffered catastrophic side effects."

CINCHONA

SCIENTIFIC NAME: *Cinchona ledgeriana,*
C. calisaya,
C. succirubra,
C. officinalis

PARTS USED: Bark

DOSAGE:

Bark: If available, the compound tincture is taken in doses of 0.65-3.9 grams. However, commercially available drugs are more reliable.

CINCHONA: *The bark of this tree is the source of the malarial cure Quinine.*

Traditional Usages

Cinchona bark was first brought to Europe in 1640 through the auspices of the Countess of Chinchon, of Peru. However, it was not until 97 years later while journeying in the Loxa province of Peru that a French naturalist identified the tree from which the bark was obtained Once Cinchona became popular as a cure for intermittent fevers, it was distributed and sold by the Jesuit fathers, who maintained missions in the area; in the latter 18th century, other sources of the bark were discovered in Columbia, central Peru, and Bolivia.

Quinine has been recognized as one of nature's most important medicinal gifts to the human race, for it has been instrumental in relieving great suffering from malaria and other intermittent fevers.

Recent Scientific Findings

The alkaloid quinine is derived from Cinchona bark and is well known for its antimalarial properties. Besides its antiperiodic action against intermittent fever, Cinchona bark has **tonic**, **antiseptic**, and **astringent** properties.

Although **quinine** and preparations containing quinine are relatively safe, one must be cautious of the amounts used. Excessive doses of Cinchona can lead to a condition known as cinchonism or quinism, marked by buzzing in the ears, deafness, headache, vertigo, and nausea. While these effects generally disappear within a few hours, they are a warning signal regarding dosage.

Nature, as in many cases, has provided a built-in warning to notify us when the safe limit of these preparations is approaching. When on experiences a ringing in the ears, the amount being taken should be reduced, and the sounds will disappear.

Recent research has only confirmed Cinchona's effectiveness against malaria and its superiority to synthetic pharmaceuticals. During the Vietnam War, a strain of malarial parasite developed which was highly resistant to both well-established and new synthetic anti-malarial drugs. It was soon found, however, that most cases of malaria caused by the new parasite could be effectively treated with the centuries-proven drug, quinine. In recent years, cases such as this have led to increased use of quinine in place of synthetic drugs.

CINNAMON

SCIENTIFIC NAME: *Cinnamonum zeylanicum*,
Cinnamonum cassia

PARTS USED: Bark, leaves, and roots

DOSAGE:

1-2 grams of the dried herb, in capsule or powdered form, 1-2 times per day with food or beverage.

CINNAMON: *This common spice has been used as a carminative for centuries and may also be an effective antibacterial agent.*

Traditional Usages

Cinnamon trees have been extensively cultivated in the tropics for the dried bark, which is the common spice. Cinnamon's use as medicinal also goes back to ancient times; it is mentioned in both early Chinese herbals and Egyptian texts. The Greeks used Cinnamon as a treatment for bronchitis. In his writings, Galen mentions that he employed five different types of Cinnamon.

Chinese Cinnamon, or Cassia (*Cinnamonum cassia*), while stronger in flavor was employed for similar ailments as *Cinnamonum zeylanicum*. Cinnamon has long been a popular carminative. It was commonly employed for most gastrointestinal problems. Most often, Cinnamon was used in conjunction with other herbs in the treatment of a variety of ailments, including **flues** and **dysentery**.

Recent Scientific Findings

Various parts of this plant have been so widely used throughout the world and have been so extensively tested, that only a brief summary will be possible. The leaves, bark, stems, and roots contain several essential oils that are used as a flavoring in food and gum as well as in perfumes and incense. In these formulas the essential oil from the flowers is used.

This essential oil has been found to stimulate the gastrointestinal tract, supporting Cinnamon's traditional use. Cinnamon also has been found to dilate blood vessels. This may explain Cinnamon's folkloric use in conjunction with other herbs since increased blood circulation may enhance the delivery of the herbs effects.

Mitogenic activity occurred in cell culture experiments as well as **antifungal** activity against *Aspergillus favus.* An estrogenic effect in animals has been demonstrated. **Antiyeast** activity also took place in Agar plate experiments, especially against *Candida, lipolytica,* and another yeast known as *Kloeckera apicultra.* Many other types of yeast have been destroyed in Agar plate experiments by extracts of the essential oil of this species.

A commercial sample of the bark has been tested in Japan and found to have anesthetic activity in animal experiments. Numerous experiments with extracts of this plant showed wide antibacterial activity against various species of bacillus. Dried bark has been tested in Japan as a decoction and found to possess anticonvulsant activity in experiments with mice. Again, **antibacterial** activity of the essential oil of the bark has been **shown to kill** *staphylococci* **and other kinds of bacteria, including *Staphyloccus aureus*.** Interesting experiments in India showed the essential oil to have **insect repellent activity** and also to have spermicidal effects. Most interestingly, extracts of the leaf juice in Agar plate experiments had strong activity against *Mycobacterium tuberculosis,* the bacteria found in **tuberculosis.**

CITRUS

SCIENTIFIC NAME: Various species
PARTS USED: Essential oils extracted from peel of lemons and oranges

DOSAGE:
1 to 5 capsules, 2 to 3 times per day.

CITRUS: *Citrus contains limonene, which may both prevent and treat cancer.*

Traditional Usages

Citrus is most well known historically as a treatment for scurvy. Though used in folk medicine for some time, it was James Lind who in 1753 conducted his renowned experiment that proved citrus fruits cured scurvy. The British Navy's requirement that ship's carry limes or lemons led to the epithet Limey.

The name citrus was first used by Pliny. Lemon juice was employed as a diuretic and astringent.

Recent Scientific Findings

In recent years, research has uncovered **anti-cancer** properties in certain essential oils. Limonene is the major component of the essential oil of orange and other citrus fruits. It also occurs widely in the plant kingdom, particularly in those species producing essential oils, flavors and spices. This compound belongs to a class of natural compounds known as terpenes, soon to equal the bioflavonoids and carotenoids in their applications.

About ten animal studies have been published which show that dietary limonene (the d-isomer, or d-limonene) lowers the incidence of chemically-induced cancers as well as delaying their appearance. Elson and colleagues at the University of Wisconsin are currently the leaders in this field. In one study, they demonstrated that dietary d-limonene markedly reduced dimethylbenzanthracene-induced mammary cancers. The dosage used in this study was 1000 parts per million, or 1 gram per kg of diet. [NOTE: humans eat about 1/2 kg per day, which translates to about 500 mg of d-limonene per day.]

Using this same model system, they subsequently showed that the essential oil of orange (85% d-limonene) was more effective than pure d-limonene in preventing tumor formation. Thus, naturally-occurring terpenes in orange oil other than d-limonenes also possess anticancer activity. Further investigations by this group revealed that dietary d-limonene is effective in reversing preformed tumors, as evidenced by an increase in the tumor regression rate. Finally, Elson and associates recently observed that dietary d-limonene was effective in reducing the number of chemically-induced mammary tumors in rats when provided either during the initiation phase or during the promotion/progression phase.

The mechanism(s) of action of d-limonene against cancer are not well understood, but may involve the enhancement of drug-metabolizing systems such as *glutathione-S-transferases*. The ability of d-limonene to **reverse preformed tumors** and to **inhibit tumor growth** during the promotion/progression phase of cancer suggests an **immunostimulating action,** and some recent evidence does support this concept.

As an added benefit limonene is a potent, **natural cholesterol-lowering compound.** It acts by inhibiting the same enzyme (HMG-coenzyme A reductase) which is the target of many prescribed **cholesterol-reducing** drugs such as lovostatin. If these actions were not sufficient, **limonene is also a powerful agent for dissolving gallstones.**

Researchers at the University of Wisconsin, Madison, confirmed d-limonene's **antitumor potential.** In a series of animal experiments, **up to 90% of tumors completely disappeared in mice fed this compound,** whereas only 15% of tumors spontaneously diminished in size in animals not given the compound. Human cancer cells have also been shrunk with d-limonene in laboratory experiments. Michael Gould, professor of human oncology at the University of Wisconsin was quoted as saying **"we can potentially use limonene to treat as well as prevent cancer."**

In another study of d-limonene it was found that **gallstones were dissolved** by this "simple, safe, and effective solvent."

CLOVER, RED

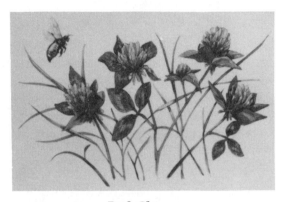

Red Clover

SCIENTIFIC NAME: *Trifolium pratense*
PARTS USED: Blossoms

DOSAGE:
1 to 2 capsules, 1 to 3 times per day taken with food or beverage.

RED CLOVER: An extract is marketed in Europe as a treatment for diarrhea.

Traditional Usages

Red Clover was used for female complaints, as an anti-diarrhetic, and to treat dysentery.

Recent Scientific Findings

An extract of Red Clover, Uzarin, paralyzes smooth musculature. It is marketed in Europe under the name UZARA in the form of drops and tablets and is recommended as an **antidote to diarrhea**.

The isoflavone biochanin A is another extract of Red Clover. It has been found to be a **potent carcinogenic inhibitor**.

CLOVES

SCIENTIFIC NAME: *Syzygium aromaticum*

PARTS USED: Flower bud

DOSAGE:
For toothache pain, drops of oil directly onto cavity.

CLOVES: *The essential oil of this common spice has shown promising anti-inflammatory effects in recent experiments.*

Traditional Usages

The dried flowerbuds of Cloves are well known as the source of this common spice. Oil of Cloves have long been employed as a mild anesthetic as well as a stimulant and carminative. Clove oil was used to alleviate nausea and stop vomiting. It has especially been used for **toothaches**, with drops of the oil placed on a cavity. Clove tea was used to relieve **nausea**.

In traditional Chinese medicine, Cloves are a common digestive remedy, used for vomiting, diarrhea, and pains in the chest and abdomen.

Recent Scientific Findings

Clove's essential oil has exhibited much promise in recent research. **Anti-inflammatory** activity of clove extract has been demonstrated in rats and adult humans.

Essential oil of Clove has been shown to **kill (in vitro)** the pathogenic yeast *Can-*

dida albicans and many older species of yeasts including *Trichophytum.* The essential oil also inhibited prostaglandin production and is therefore an **anti-inflammatory. Antifungal** activity against *Trichophytum pubrum* has been shown in humans.

Clove oil demonstrated in vitro **antibacterial activity against** *Bacillus subtilis* (one causative agent of food poisoning). Other susceptible organisms are *E. coli, pseudomonas aurginosa* and *Staphylococcus aureus.* **Clove oil was also active against** *Mycobacterium tuberculosis* in vitro. **Antiviral activity has been shown against herpes simplex virus.**

Extract of clove suppresses dental plaque formation, specifically by being active against *streptococcus mutans,* a causative agent in dental carey formation. Clove's essential oil showed activity as an **inhibitor of platelet aggregation.**

COHOSH, BLACK

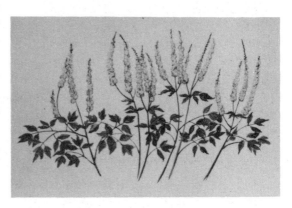

Black Cohosh

SCIENTIFIC NAME: *Cimicifuga racemosa*
PARTS USED: Rhizome and root

DOSAGE:

Root: When used in medicine, the usual dose is 2 teaspoons of powdered root per 1½ pints of boiling water, boiled in a covered container for about ½ hour, at a slow boil. Allow the liquid to cool slowly in the *closed* container. Drink cold, 2 to 3 tablespoons 6 times a day.

BLACK COHOSH: *Used for centuries by Native Americans, an extract of Black Cohosh was recently approved by the Russians as a central nervous system tonic and as a treatment for high blood pressure.*

Traditional Usages

Native American tribes used this plant for "women's problems," hence the Anglicized named "squawroot." The Black Cohosh, or Black Snakeroot, is a native of the United States, growing in shady and rocky woods from Canada to Florida, and flowering in June and July. The root is the part employed.

This, as found in the shops, consists of a thick, irregularly bent or contorted body or caudex, from 1/2 inch to 1 inch in thickness, often several inches in length, furnished with many slender radicles, and rendered exceedingly rough and jagged in appearance by the remains of the stem of successive years, which to the length of 1 inch or more are frequently attached to the root. The color is externally dark brown, almost black, internally whitish. The odor is feeble, the taste bitter, herbaceous and somewhat astringent, leaving a slight sense of acrimony. The root yields its virtues to boiling water.

Collected in the autumn, particularly in the Blue Ridge mountains, this interesting root has been used as **relaxant, antispasmodic,** and sedative. In the course of its employment as a treatment for chorea, or St. Vitus' dance, it was reported to have the undesirable side effects of inducing vomiting, giddiness, headache, and prostration. Between 1820 and 1936, when the plant was official in the *U.S. Pharmacopoeia*, the rhizome and root were utilized in the U.S. as a **sedative,** for **rheumatism,** and to **promote menstruation.**

Recent Scientific Findings

Acetin, one of Black Cohosh's active principles, has been shown to **lower blood pressure in experiments with rabbits and cats,** and experiments with dogs have shown **significant peripheral vasodilation.** Furthermore, Black Cohosh extracts have been proven antimicrobial in *in vitro* experiments. This **bacterial and yeast-killing activity may support the folkloric use of Squawroot for a myriad of "women's complaints."**

Extracts of Black Cohosh rhizomes and roots have been shown to decrease experimental inflammation by one third in laboratory animals, although the constituents responsible for this effect have not yet been identified. **Thus, it appears that the use of this plant for neuralgia and rheumatism has a rational basis.**

Extracts of Black Cohosh also have been tested for estrogenic effects in mice and are devoid of this activity. Since this type of biological test is most always predictive for humans, it must be presumed that the use of Black Cohosh for dysmenorrhea cannot be based on an estrogenic effect. Other experiments have shown that **Black Cohosh reduces hypertension and acts as an anti-inflammatory and hypoglycemic.** In one experiment, it was found that Black Cohosh had a **hypotensive effect.**

Investigations have also verified the use of Black Cohosh as a **smooth muscle and nerve relaxant.** Recently, the Russians approved an extract of Black Cohosh as a **central nervous system tonic** and as a **treatment for high blood pressure.**

Caution: Persons taking other drugs of either pharmaceutical or herbal origin to lower their blood pressure are warned against the use of Black Cohosh concurrent with these other medications.

COHOSH, BLUE

SCIENTIFIC NAME: *Caulophyllum thalictroides*

PARTS USED: Root stock

DOSAGE:

Root: The medicinal preparation consists of 1 teaspoon of granulated root boiled with 1½ pints of slowly boiling water for ½ hour, in a covered container. This is drunk cold, a mouthful at a time, a total of 1 cupful per day.

BLUE COHOSH: *Scientific investigations have confirmed this root's use by Native American women as an aid in child delivery.*

Traditional Usages

Like the May-Apple, this plant is quite bitter, and is therefore avoided by grazing animals. The thickened rootstocks have been used in medicine. Some persons are susceptible to handling the plant and develop a dermatitis.

Blue Cohosh was widely as utilized an **aid to parturition**, first by Native Americans and then by the early white settlers who called it squawroot and papoose root. **To promote a rapid delivery**, an infusion of the root in warm water was drunk as a tea for a week or two prior to the expected delivery date. Various tribes took this same preparation for other purposes as well. The Menominees, Ojibwa, Meskwakis, and Potawatomis used it for "female troubles." The Omahas boiled a decoction of the root as a fever remedy.

Reportedly, Blue Cohosh has also been employed to **purge the intestinal tract of infestations of worms**. The root is a **diuretic** as well, **promoting urination**; it has also been used medicinally for its ability to **produce sweating**.

The dried root was official in the *U.S. Pharmacopoeia* from 1882 to 1905 when it was used for **antispasmodic, emmenagogue**, and **diuretic** purposes. At the turn of the century, Blue Cohosh root was actively collected and traded, bringing a wholesale price of from two and one-half to four cents a pound. One clinician found that an extract of the root has a **pronounced stimulating effect on the uterine muscle.**

Recent Scientific Findings

Scientific investigations with a fluid extract of Blue Cohosh have **confirmed folkloric claims to stimulate the uterus**. Other findings include **anti-inflammatory activity. Antihypertensive activity** was observed in adult humans. It is reported that this preparation is **useful in the treatment of cirrhosis of the liver.**

COLTSFOOT

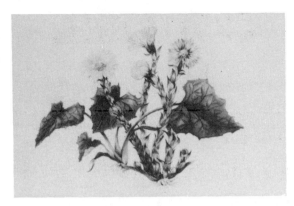

Coltsfoot

SCIENTIFIC NAME: *Tussilago farfara*
PARTS USED: Leaves

DOSAGE:
   Caution: See articles on *Borage* and on *Comfrey.* Coltsfoot preparations should be approached cautiously for the same reasons.

COLTSFOOT: *For centuries, this has been a respiratory remedy.*

Traditional Usages

Coltsfoot has been recognized as a **remedy for coughs** and **respiratory ailments** since antiquity. An **external emollient** and **internal demulcent**, Coltsfoot has been considered very helpful in relieving the coughs of colds and was applied externally as a poultice for relief of chest congestion. In **traditional Chinese medicine, Coltsfoot has long been used to treat various respiratory conditions.** Hippocrates recommended mixing the root with honey for ulcerations of the lungs, while other classical Greek physicians reported that the smoke of the leaves was helpful for coughs and difficult breathing. Reportedly the fumes of the burning leaves relieved toothache.

Containing an acrid essential oil, a bitter glucoside, a resin, and gallic acid, the leaves are often used as a tobacco substitute and are sometimes smoked in an herbal blend for **asthma.**

Among Native American tribes in Northern California Sweet Coltsfoot was a salt substitute that became so important that it led to intertribal warfare.

Recent Scientific Findings

Test-tube and culture studies have shown Coltsfoot extracts to have **anti-inflammatory, antispasmodic**, and **anti-tuberculousis** properties. In a mixture with other plants, Coltsfoot leaves, when smoked by human subjects, had **anti-asthmatic activity.** However, it is not known whether it was the Coltsfoot or other plants in the mixture that accounted for these results.

In animal studies in China, Coltsfoot flowers, when added to the diet, were observed to be strongly active in producing liver tumors in rats; because of this finding, Coltsfoot should probably not be used internally until further research has been done on its possible carcinogenic properties.

Recently, an extract of Coltsfoot has been found to be a **potent cardiovascular and respiratory stimulant**. In animal experiments, it's effect has been similar to dopamine without tachyphylaxis.

COMFREY

SCIENTIFIC NAME: *Symphytum officinale*
PARTS USED: Leaf/root

DOSAGE:

Leaf: Approximately ½ ounce of leaves to 1 pint of water. Boil water separately and pour over the plant material and steep 5-10 minutes, depending on the desired effect. Drink hot or warm, 1 to 2 cups per day, at bedtime and upon awakening.

Root: 1 teaspoon of granulated root boiled with 1½ pints of slowly boiling water for ½ hour, in a covered container. This is drunk cold, a mouthful at a time, a total of 1 cupful per day.

COMFREY: *The roots of this plant help heal wounds and broken bones.*

Traditional Usages

This popular herb has been widely utilized for a variety of medical problems. Dioscorides prescribed Comfrey to aid the **healing of broken bones and wounds.** The juice of the crushed root, mixed with wine, was drunk to **stop internal bleeding,** particularly **uterine hemorrhaging.** Similarly, the powdered root was snuffed up the nostrils to prevent or allay nosebleeds. The root, crushed and boiled, has been drunk to relieve chest congestion.

Perhaps its most common use was to promote tissue healing. Plasters made from decoctions of the glutinaceous root were applied externally and reportedly

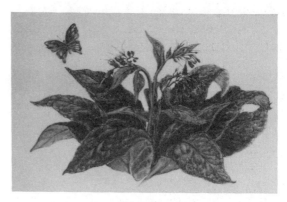

Comfrey

aided the knitting of tissues cut during surgery or torn apart from injury. Comfrey was often employed to aid the union of fractured bones.

Recent Scientific Findings

Comfrey is another example of a popular herbal preparation that should not be taken regularly by humans, for the same reason that Borage should not be used, i.e., they both contain chemical compounds that are known to be potentially toxic and/or carcinogenic.

Recently, Comfrey has been subject of controversy due to claims that it is carcinogenic and toxic to the liver. Comfrey contains pyrrolizidine alkaloids (PAs). These alkaloids cause a liver disease known as hepatic veno-occlusive disease (HVOD). However, different PAs possess different levels of toxicity and the risk to humans is still not established. Currently, the USFDA is analyzing Comfrey while Australia has banned it and Canada has restricted it to medical use. Comfrey roots contain higher amounts of PAs than the leaves and therefore manufacturers have been told to refrain from using the root in herbal preparations.

The most toxic of Comfrey's PAs, echimidine, is only found in Prickly Comfrey (*Symphytum asperum*), not *Symphytum officinale*. One of Prickly Comfrey's hybrids is Russian Comfrey (*Symphytum x uplandicum* Nyman), which is commonly sold in commercial preparations and contains echimidine. Unfortunately, the species of Comfrey products is often not on the label of commercial products. When Canadian researchers studied 13 Comfrey products, they found six contained echimidine. Yet all were labelled either as *Symphytum officinale* or simple as "Comfrey." In fact, three of the six containing echimidine were labeled as *Symphytum officinale*. Examiners of commercial preparations sold in the United States found the PAs to be consistent with *Symphytum officinale*.

This confusion of species identification has carried over into the scientific research. For instance, a team of Japanese researchers in an article on the constituents of *Symphytum officinale* stated that the species they were examining "is called Comfrey or Russian Comfrey." The *British Medical Journal* claimed they were nine PAs in *Symphytum officinale*, basing their claim on an investigation that analyzed plants from four different geographic locations.

> So where does this leave consumers? At this time, one must assume that the type of PAs found in Comfrey have the potential for liver damage. While the plant may be safe in small doses, it is advisable to restrict its use until the controversy surrounding its toxicity is resolved.

On the other hand, many herbal manuals allude to the fact that Comfrey promotes the growth of healthy cells, both externally and in mucous membranes, owing to its component allantoin. Because the toxic reaction of PAs seems to occur during metabolism in the liver, it may be reasonable to suggest that *external* applications of the leaves are still useful to heal wounds and broken bones, and to diminish various skin growths. **Animal experiments have found wound healing acceleration and anti-inflammatory activity.** A 1989 study found that Comfrey extracts aided repair, especially after surgery.

Caution: **See above discussion.**

CORN

SCIENTIFIC NAME: *Zea mays*
PARTS USED: Silk and oil

DOSAGE:
   Silk: Steep a handful of the silk. Can be drunk or administered as an enema.

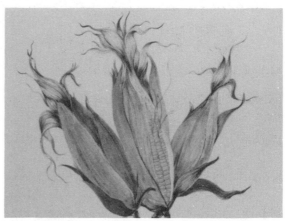

CORN: *This staple food may also have cancer reducing effects.*

Traditional Usages

Maize was eaten throughout much of North America. It is thought to have originated in Mexico. This crop became the center of art and religious life for many tribes. Countless ceremonies were performed for this food, so that by the time the Europeans arrived, some tribes referred to maize by words that mean "our life" or "it sustains us" or "giver of life."

Amerind tribes utilized the corn plant in several medicinal ways. The Chickasaws squeezed the oil from the grains and rubbed it directly into the scalp as a **dandruff remedy**. Eastern tribes used the oil in poultices for **boils, burns,** and **inflammations.** Corn meal has also been used as an **emollient** for **skin problems.** Corn starch is an effective antidote for iodine poisoning, simply swallowed.

Recent Scientific Findings

Corn has exhibited hypocholesterolemic activity in adult humans. It has also been found to contribute to the **dissolution of kidney stones** in humans. An estrogenic and ovulation induction effect was observed in animal studies. **Preliminary animal experiments with an aqueous extract have found immunostimulant activity,** as well as the stimulation of interferon induction and macrophage migration.

Though at this time there is no laboratory studies to confirm or deny whether Corn prevents cancer, a 1981 investigation by the Louisiana State University Medical Center found that the death rates from colon, breast, and prostate cancer were lower among populations with increased per capita consumption of Corn.

COTTON

SCIENTIFIC NAME: *Gossypium herbaceum*
PARTS USED: Root bark (inner)

DOSAGE:

Not recommended. Very strong.

Root Bark: A decoction was prepared using 1 teaspoon of the root bark per 1½ pints of water, boiled in a covered container, at a slow boil, for about ½ hour. Liquid was allowed to cool slowly in the closed container and was drunk cold, 1 swallow or 1 tablespoon at a time, 1 to 2 cups per day.

COTTON: *The root bark of this popular crop causes uterine contractions.*

Traditional Usages

The inner root bark of the Cotton plant, the most common crop in the southern United States, was used in that region instead of Ergot of rye to promote uterine contractions. It was reported to act as a **stimulant for menstruation** and to **arrest uterine hemorrhage.** The Alabama and Koasati tribes made a tea of cotton roots, which was taken to ease labor. In 1840, a French writer reported that Southern slaves utilized the root bark to **produce abortion. Cotton was employed during labor, childbirth, and delivery of the placenta.** Southern practitioners employed the plant from 1840 well into the 20th century. In unskilled hands, however, it was considered a dangerous remedy, causing nausea and vomiting when taken in large doses. The root bark was officially recognized in the *U.S. Pharmacopoeia* from 1863 to 1950 for its effects on the uterine organs.

Recent Scientific Findings

Experimentally, extracts of Cotton root bark have been well established as **causing contractions of the uterus,** not only in test tube experiments, but by administration to animals as well. **This effect, if similar in humans, would result in abortions,** and would also constricted blood vessels in the vaginal tract, thus resulting in a diminution of blood flow in cases of menorrhagia. These findings support folkloric claims.

COWSLIP

SCIENTIFIC NAME: *Primula veris,*
P. officinalis
PARTS USED: Flowers, roots, and leaves

DOSAGE:

Leaves   and   Flowers:
Approximately ½ ounce of leaves or flowers to 1 pint of water. Boil water separately and pour over the plant material and steep for 5-20 minutes, depending on the desired effect. Drink hot or warm, 1 to 2 cups or more per day, at bedtime and upon awakening.

COWSLIP: *Once a renowned remedy for paralysis and headache, now the leaves are used to make a pleasant relaxing tea.*

Traditional Usages

Once high renowned as a narcotic and sedative, by 1837 Cowslip had ceased to be much more than a rustic remedy. Linnaeus deemed it useful as an **analgesic** and as a **sleep inducer**, as did many of the old herbalists.

At one time Cowslip was the chief plant **employed to treat paralysis and headache.** All parts of the plant were used, but the dried flowers were believed to be most potent.

In some countries fermented beverages are made from the flowers with sugar, honey, and lemon juice, while the roots are also put into casks of wine or beer to enhance the strength and flavor of those beverages.

From all accounts it appears that Cowslip was an **extremely gentle pain reliever and sleep inducer,** which caused none of the undesirable side effects that are encountered in some other such remedies.

Recent Scientific Findings

Containing primulin and cyclamin, Cowslip leaves are a good substitute for tea used to improve various nervous conditions.

CRAMP BARK

or

HIGHBUSH CRANBERRY

SCIENTIFIC NAME: *Viburnum opulus*
PARTS USED: Bark

DOSAGE:
> **Bark:** 1 to 4 grams dried bark three times a day

CRAMP BARK: *True to its name, this bark has been found to be a uterine relaxant.*

Traditional Usages

Indigenous to southern Canada and the northern United States, the Highbush Cranberry was a popular remedy among the tribes of those regions. The Malecites and the Penobscots drank an infusion of an unnamed part of the plant as a treatment for **mumps**. Since the bark most clearly holds the medicinal properties, one can assume that these people discovered this remedy through their own methods. One early 20th century writer stated that Native Americans used Cramp Bark as a **diuretic**, which is interesting since the excretion of liquids is desirable during mumps.

From 1894 to 1916, Cramp Bark was listed in the *U.S. Pharmacopoeia*. It was a popularly employed as a **sedative** and **antispasmodic**. It is claimed that its use during pregnancy tends to diminish miscarriage, especially if used with equal parts of button snakeroot.

Recent Scientific Findings

As its name indicates, this bark is very effective in **relieving cramps** and **spasms** of all kinds. As it also exerts a decided influence upon the **reproductive organs**, it is especially useful in **menstrual cramps** and pains, giving tone and energy to the uterus.

Research supports Cramp Bark's folkloric reputation. Test-tube studies have shown cramp bark to have both **uterine-stimulant** and **uterine-relaxant properties**. Other studies show Cramp Bark to be active as a **smooth muscle relaxant** and as a **cardiotonic**.

Animal studies have shown *Viburnum* species extracts to reduce blood pressure in the dog and lower body temperature in the mouse. **Cardio activity (strengthening heart muscle contraction)** of aqueous extract was observed in both the dog and frog model.

Antiviral activity of aqueous extract of Cramp Bark was observed in cell culture **against influenza virus**. **Cytotoxic activity** of aqueous extract was observed in cell culture against the HELA cancer cell line.

Preparations of a related species, *V. prunifolium*, have been shown **to produce abortion** and to stimulate gastric secretions in humans.

CRANBERRY

SCIENTIFIC NAME: *Vaccinium macrocarpon*
PARTS USED: Berry

DOSAGE:
1 to 3 grams, 2 to 3 times per day.

CRANBERRY: *This common berry has shown remarkable properties in combating urinary tract infections.*

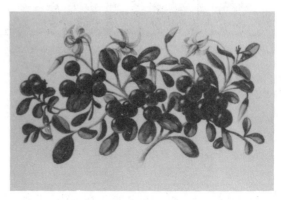

Cranberry

Traditional Usages

Traditionally Cranberry was used for **urinary tract infections** and for **dissolving kidney** and **gall stones.**

Recent Scientific Findings

The folkloric claims of Cranberry's effectiveness against urinary tract infections has been confirmed by several studies. In one study, cranberry juice was given to a group of people with urinary tract infections. After drinking the juice for 21 days, **70% of the individuals improved.**

Cranberry's chemical constituents are anthocyanins, catechin, and triterpenoids. Cranberry contains 10% carbohydrate, protein, fiber, vitamin C, and citric acid. The high acid content also increases urine's acid content, **killing the bacteria that causes urinary infections.** Interestingly, **Cranberry also prevents the bacteria from adhering to cells, allowing the bacteria to be flushed from the system.** Dr. Anthony Sobota discovered this property of Cranberry when he observed this effect under the microscope. He even found that **commercial Cranberry juice was strong enough to achieve this effect.** Sobota also analyzed the urine of individuals after having them drink Cranberry juice. The amount of antibacterial chemical present in the urine was significantly higher. Though further research continues on the specifics of Cranberry's properties, it appears that **this common drink is a simple and effective means for combating urinary infections.**

DAMIANA

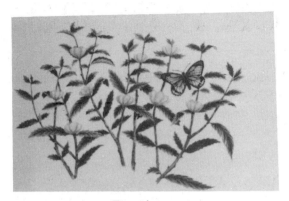

Damiana

SCIENTIFIC NAME: *Turnera aphrodisiaca*
PARTS USED: Leaves

DOSAGE:

> **Leaves:** 2-4 grams of the leaves in the form of an infusion of fluidextract.

DAMIANA: *This is one of the most popular and safest of the plants claiming to be aphrodisiacs.*

Traditional Usages

About 60 species of Damiana occur, mainly in tropical and subtropical America. The two *Turnera* species which yield Damiana are small shrubs indigenous to southern California, Mexico, and Antilles. The leaves are reputedly **aphrodisiac**, and have also been utilized for **tonic**, **stimulant**, and **laxative** purposes.

Damiana acquired a reputation for **curing sexual impotence**; however, in these treatments it was generally administered in conjunction with a more powerful stimulant such as strychnine or phosphorous and so it is difficult to assess the degree to which Damiana alone contributed to the results.

In Mexico, the leaves are used as a substitute for Chinese tea and also to flavor liqueurs.

Recent Scientific Findings

Damiana is one of the most popular and safest of all plants claimed to have an aphrodisiac effect. Although some sources claim that caffeine is present in this plant, we have been unable to substantiate this claim from an exhaustive search of the literature. In fact, there are no animal experiments that have been reported which would lead one to believe that Damiana has an aphrodisiac effect, and no chemical compounds have been found in this plant that would be expected to cause such an effect. **Clearly, this is a plant that needs and deserves a careful chemical and pharmacological study.**

DANDELION

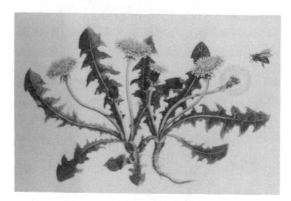

Dandelion

SCIENTIFIC NAME: *Taraxacum officinale*
PARTS USED: Rhizome and root

DOSAGE:

Leaves: Approximately 1 ounce of leaves to 1 pint of water. Boil water separately and pour over the plant material and steep for 5 to 20 minutes, depending on the desired effect. Drink hot or warm, 1 to 2 cups per day, at bedtime and upon awakening.

Root: 1 teaspoon, boiled in a covered container of 1½ pints of water for about ½ hour, at a slow boil. Allow liquid to cool slowly in the *closed* container. Drink cold, 1 swallow or 1 tablespoon at a time, 1 to 2 cups per day.

DANDELION: *A German over-the-counter preparation containing this common weed has been found effective against gallstones.*

Traditional Usages

This species grows spontaneously in most parts of the globe. It is abundant in the U.S., adorning our grass plots and pasture grounds with its bright yellow flowers. All parts of the plant exude a milky bitter juice when they are broken or wounded.

Although introduced to North America from Europe, many tribes soon learned to enjoy eating Dandelion. The Iroquois preferred the boiled leaves with fatty meats. It was used in Native American medicine soon after it was introduced to this country. No doubt Native Americans "borrowed" the recipes for this plant from colonial settlers.

A tea from the roots was drunk for **heartburn** by the Pillager Ojibwas, while the Mohegans and others tribes drank a tea of the leaves for their tonic properties. Kiowa women boiled Dandelion blossoms with Pennyroyal leaves and drank the resulting tea to **relieve cramps and pain associated with menstruation.** The dried rhizome and roots were official in the *U.S. Pharmacopoeia* from 1831 to 1926.

Recent Scientific Findings

Best prepared by boiling in water and then chilling, the leaves are used throughout the world as greens. They are rich in vitamins A and C and should be considered an important survival food. To verify the value of this common weed, we are told that many of the inhabitants of Minorra, one of the Balearic Islands in the Mediterranean, subsisted on Dandelion roots after their harvest had been entirely destroyed by locusts.

A **mild laxative** and **tonic medicine,**

Dandelion is commonly administered as a home remedy for mild constipation and stomach ache. Dandelion leaf tea, drunk often, is **recommended as an aid for promoting digestive regularity**. The plant was noted to have an almost specific affinity for the liver, modifying and increasing its secretions; hence it has been used in **chronic diseases of the digestive organs, especially hepatic disorders**, including jaundice and **chronic inflammation and enlargement of the liver**.

The young leaves of Dandelion, collected in the spring, make a healthful and tasty addition to salads. The root, dried and powdered, may be added to coffee for its medicinal value or used as a coffee substitute.

Experimentally, extracts of Dandelion rhizomes and roots have been shown to increase the bile flow in animals when administered orally, and thus might have **beneficial effects in hepatic disorders**. The specific substance responsible for this reported cholagogue effect has not yet been identified, but it is known that the roots contain inulin, an essential oil and a bitter compound.

The German over-the-counter preparation, "Hepatichol," which contains Dandelion and other herbs, has **proven effective against gallstones**. Further testing found the preparation significantly enhanced the concentration and secretion of bilirubin.

Dandelion has also been found effective in **relieving chronic arthritis**. Although some herbalists have claimed that the plant has **diuretic effects**, we are unable to confirm that Dandelion has such properties on the basis of laboratory research.

DEVIL'S CLAW

SCIENTIFIC NAME: *Harpagophytum procumbens*

PARTS USED: Tuber and root

DOSAGE:
Unknown

DEVIL'S CLAW: *Modern research confirms this South African plant's effectiveness against arthritis and rheumatism.*

Traditional Usages

For more than 250 years decoctions of the roots of this plant were popularly embraced by various cultures in South Africa, including the Hottentots, Bantus, and Bushmen. The claims for Devil's Claw root are as a tonic and for **arthritis** and **rheumatism**. To reduce fevers an infusion of the roots is employed, while an ointment is applied to **ulcers, sores, and boils**.

Recent Scientific Findings

Devil's Claw root has been introduced into North America as an herbal remedy during recent years. It is also currently very popular in Europe. This plant has been found to contain at least three bitter principles, the main one being an **iridoid glucoside** named **harpagide**. In animal studies harpagide has shown anti-inflammatory activity in a number of different types of animal models in which inflammation was induced by the injection of various types of agents.

Harpagide and other extracts of Devil's Claw have been evaluated in recent times in clinical trials involving human subjects with **arthritis** and have shown a beneficial effect. There have been no adverse effects published for extracts of Devil's Claw root; thus the folkloric claims seem to be justified.

In many excellent animals studies, Devil's Claw has shown **analgesic activity, anti-inflammatory activity, smooth muscle relaxant activity,** and **antihypertensive activity.** In rat and rabbit studies, cardiac effects included **antiarrhythmic activity,** no inotropic effect, and bradycardia activity

One study treated patients with metabolic diseases with the tea of Devil's Claw root. **Cholesterol and neutral fat levels were lowered.** Currently the drug is quite popular in Europe.

DOGWOOD

SCIENTIFIC NAME: *Cornus florida* and other *Cornus* species

PARTS USED: Bark

DOSAGE:

Bark: 1/2 ounce of the dried powdered bark; or 1.8-3.8 milliliters of the fluidextract.

DOGWOOD: *The bark of this lovely tree was once a common substitute for Cinchona.*

Traditional Usages

In folk medicine, Dogwood is esteemed for its tonic properties. Numerous Native American tribes used Dogwood for fevers. The Delawares called the tree *Hat-ta-wa-no-min-schi* and boiled the inner bark in water to make a fever-reducing tea. Flowering Dogwood bark was similarly utilized by the Alabamas and the Houmas. Young branches were stripped of their bark and used to clean teeth.

During the last century, Dogwood bark was often substituted for Cinchona bark. When the alkaloid quinine was successfully isolated from Cinchona and administered as a sulfate, the use of both Cinchona and Dogwood for **intermittent fevers** ceased almost completely. Up until that time, Dogwood bark had also been given for typhoid fevers and other disorders.

Recent Scientific Findings

Dogwood bark contains cornin, a bitter principle, and high concentrations of tannin, which explains its **astringent** effect.

ECHINACEA

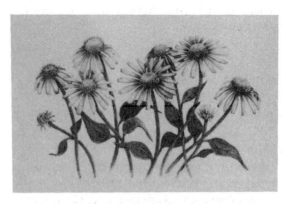

Echinacea

SCIENTIFIC NAME: *Echinacea angustifolia, E. purpurea, E. pallida*

PARTS USED: Root and rhizome

DOSAGE:

Root: 1 teaspoon root stock with 1 cup of water. Take 1 tablespoon 3 to 6 times per day.

ECHINACEA: *Native Americans believed this plant possessed almost magical healing properties; recent scientific documentation reveals startling immune-enhancing effects.*

Traditional Usages

Sometimes known as Coneflower, this perennial grows from the prairie states north and eastward to Pennsylvania. Its distinctive spiny appearance led the German botanist Conrad Moench in 1794 to name the purpurea species of this plant *Echinacea—echinos* is the Greek word for sea urchin or hedgehog.

Long considered a panacea by Amerind tribes, they utilized Echinacea to treat abscesses, boils, gangrenous wounds, septicemia, scarlet fever, ivy poisoning, spider bites, and ulcers. The tribes of the western plains applied Echinacea to insect bites, stings, and snakebites. A piece of the plant was used for toothache and mumps. The Sioux drank a root decoction as a remedy for hydrophobia and snakebites. By the 1880's it became the most widely prescribed agent among medical practitioners for infections and inflammations. Echinacea was used to treat common fevers and minor infections, as well as typhoid, meningitis, malaria, diphtheria, etc.

In 1906 a report was published by Hewett describing several case reports on the treatment of various conditions such as **abscesses**, boils, gangrenous wounds, septicemia, scarlet fever, ivy poisoning, spider bites, and **ulcers**. The dried roots and rhizome of the coneflower were official in the National Formulary (NF), from 1916-1950.

Recent Scientific Findings

This plant of the western plains will serve mankind well into the future, based on recent scientific documentation of its immune-enhancing effects. Current pharmacology indicates Echinacea is **antitumor, anti-viral**, and an **immunostimulant**. It also is effective against **herpes** and **influenza**, is used for **wound healing**, has been proven to activate reticulo-endothelial layer to increase alpha, beta, and gamma globulin (which is the formation of antibodies), and to increase the rate of phagocytosis.

In the 1960's reports from Eastern Europe were published on the plant's **immunostimulant** activity. A polysaccharide fraction increased the rate of phagocytosis. An aqueous extract used internally was found to activate reticulo endothelium to increase alpha, beta and gamma globulin, and promote the formation of antibodies.

In 1972 an extract of Echinacea root was shown to possess significant antitumor activity in experiments with rats. **Antiviral activity** was reported in 1978, showing that a root extract was **effective in destroying herpes influenza viruses**. Work in the previous decade (1956) demonstrated the powerful **antibacterial** properties of coneflower. By adding an aqueous extract of the root to suspensions of penicillin, activity levels of the drugs were increased.

In Germany in the 1980's, Wagner and co-workers reported on immunologically active polysaccharides derived from tissue cultures of this beautiful plant. Other European laboratories reported the activation of human lymphocytes, increased rate of phagocytosis and macrophage activation.

An extract of Echinacea also revealed **anti-viral activity**. In extensive experiments the extract exhibited an action similar to interferon except, unlike interferon, the drug remains active even when stored at room temperature. Since interferon is difficult to obtain, Echinacea could prove to be a very important aid in **increasing immunoproduction**.

Here we have a biologically active plant, known to the Native American to possess almost magical healing properties and now proving itself worthy of acceptance as a world-class medicine.

ELDER

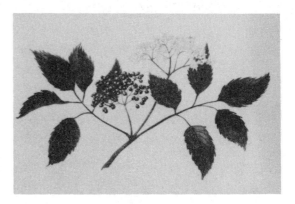

Elder

SCIENTIFIC NAME: *Sambucus canadensis, Sambuscus nigra, Sambuscus racemosa*

PARTS USED: Flowers, berries, root, and inner bark

DOSAGE:

Leaf buds: Do not use.

Berries: Fresh juice, 1 ounce, is a strong purgative.

Inner bark and root juice: Mild decoction of 1 teaspoon of plant material boiled in a covered container with 1 pint of water for only 5 minutes, cool slowly in closed container and drink cold, 1 swallow or 1 tablespoon at a time, 1 to 2 cups per day.

Dried root: 1 teaspoon of root, boiled in covered container with 1½ pints of water for about ½ hour, at a slow boil. Allow liquid to cool slowly in the *closed* container. Drink cold, 1 swallow or 1 tablespoon at a time, no more than ½ ounce dose daily.

ELDER: *Since the ancient Greeks, this plant has been utilized as a laxative.*

Traditional Usages

The medicinal properties of the Elder have been recognized since the time of the ancient Greeks. Hippocrates mentions its employment as a **purgative**. One ounce of pure juice squeezed from the berries will strongly **purge**. A tea made from the root of the Elder taken daily in half-ounce doses, performed as a **gentle laxative**. The juice from the berries was also used as a remedy for **rheumatism, gout, external skin eruptions,** and **syphilis**. The berries are also the source of the popular elderberry wine, as well as a jam.

The inner bark and the young leaf buds, as well as the juice of the root, are also considered active hydragogue cathartics, promoting the watery evacuation of the bowels. The plant was therefore used to treat dropsical affections. The inner bark was considered **emetic** in strong doses. **The young leaf buds are so violent in their purgative action that they are considered unsafe.**

American Elder was widely utilized by various Native Americans tribes. The Menominees used the dried flowers in a tea to **reduce fevers**. The Meskwakis made a tea from the root bark for the **expulsion of phlegm, to treat headache, and to encourage labor.** The Houmas employed the **boiled bark in a wash for inflammations.**

Probably due to this wide usage, Elder became an important ingredient in the home remedies of whites. The flowers were utilized in the form of poultices, fomentations, and ointments for topical application to lesions, tumors, and rheumatic limbs. They were considered gently excitant and sudorific, although they were rarely taken internally.

Elderberries were listed in the *U.S. Pharmacopoeia* from 1820 to 1831, while Elder flowers were listed from 1831 to 1905 when they were used to make a flower water and as a flavoring.

Recent Scientific Findings

Though still used in some European countries as a home remedy, Elder is not used as a laxative due to the preference for other agents. The plant contains glycosides; the exact constituent that causes Elder's purgative effects is unknown. When taken in moderate amounts, **Elder can be an effective purgative and laxative.** However, there are negative effects, including dizziness and even stupor. **The fresh plant is poisonous.** American Elder's toxic content is higher than the European variety. However, when cooked, the berries are harmless. Indeed, the cooked berries are a common ingredient in jams.

Caution: **See above.**

ELECAMPANE

SCIENTIFIC NAME: *Inula helenium*
PARTS USED: Root stock

DOSAGE:

> **Root:** 1 teaspoon of root, slowly boiled in a covered container of 1½ pints water for about ½ hour. Allow liquid to cool slowly in the *closed* container. Drink cold, 1 swallow or 1 tablespoon at a time, 1 to 2 cups per day.

ELECAMPANE: *A folk medicine for thousands of years, modern research supports this plant's usefulness as an expectorant.*

Traditional Usages

Elecampane has been used in folk medicine for thousands of years. The species name *helenium* comes from Helen of Troy, who supposedly was carrying the plant when abducted by Paris. Well known to the ancient Greeks, Elecampane was valued for its ability to promote **menstruation**, as a tonic and gentle **stimulant**, and as a means of promoting perspiration, particularly to **relieve the common cold.** Hippocrates maintained that Elecampane stimulated the uterus, kidneys, stomach, and brain. Elecampane may also be the *Helenium folis verbasci* employed by Dioscorides and Pliny's *Inula.*

At one time, Elecampane was widely used in English medicine as a **diuretic** and to induce profuse sweating, but later fell into disuse. In France, Elecampane was one of the ingredients of absinthe. The root was also used as an expectorant; it was valued when lung ailments were accompanied by gastric complaints, since it was the one medicine applicable for both conditions.

Official in the *U.S. Pharmacopoeia,* the dried root was employed in **"affections of the respiratory organs,"** skin diseases, **and digestive and liver disorders.** A 1936 textbook on plant drugs states that Elecampane is a stimulant that promotes the expulsion of phlegm (**expectorant**), induces sweating (**diaphoretic**), and promotes the excretion of urine (**diuretic**). Externally it was employed for a variety of skin eruptions. After its use in human medicine declined, Elecampane remained popular in veterinary practice.

Recent Scientific Findings

Evidence supports the traditional claims that Elecampane is a **very useful remedy** for **coughs** and **colds** in bronchial tubes and lungs. It assists in loosening phlegm and relieves irritation in the air passages. The rhizomes and roots contain several sesquiterpene lactones, which have varying degrees of antiseptic properties. They are also all bitter substances, and thus produce a tonic effect if extracts are taken orally.

Clinical experiments indicate an extract is a powerful **antiseptic** and **bactericide,** which is **particularly effective against the organism that causes tuberculosis.** Other experiments suggest Elecampane possesses **antibacterial** activity against several pathogens and **antiyeast** activity against *Candida albicans.* **Anti-ulcer** activity has been observed in adult humans.

Caution: Overdose may cause dizziness, nausea, vertigo, and abdominal pain. External contact may cause contact dermatitis or allergy in humans.

EPHEDRA

or

"Ma-Huang"

SCIENTIFIC NAME: *Ephedra,* various
species
PARTS USED: Branches

DOSAGE:

Herb: Approximately ½ ounce of herb to 1 pint of water. Boil water separately and pour over the plant material and steep for 5 to 20 minutes, depending on the desired effect. Drink hot or warm, 1 cup per day upon awakening

EPHEDRA: *Used in Chinese medicine for over 5,000 years, modern medicine continues to find beneficial both synthesized compounds and the natural herb.*

Traditional Usages

The genus *Ephedra,* of which there are approximately 40 species all over the world, may be one of the most effective of all plants used to treat allergy. The plant's yellow color and its numbing of the tongue led the Chinese to name it *Ma-Huang.* Ephedra has been in use in Chinese medicine as a crude drug for over five thousand years. It was recommended by herbalists as a **bronchodilator**, especially for conditions such as bronchial asthma (but *not* as a "simple nonspecific bronchodilator"). In China it has also been employed to **relieve cough** and reduce fevers, and even allergic skin reactions. **Widely utilized for pain or inflammatory conditions**, the herb was never given alone but always in combination with other herbs. Topically, Ephedra has been used as an **eyewash**.

Recent Scientific Findings

The interest in Oriental herbal medicine is most readily traced to the story of ephedrine from the Ephedra Herb. During his investigation of the pharmacological mechanisms of herbal medicines, N. Nagamine isolated the alkaloid ephedrine from the herb Ephedra, in 1885. Three years later Takahasi and Miura discovered the mydriatic action (i.e., it dilates the pupil) of this chemical extract. At the University of California, San Francisco, School of Medicine, in 1924, Chen and Schmidt demonstrated that ephedrine had **powerful bronchodilatory activity**. Finally, in 1927 ephedrine was synthesized and rapidly accepted by western physicians as a new pharmacologic agent. Both ephedrine and pseudo-ephedrine (ex: Sudafed™) are still widely utilized for their **anti-asthmatic**, and **anti-allergic** properties.

Modern research has tried to elucidate the varied actions of "Ephedrae Herba," but its complete profile is still undefined. Many compounds are found in this genus, most notably ephedrine and pseudo-ephedrine. The Ephedras contain 0.5-20% alkaloids with most Ephedra species containing the alkaloid ephedrine in all parts of the plant. Ephedrine may account for 30-90% of this alkaloid content. Some plants also contain pseudoephedrine, which is an isomer of ephedrine. Pseudoephedrine and ephedrine may be naturally derived or produced synthetically. Ephedrine and pseudo-ephedrine are **potent sympathomimetics**, which means they excite the sympathetic nervous system causing the vaso-constriction of the nasal mucosa, dilation of the bronchioles, as well as cardiac stimulation.

Other compounds found in Ephedra include phenylaline, ascorbic acid, catechin, cinnamic acid, quercetin, leucodelphinidin, quercitin, rutin, tannic acid, tannin, and terpinen-4-oL. All of these compounds exhibit **anti-inflammatory** or **antiallergic** activity.

Ephedrine produces many effects when taken orally by humans, the most important being dilation of the lung bronchioles and increase in blood pressure. Ephedrine is employed as a **vasoconstrictor** and **cardiac stimulant** and as a **bronchodilator** in the treatment of **hayfever, asthma**, and **emphysema**. It should be noted that the effects of either alkaloid last a few hours and that side effects may appear, including nervousness, insomnia, and vertigo.

We have all heard of pseudoephedrine because it is often in over-the-counter (OTC) products. Some confusion surrounds this alkaloid; people are unsure if it is made in the laboratory or extracted from Ephedra. Both may be so! Pseudoephedrine may have certain advantages. Compared to ephedrine, it causes fewer heart symptoms such as palpitation, but is equally effective as a bronchodilator.

This is but one example of the transition of a "folk-remedy" into the annals of world medicine. There are dozens of other current prescription and over-the-counter drug preparations that owe their existence to the tireless efforts of a succession of investigators, but all leading to their original usage as herbal treatments.

The story is simple enough, but subtle clinical twists explain why the herbs themselves are still used today, *not* having been rendered obsolete by their modern, synthesized cousin compounds. If ephedrine produced all the effects associated with Ephedrae Herba, then Ephedrae Herba would have fallen out of use; however, this has not happened. These natural substances produce effects similar to epinephrine (adrenaline), but are, of course, *less* stimulating to the central nervous system than amphetamine. This is why Ephedra is such a useful plant. It is extremely effective without being too strong in its actions, when properly utilized.

Ephedra has also been found to **promote weight loss** due to its **thermogenic** and **fat-metabolizing effect**. Ephedrine also exhibits **anorectic properties** (reducing the desire for food). The alkaloid is thought to activate both alpha and beta adrenoceptors, which elevate metabolic rate, increase calorie expenditure and result in weight loss. When combined with caffeine, a synergism results, yielding a greater increase in metabolic rate than ephedrine or caffeine alone. For those interested in increased energy, endurance, alertness, and weight loss, this ancient remedy from China may hold a key.

> **WARNING:** Do not use if you have high blood pressure, heart or thyroid disease, diabetes, or if you are specifically taking an MAO inhibitor or *any* prescription drug. Do not use if you are pregnant or nursing. Not for children under 18. Do not take after 4:00 p.m., as this herb may cause sleeplessness.

ERGOT

SCIENTIFIC NAME: *Claviceps purpurea*
PARTS USED: Sclerotium of fungus

DOSAGE:
> *Caution: Only prepared pharmaceutical preparations are advised.* Avoid self-medication.

ERGOT: *This fungus has long been used by midwives to promote contractions during birth.*

Traditional Usages

In all the grass family, the place of the grains or fruits is sometimes occupied by a morbid growth that due to its resemblance to the spur of a cock received the name Ergot (adapted from the French). This product is most frequent in the rye, *Secale cereale*, and from that grain it was adopted in the first edition of the *U.S. Pharmacopoeia* under the name of *Secale cornutum*, or Spurred Rye.

In the Middle Ages epidemics of ergotism from eating contaminated rye flour were characterized by both gangrenous and convulsive symptoms. Ergot's principal uses were as a **uterine stimulant** and a vasoconstrictor.

It was long **used by midwives to promote contraction of the uterus during labor**, particularly at the end of the second stage, as well as to **speed childbirth** and **prevent possible postpartum hemorrhage**. Ergot was **also utilized in the nonpregnant uterus to check excessive menstrual bleeding** or other uterine hemorrhaging. A common belief was that Ergot extracts when taken orally are useful to induce abortion.

Additionally, Ergot alkaloids have important applications in the treatment of **migraine**. This medicinal fungus stimulates other involuntary muscle fibers, including the heart and the arteries.

Recent Scientific Findings

Investigation has revealed that Ergot is not the diseased grain of rye, but the sclerotium of a fungus, the *Clavices purpurea*. This fungus has three stages in its life history.

This sclerotium of Ergot contains a number of complex and potent alkaloids, some of which have the lysergic acid (LSD-like) basic skeleton. There are two major indole alkaloids. The first, ergonovine, acts primarily to contract uterine muscle and to constrict blood vessels of the endometrium of the uterus. The second, Ergotamine, acts primarily on the blood vessels of the brain, with minimal effects indicated here for ergonovine. **This explains why Ergot (or ergonovine) has been an indispensable drug for centuries in obstetrics.** It initiates contractions of the pregnant uterus, primarily at the time of delivery, and is **used to aid difficult deliveries.** Of great importance is the fact that Ergot constricts blood vessels of the endometrium, and prevents the hemorrhaging that often accompanies childbirth.

There is no evidence that supports the belief Ergot induces abortion, since Ergot only acts in the terminal stages of pregnancy, when abortion is not desired. Thus **Ergot preparations do not usually induce abortion**, but are extremely useful to aid in term delivery of the fetus, to expel the placenta, and to prevent hemorrhage after delivery. Maximum labor-induction effect is attained only by injection of Ergot extract or ergonovine.

The other useful alkaloid of Ergot, ergotamine, is used extensively to relieve the symptoms of **migraine headaches.** Ergot itself is not utilized for this purpose, because of the predominant effects of this drug in the crude form on the uterus.

It must be pointed out that **regular use of Ergot preparations must be avoided,** since the blood vessels of the extremities, i.e., fingers and toes, will be constricted. This constriction restricts the blood supply to the extremities, and the end result is gangrene.

As with any drug plant, when used properly and in the correct amount, its virtues are an asset. When misused, the attributes are changed to the detriment of the health and well-being of the user.

EUCALYPTUS

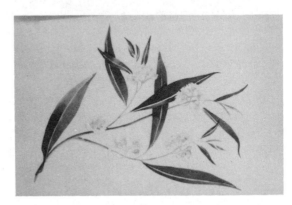

Eucalyptus

SCIENTIFIC NAME: *Eucalyptus globulus*
PARTS USED: Leaves, also oil distilled therefrom

DOSAGE:

Leaves: 0.65-2 grams of the leaves to 1 pint of water. Boil water separately and pour over the plant material and steep 5-20 minutes, depending on the desired effect. Drink hot or warm, 1 to 2 cups per day. The oil may be used in the amount of 0.3-0.6 milliliter in water.

EUCALYPTUS: *The essential oil of the leaves of this tree is an effective expectorant.*

Traditional Usages

Eucalyptus was commonly used to treat respiratory ailments. The leaves were **smoked for relief of bronchitis** and asthma. A mixture of a few drops of the oil to a gallon of water was boiled and the steam inhaled as a stimulating expectorant to treat **chronic bronchitis** and **tuberculosis** as well as **asthma**.

The volatile oil, distilled from the leaves has also been used as a **germicide** and has been applied locally as an **antiseptic**; in this connection it has been employed to treat both skin diseases and upper respiratory infections.

Eucalyptus oil was sometimes utilized as a substitute for quinine in the treatment of malaria and other intermittent fevers. The leaves have a characteristic aromatic odor that is due to an essential oil made up almost entirely of a monoterpene compound known as eucalyptol.

Recent Scientific Findings

Human and animal testing has shown that Eucalyptus essential oil and eucalyptol both dilate the bronchioles in the lungs, and have **antiseptic** effects against a variety of microorganisms. Experiments have also shown that Eucalyptus preparations have stimulating expectorant properties.

A combination of Eucalyptus and Peppermint has shown promise as an external application for **pain relief** in a 1991 study. The researchers concluded that the application "may be beneficial for pain relief and/or useful to athletes."

EYEBRIGHT

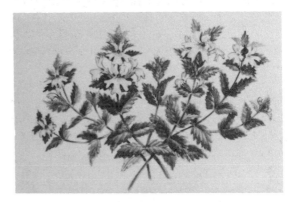

Eyebright

SCIENTIFIC NAME: *Euphrasia officinalis*
PARTS USED: Herb

DOSAGE:

Herb: Approximately ½ ounce of herb to 1 pint of water. Boil water separately and pour over the plant material and steep 5-20 minutes, depending on the desired effect. Drink hot of warm, 1 to 2 cups per day, at bedtime and upon awakening. As an eyewash (when cool) its action is healing and strengthening one part of the herb to 6 parts of water).

EYEBRIGHT: *For centuries, this herb has been an eye treatment.*

Traditional Usages

Eyebright is a very old and revered folk medicine for **eye troubles**. It was first mentioned as a medicinal plant in a 1305 herbal. The powers of Eyebright, or Euphrasy as it was also commonly called, are even recorded by the poet Milton:

Michael from Adam's eye the
film removed,
Which the false fruit, that
promised clearer sight,
Had bred; then purged with
"euphrasy" and rue
The visual nerve, for he had
much to see.
— *Paradise Lost*, Book XI, line 412

Shenstone exclaims:

Famed *euphrasy* may not be left
unsung,
That gives dim eyes to wander
leagues around.

Eyebright had the reputation of being able to **restore sight** to persons over seventy years of age. It was also used to treat **cataracts, inflammation,** and **irritation.** In Iceland, the expressed juice of the plant was employed to treat a variety of eye complaints. The Scottish Highlanders mixed the juice with milk and used a feather to apply the lotion to the eyes. The herb also was occasionally employed to treat jaundice, loss of memory, and vertigo.

Recent Scientific Findings

When given internally, Eyebright's mechanism of action is not yet known. **Externally, compresses relieve conjunctivitis and blepharitis along with other eye inflammations.** A mixture of Eyebright along with Fennel, Chamomile, and walnut leaf is a useful application for scrofulous eye conditions in children.

FALSE UNICORN (HELONIAS ROOT)

SCIENTIFIC NAME: *Chamaelirium luteum*
PARTS USED: Rhizome

DOSAGE:

Rhizome: Boil 1 teaspoon of plant material in a covered container of 1½ pints water for about ½ hour, at a slow boil. Allow liquid to cool slowly in the *closed* container. Drink cold, 1 swallow or 1 tablespoon at a time, 1 to 2 cups per day.

FALSE UNICORN: *Also named Devil's Bit, this was at one time a popular liver remedy.*

Traditional Usages

It was sometimes called Devil's Bit because certain Native American tribes considered this root a cure-all. The name came from the belief that the root's healing properties angered a bad spirit who bit off a portion of the root to prevent its use.

False Unicorn was considered a **diuretic** and **emetic,** and was used for **colic, worms,** and **fevers.** The root was also chewed as a **cough remedy.** In the 19th century domestic American medicine it was considered an **effective liver remedy.**

The rhizome was used in cases of **infertility** and **menstrual irregularities**.

Recent Scientific Findings

Current pharmacology indicates that the steroidal saponins have **adaptogenic effect on ovaries (normalizing function)**.

FENNEL

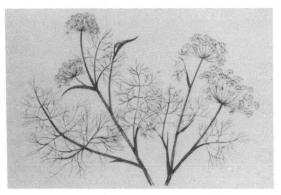

Fennel

SCIENTIFIC NAME: *Foeniculum vulgare*
PARTS USED: Seeds

DOSAGE:

    Seeds: In its fresh state, the drug is too irritant. A decoction is prepared, using ½ ounce of crushed dried plant material (at least 1 year old) to 1 pint of water, boiled in a covered container for about ½ hour, at a slow boil. Allow liquid to cool slowly in the *closed* container. Drink cold, 1 swallow or 1 tablespoon at a time, 1 to 2 cups per day.

FENNEL: *This popular food flavoring also soothes gastrointestinal upsets.*

Traditional Usages

The ancient physicians Hippocrates and Dioscorides employed Fennel to **increase milk secretion in nursing** mothers. On the basis of the old observation that when they shed their skins serpents eat Fennel to restore their sight, Pliny recommended it for **visual problems**, including blindness.

The gum-resin from the cut stems was applied topically to **indolent tumors** and **chronic swellings**. The juice expressed from the root was considered a **diuretic** and was given for intermittent fever. Externally, Fennel was a popular remedy for **toothache** and **earache**.

The main applications of the plant were as an **aromatic, stimulant**, and **carminative**, and especially to **prevent colic in infants**. It is often combined with Senna or Rhubarb to make these stronger-tasting medicinals more palatable as well as more tolerable to the upset gastrointestinal tract. An infusion of Fennel seeds was administered as an enema to infants to aid expulsion of flatus. Fennel remained an important element of veterinary medicine long after its use in human ailments declined.

The entire plant has a fragrant, aromatic odor; it has been widely employed in foods, both for flavoring and as a vegetable, both raw and cooked. Fennel is used to flavor absinthe and other liquors.

Recent Scientific Findings

Oil of Fennel is known to contain 50 to 60 percent anethole, and 20 percent fenchose, chavicol, and anisic aldehyde. It is **soothing for gastrointestinal upsets** as well as being an **appetite stimulant**. One experiment on adult humans found a kidney stone dissolution effect.

Other studies have observed **antimutagenic** activity in bacteria as well as **antifungal** activity against *Aspergillus* and Trichophytum in cell culture studies. **Antibacterial** activity in vitro against several human pathogens has been observed. Fennel exhibited **anti-yeast** activity against *Candida albicans,* and **anti-inflammatory** activity in humans and rats. The fruit has been shown to be effective as an **insect repellent**.

In an animal study, a boiled water extract of Fennel leaves produced a significant dose-related **reduction in arterial blood pressure**. Heart and respiratory rates were not effected. Interestingly, a non-boiled extract showed no effect.

FENUGREEK

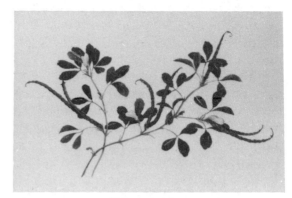

Fenugreek

SCIENTIFIC NAME: *Trigonella foenumgraecum*

PARTS USED: Seed

DOSAGE:

Seeds: Place 2 teaspoon seeds per 1 cup of water and let stand for 5 hours. Boil for 1 minute. 2 to 3 cups per day.

FENUGREEK: *Used by the ancient Egyptians and Greeks, the seeds have been found to reduce blood glucose in diabetics.*

Traditional Usages

The ancient Egyptians and Greeks both used Fenugreek for respiratory problems. It was also considered a restorative and so given to people recovering from a variety of illnesses.

In traditional Chinese medicine, Fenugreek's recorded use dates back a thousand years. The dried seeds are used to treat the **kidney** meridian. The bitter seeds are dried and given for **hernia, beriberi, abdominal pains,** and **impotence**.

Fenugreek has also been utilized as an **anti-inflammatory** agent and as a muciliganous poultice. In some societies, it was believed to be an **aphrodisiac**.

Recent Scientific Findings

Fenugreek is rich in steroid saponins, especially diosgenin. French researchers found that Fenugreek **reduced blood glucose and plasma cholesterol levels** in diabetic dogs.

Human experiments confirmed the animal research. Defatted Fenugreek seed powder was added to the diet of **diabetic patients** and served with both lunch and dinner. This **resulted in a 54% percent reduction in urinary glucose**. Blood sugar levels decreased. **Cholesterol was also significantly reduced**.

Another study with non-insulin dependent diabetics produced similar results. Powdered Fenugreek seed soaked in water significantly reduced glucose levels and lowered plasma insulin. These studies indicate that **Fenugreek may be beneficial in the treatment of diabetes**.

FEVERFEW

SCIENTIFIC NAME: *Tanacetum parthenium, or Chrysanthemum parthenium*

PARTS USED: Herb

DOSAGE:

Flowering tops: Approximately ½ ounce of flowering tops of whole herb to 1 pint of water. Boil water separately and pour over the plant material and steep for 5 to 20 minutes, depending on the desired effect. Drink hot or warm, 1 to 2 cups per day, at bedtime and upon waking.

FEVERFEW: *In use since the time of the ancient Greeks, this aptly named herb has been found to eliminate migraine headaches.*

Traditional Usages

This plant's action against **fevers** earned it its name. Physicians dating back to Dioscorides have considered Feverfew to be especially valuable for its action on the **uterus**. It was employed to stimulate menstruation and in childbirth to aid expulsion of placenta after birth. Herbalist John Parkinson in 1629 wrote "It is chiefly used for the diseases of the mother, whether it be the rising of the mother, or the hardness or inflammations of the same."

However, it is a remedy for **headaches** that Feverfew is most noted. Gerard wrote

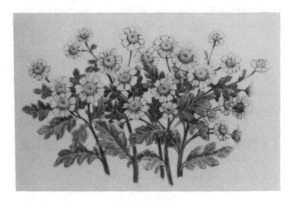

Feverfew

in 1633 that Feverfew is "very good for them that are giddie in the head." Echoing that endorsement in 1772, John Hill declared that "in the worst headache this herb exceeds whatever else is known."

Other uses were as an antispasmodic, stomachic, diuretic, and rheumatism. A Cuban variety of the plant was used by local practitioners as a febrifuge and antiperiodic to treat intermittent fevers; an American variety was used in the southwest United States as a tonic and antiperiodic.

Feverfew smells, tastes, and looks like Roman Chamomile (Anthemis nobilis). In France the two plants were at one time used interchangeably. This perennial herb is sometimes added for its flavor in wine making and certain pastries.

Recent Scientific Findings

At my herbal seminars people often ask if Feverfew (*Tanacetum parthenium*) is as effective for treating *regular* headaches as it is for its accepted use in the treatment of *migraine* headaches.

A 1988 study may help us to

understand **why feverfew "works" only for migraine headaches.** The researchers reported that crude extracts of the plant both inhibit platelet aggregation and also inhibit secretory activity in platelets, most cells, and PMN's (polymorphonuclear leucocytes). They speculate that such activities are relevant to the plant's medicinal properties.

Feverfew contains the sesquiterpene lactones (parthenolide and parthenolide-like compounds). These compounds bring about the anti-clotting effects of extracts. Blood platelets are so affected because the cellular sulphydryl groups they contain are "neutralized" by this herb. Feverfew extracts also slow the spread of platelets and the formation of clot-like substances on collagen. In a series of novel experiments the authors demonstrated that extracts of this plant protected the endothelial layer of rabbit aorta from laboratory induced injury (i.e., perfusion with a salt solution).

As for headaches, it is interesting to note that by inhibiting the secretion of histamines from mast cells, migraine type pain is controlled or eliminated. In conclusion, Voyno-Yasenetskaya and colleagues reconfirmed **"feverfew being of value as an antithrombotic agent as well as being of value in migraine and arthritis."**

The renewed used of Feverfew to treat migraines came about not by laboratory research but because of a woman in England. For years she had suffered from severe migraines. On the advice of a friend's father, the woman began eating Feverfew leaves. Gradually the headaches disappeared. The woman became convinced of Feverfew's healing properties and passed on her experience to other migraine sufferers. Finally,

the media paid attention, which led to the involvement of Dr. Stewart Johnson of King's College. Overcoming his initial skepticism, over eight years of research, Dr. Johnson also became convinced.

During the course of his investigation, Johnson conducted a double-blind study with 20 patients who had a history of suffering from migraine. All the subjects ate the leaves for at least three months prior to the study. However, once the study began, the placebo group underwent a "significant increase in the frequency of headache, nausea, and vomiting." The Feverfew group showed no change in severity or frequency of migraine.

Subsequent research by other investigators has confirmed Feverfew's efficacy in treating migraine. In 1988 a randomized, double-blind, placebo controlled study with 72 human volunteers was carried out over an eight month period. The researchers found Feverfew significantly reduced migraine attacks.

FLAX

SCIENTIFIC NAME: *Linnum usitatissimum*
PARTS USED: Seeds

DOSAGE:

Seeds: Infusion of seeds—½ ounce of seeds to 1 pint of water. Boil water separately and pour over the seeds and steep for 5 to 20 minutes. Drink hot or warm, 1 to 2 cups per day. As a laxative, 1 tablespoon of the seeds is taken orally.

FLAX: *For centuries, the seeds have provided a soothing mucilage.*

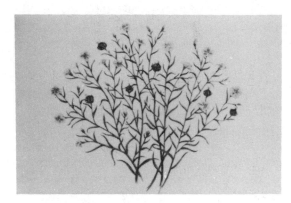

Flax

Traditional Usages

It is estimated that Flax has been grown as a fiber crop for weaving into fabric since the 23rd century B.C. Medicinally, the seeds are a valuable demulcent and emollient, with soothing qualities both internally for coughs and externally for skin irritations. The soothing mucilage is obtained by infusing the seeds in water. This infusion is valuable in treating irritations and inflammations of the mucous membranes, particularly of the **lungs, intestines,** and **urinary passages**; it has therefore been used for **pulmonary catarrhs, dysentery, diarrhea, urinary infections, kidney diseases,** and **urinary stones.** A **laxative enema** is derived from the decoction.

The meal from the pressed seeds mixed with hot water makes an excellent emollient poultice. **Linseed** oil, expressed from the seeds, also **has emollient properties and is applied externally for burns and scalds,** mixed with lime water or oil or turpentine; this treatment is said to reduce the pain considerably and prevent undue blistering.

Recent Scientific Findings

Flax seeds have a thick outer coating of mucilage cells. When water comes in contact with these cells they swell and give rise to a **soothing demulcent** and/or **emollient protective effect.** When the skin or mucous membranes are coated with this mucilage, this effect becomes evident.

The seeds also contain a high concentration of fixed oil, which explains the **laxative** effect when taken internally.

FO-TI
(HO SHOU WU)

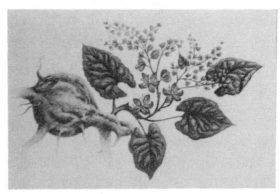

Fo-ti

SCIENTIFIC NAME: *Polygonum multiflorum*

PARTS USED: Root

DOSAGE:

Root: 1 teaspoon of root, boiled in a covered container of 1½ pints water for about ½ hour, at a slow boil. Allow liquid to cool slowly in the *closed* container. Drink cold, 1 swallow or 1 tablespoon at a time, 1 to 2 cups per day.

FO-TI: *Second only to Ginseng in traditional Chinese medicine, this plant has shown positive results in eliminating the symptoms of heart disease.*

Traditional Usages

Fo-Ti is **one of China's main herbal tonics,** second only to Ginseng in reputed benefits. Its use was first recorded in a herbal written in 973 A.D. It is a key herbal remedy for the elderly. Said to nourish yin, Fo-Ti is utilized to **"replenish sperm," reverse hair graying,** and for "pain in the knees and loins." In other words, all the sins that aging flesh is heir to!

The Chinese name, *Ho-shou-wu,* has a colorful history. According to legend, *Ho-shou-wu* was the grandson of a man who at age 58 had been unable to father a child. A monk advised him to eat the *chiao-teng* he gathered on the mountain. He then fathered several children. His hair turned from gray to black and his body became more youthful. He lived to the age of 160, still with black hair, while his child lived to be 130. From that time on, Fo-Ti has been used to strengthen the body and to nourish vital essence.

In Ayurvedic medicine, Fo-Ti is utilized as a remedy for **colic** and **enteritis,** while in Brazil it is employed for **gout** and **hemorrhoids.**

Recent Scientific Findings

Chemically, this species of *polygonum* contains phospholipids, anthraquinones and bianthraquinonyl glucosides. The principle actions of the major constituents are **purgative, cholesterol lowering, anti-inflammatory, cardiotonic,** and **antiviral.** These effects are thought to be owing to the plant's leucoanthocyanidins (LAC) (NAS).

In human studies, Fo-Ti has **reduced hypertension, cholesterol levels, and the incidence of heart disease among those prone to the condition.** A 1991 study found that emodin, one of Fo-Ti's active principles, served as an **effective immunosuppressive agent** in human cells. The authors speculate that emodin may be **useful against transplantation rejection and autoimmune disease.**

In what appears to be an attempt to *discredit* Chinese herbal remedies, an investigator at the University of California, Berkeley, published an article in 1981 which instead exonerated Fo-ti. Calling the article "Mutagenic Activity of Ho Shou Wu (*Polygonum Multiflorum*)," I had to read this brief entry three times to realize that the title held the opposite meaning of the findings. The author subjected this herb to the by now infamous "Ames-test" and discovered "that the herb is not mutagenic," and that ". . . a positive dose-response relationship did not exist." Instead of stating this at the outset, the author saved this for the end, even adding the caveat, "Oxidation and pyrolytic products could be created during the long simmering process. Especially when other herbs are present, molecular recombination and alteration of functional groups may occur." Unable to nail this herb to the cross of scientific bias, he concludes, "pinpointing herbs with mutagenic potential awaits further investigation." Amen!

FOXGLOVE

SCIENTIFIC NAME: *Digitalis purpurea*
PARTS USED: Leaves

DOSAGE:

Digitalis preparations are very powerful medicines, and should only be used cautiously, under proper medical supervision. An overdose could be fatal.

FOXGLOVE: *The leaves of this plant are the source of the well-known heart medicine digitalis.*

Traditional Usages

Probably the best example of a herbal remedy that eventually became an indispensable drug to the medical profession are the leaves of Foxglove (*D. purpurea*). The point of departure was that Foxglove was being used by a Welsh woman as one of several plants in a tea for the treatment of **dropsy.** (Dropsy is a symptom of a poorly operating heart, with a resulting accumulation of fluid in the body, particularly in the legs and ankles.) The English botanist Dr. William Withering observed this use in 1775. Through experimentation he found that the major plant in the mixture responsible for this effect was *Digitalis purpurea* leaves. Withering then used an infusion of the leaves of this plant in his medical practice for the treatment of dropsy. For over a decade Withering recorded his clinical observations and so established guidelines for use of the drug.

Prior to the discovery of its cardiac applications in 1775, Foxglove was utilized as an expectorant, in **epilepsy**, and to reduce glandular swellings. The juice obtained by bruising the leaves was mixed with honey and drunk to purge the gastrointestinal tract in both directions. Culpepper recommended that Foxglove be used to treat obstructions of the liver and spleen, as well as externally for scabies. The plant was **used externally in Italy to heal wounds and reduce swellings**.

Recent Scientific Findings

Digitalis, the active principle of Foxglove, came to be employed as a **stimulant in acute circulatory** failure, as a **diuretic**, and as a **cardiac tonic in chronic heart disorders.**

Both powdered Foxglove leaves and digitalis are currently widely used for the treatment of **congestive heart failure.** A symptom of overdose is vomiting, but when taken in proper amounts Foxglove causes the heart to beat slower and stronger, which then causes fluids to be excreted from the body more efficiently, resulting in a **secondary diuretic effect.**

The **cardiotonic and diuretic effects of digitalis** make Foxglove very useful in cases of dropsy associated with heart disease. The drug reduces the force and velocity of the circulation and helps to **regulate irregular heartbeats.** In recent years, some cardiologists have curtailed use of digitalis except for specific heart rate conditions.

GARLIC

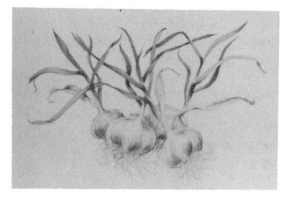

Garlic

SCIENTIFIC NAME: *Allium sativum*
PARTS USED: Cloves

DOSAGE:
    1/2 teaspoon of the juice 3 times daily

GARLIC: *This commonly used plant may help prevent cancer.*

Traditional Usages

The Egyptians employed Garlic to give strength and nourishment to the slaves constructing the pyramids. The Romans also gave Garlic to their laborers, while Roman soldiers believed that Garlic inspired courage and dedicated the plant to Mars, the god of war.

In the Middle Ages, Garlic was used to ward off demons and the evil eye. Because of the belief that evil spirits caused diseases, Garlic was held to have magical powers.

Garlic also has been utilized for thousands of years as a **cancer treatment.** Hippocrates wrote about a steam fumigation of Garlic to treat cancer of the uterus. Similar usage against various forms of cancers are recorded in ancient Egypt, Greece, Rome, India, Russia, Europe and China. Pliny wrote that Garlic was a useful remedy for a variety of conditions including ulcers, asthma, and rheumatism.

In Japan, Garlic has been a folk medicine for centuries, most commonly for various gastrointestinal ailments.

Recent Scientific Findings

As knowledge about the benefits of Garlic continues to spread from folklore into mainstream medicine, numerous claims are being made regarding various Garlic products. Before looking at some of these claims we should summarize the health significance of Garlic and Garlic constituents.

One of the world's leading authorities on this subject is Dr. Eric Block, a professor of chemistry at the State University of New York at Albany. His review article published in *Scientific American* (Volume 252, pp. 114-119, 1985) remains an important summary of the chemistry of this fascinating plant.

To summarize, here are some of the claimed nutritional and pharmacological properties of Garlic:

1. **Lowers** serum total and low density lipoprotein cholesterol in humans.

2. **Raises** high density lipoprotein cholesterol (HDL's), in humans.

3. **Reduces** the tendency of blood to clot, and the aggregation (i.e. clumping) of blood platelets.

4. **Inhibits** inflammation by modulating the conversion of arachidonic acid (A.A.) to eicosanids.

5. **Inhibits** cancer cell formation and proliferation by inhibiting nitrosamine formation, modulating the metabolism of polyarene carcinogens, and acting on cell enzymes which control cell division.

6. **Protects** the liver from damage induced by synthetic drugs and chemical pollutants.

7. **Kills** intestinal parasites and worms, as well as gram-negative bacteria.

8. **Protects** against the effects of radiation.

9. **Offers** anti-oxidant protection to cell membranes.

Some of these health effects are worth looking at in more detail.Perhaps most significant is the effect of Garlic and onion and their extracts on the lipid profile of blood and tissues. They **lower cholesterol, triglycerides and LDL cholesterol levels while also increasing the beneficial cholesterol, HDL.**

Both Garlic and onion oils inhibit the enzymes lipoxygenase and cyclooxygenase. Each of these enzymes is known to act on one of two parallel biochemical pathways (within the arachidonic acid cascade) and only by inhibiting these enzymes can this pathway be arrested. When arrested, the production of prostaglandin is slowed. Since many cancers are prostaglandin dependent, this may explain why the *allium* oils have **antitumor properties.**

Garlic and onion contain over 75 different sulfur-containing compounds. While most of the medical benefits derived from supplementation with extracts of these plants are a result of these sulfurous compounds, recent studies show the additional presence of the bioflavonoids quercetin and cyanidin.

The cellular antioxidant Selenium is another constituent found in the *allium* vegetables and their extracts. The antitumor effects claimed for selenium may be based on its ability to replace the sulphur in the amino acid l-cystine. Leukemic white blood cells have a rapid turnover of l-cystine, a similar amino acid, and by substituting selenium for sulphur, leukemia can be suppressed, in animals.

Recent research in China demonstrated a significant inverse relationship between the incidence of stomach cancer and the intake of Garlic and related *allium* vegetables. The researchers interviewed 1131 controls and 564 patients with stomach cancer and found that people with no stomach cancer ate significantly higher amounts of *allium* vegetables (a mean intake of 19.0 kg/year) than did the cancer patients (a mean intake of 15.5 kg/year). Those people who ate less than 11.5 kg/year were more than twice as likely to develop stomach cancer than were people who ate more than 24 kg/year.

Researchers at the Garlic Research Bureau in Suffolk, England, recently found "that even small amounts of Garlic, say 3 or 4 grams, will have a pronounced effect on fibrinolytic activity . . . in doses from 25 grams (10 cloves) to 50 grams Garlic seems to be highly effective in promoting beneficial changes in blood fat composition and in platelet adhesiveness."

To understand which type of Garlic—the raw, the cooked, or the preserved—may be most beneficial, we must look at the chemical changes which occur inside a Garlic clove. Fresh whole Garlic is pharmacologically inactive. When crushed, an internal enzyme acts on *alliin,* a sulphur-containing amino acid, to produce the reactive compound known as *allicin.* Left to stand in the air or when cooked, allicin is destroyed.

While there is no final scientific agreement on the therapeutically active component of Garlic, there is a consensus that allicin is very important, both as an active component itself or as a precursor of other active components. Because it is unstable, it has been difficult to manufacture a Garlic product with significant amounts of allicin. The term "allicin potential" has been created to refer to the established standard of activity found in fresh Garlic. Obviously, fresh Garlic is highly desirable, for those who can tolerate the strong taste and aroma.

To receive Garlic's benefits without consuming cloves and cloves each day, utilize the product form. The minimum effective dosage for benefiting the cardiovascular system is one clove (3 grams of fresh or 1 gram of dried) per day. Obviously, more would increase these benefits.

To prevent the pungent odor from seeping out in the breath some manufacturers are utilizing enteric coating. This moves the breakdown of alliin and alynase from the stomach to the small intestine.

GENTIAN

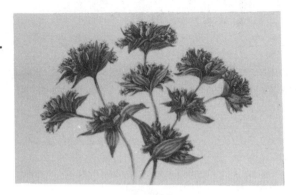

Gentian

SCIENTIFIC NAME: *Gentiana lutea*
PARTS USED: Root and rhizome

DOSAGE:

Root: Boil 1 teaspoon of powdered root in a covered container of 1½ pints of water for about ½ hour. Allow liquid to cool slowly in the *closed* container. Drink cold, 1 swallow or 1 tablespoon at a time, 1 to 2 cups per day. (To reduce the desire for cigarettes chew the root.)

GENTIAN: *Used as a medicinal by the ancient Greeks, modern German research confirms this plant's use as a digestive aid.*

Traditional Usages

Gentian is said to have derived its name from Gentius, a king of Illyria. Since ancient times it has been used medicinally. It appears in the early Greek and Arabic herbals and was known to Pliny and Dioscorides. Gentian was a common medicine during the Middle Ages.

European and American Gentian are chemically similar. The Catawbas steeped the roots of American Gentian in hot water and applied the resulting liquid on **aching backs.** European Gentian has long been utilized as a bitter **digestive tonic to stimulate gastric digestion.** From 1820 to 1955, European Gentian was official in the *U.S. Pharmacopoeia* as a **gastric stimulant.**

Gentian has also been given to treat problems arising from weakened muscular tone of the digestive organs. It is a useful **appetite stimulant for convalescing** and weak patients. It **invigorates digestion, relieves gases, and reduces excessive acid produced by faulty digestion.** At one time, Gentian was used as a remedy for intermittent (malarial) fevers, and for **gout.**

Recent Scientific Findings

Yellow Gentian contains a complex mixture of chemical substances of the xanthone, iridoid, and monoterpenoid alkaloid type. All of these are extremely bitter substances. Thus, it is clear that Gentian preparations owe their bitter tonic effect to one or more of these substances.

German scientists have been studying Gentian root for decades. Their findings confirm that Gentian is an **effective appetite stimulant** and **digestive aid.** Other experiments have found a **hair stimulant** effect in human adults, **antispasmodic** activity, and **antifungal** activity in vitro against *Aspergillus niger.*

Caution: **Overdosing may produce nausea and vomiting.** If collected in late summer or autumn, the roots must be cured prior to use.

GINGER

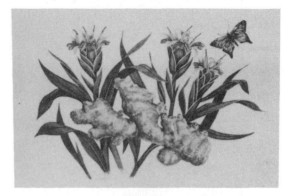

Ginger

SCIENTIFIC NAME: *Zingiber officinale*
PARTS USED: Rhizome

DOSAGE:

Root: 1 ounce of rhizome to 1 pint of water. Boil the water separately, then pour over the plant material and steep for 5 to 20 minutes, depending on the desired effect. Drink hot or warm, 1 to 2 cups per day.

GINGER: *For centuries this popular condiment has also been an effective medicinal whose properties continue to be confirmed in clinical research.*

Traditional Usages

There are more than 80 species of Ginger spread throughout tropical Asia, east to Australia and north to Japan. To encounter *Zingiber zerumbet,* or wild ginger, in full bloom in a Hawaiian rainforest and to drink the sweet juice from the stems of flower heads after a long hike, as did the ancient Hawaiians, is the stuff that dreams are made of.

This widely used condiment has a recorded history of medicinal usage in China dating from the 4th century B.C. Today, the condiment is commonly found in many Chinese food preparations, indicating well established culinary as well as medicinal uses.

It is mainly employed in **gastrointestinal upsets.** As a **stimulant** and **carminative** (removing gas from the gastrointestinal tract) it is used to treat **indigestion** and **flatulence.** Because of these properties, as well as its aromatic qualities, it is often combined with bitters to make them more palatable; Ginger adds an agreeable, warming feeling.

In Ayurveda, the traditional Indian System, Ginger is employed to **treat arthritis, pain, fever, and blood clumping**—all related to the metabolism of arachidonic acid (AA) as it affects various eicosanoids.

Recent Scientific Findings

Currently, Ginger has received new attention as an aid to **prevent nausea from motion sickness.** Ginger tea has long been an American herbal remedy for **coughs** and **asthma,** related to allergy or inflammation; the creation of the soft drink ginger ale, sprang from the common folkloric usage of this herb, and still today remains a popular beverage for the relief of stomach upset. Externally, Ginger is a rubefacient, and has been credited in this connection with **relieving headache and toothache.**

The mechanism by which Ginger produces **anti-inflammatory activity** is that of the typical NSAID (non-steroidal anti-inflammatory drug). This common spice is a more biologically active prostaglandin inhibitor (via cyclo-oxygenase inhibition) than onion and Garlic.

By slowing associated biochemical pathways an **inflammatory reaction is curtailed.** In one study, Danish women between the ages of 25 to 65 years, consumed either 70 grams raw onion or 5 grams raw ginger daily for a period of one week. The author measured thromboxane production and discovered that ginger, more clearly than onion, reduced thromboxane production by almost 60%. This confirms the Ayurvedic "prescription" for this common spice and its anti-aggregatory effects.

By reducing blood platelet "clumping," Ginger, Onion and Garlic may reduce our risk of heart attack or stroke. In a series of experiments with rats, scientists from Japan discovered that extracts of Ginger inhibited gastric lesions by up to 97%. The authors conclude that the folkloric usage of Ginger in stomachic preparations were effective owing to the constituents zingiberene, the main terpenoid and 6-gingerol, the pungent principle.

In an earlier look at how some of the active components of Ginger (and onion) act inside our cells, it was found that the oils of these herbs inhibit the fatty acid oxygenases from platelets, thus decreasing the clumping of these blood cell components.

A 1991 double-blind, randomized cross-over trial involved thirty women suffering from hyperemesis gravidarum. Ginger was alternated with a placebo.

Seventy percent of the women confirmed they subjectively preferred the period in which they took the Ginger. More objective assessment verified the subjective reactions, as significantly greater relief was found after the use of the Ginger.

In a series of experiments with rats, scientists from Japan discovered that extracts of ginger inhibited gastric lesions by up to 97%. The authors concluded that the folkloric usage of Ginger in stomachic preparations was effective due to the constituents zingiberene, the main terpenoid, and 6-gingerol, the pungent principle.

GINKGO

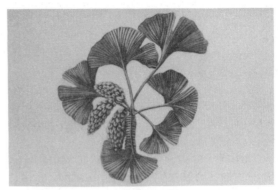

Ginkgo

SCIENTIFIC NAME: *Ginkgo biloba*
PARTS USED: Leaves

DOSAGE:

Leaves: Approximately ½ ounce of leaves to 1 pint of water. Boil water separately and pour over the plant material and steep for 5 to 20 minutes, depending on the desired effect. Drink hot or warm, 1 to 2 cups per day, at bedtime and upon wakening.

GINKGO: *For thousands of years the leaves of this ancient tree have been recognized for their benefits as a geriatric drug.*

Traditional Usages

Ginkgo, also known as maidenhair, is the oldest living tree, dating to the age of the dinosaurs. A common tree, it can live a thousand years! It has been recognized in Chinese medical practice for nearly 3,000 years. In Japan it has long been planted in temple gardens since antiquity. In 1730 the tree was introduced to Europe.

In traditional Oriental medicine, Ginkgo was used to for a variety of respiratory ailments including **asthma**. It was also employed for urinary problems.

Recent Scientific Findings

Ginkgo research has proceeded in many different areas. The most interesting and important relate to **vascular diseases, brain function, impotency, dopamine synthesis, inflammation**, and asthma.

An extract from Ginkgo leaves is marketed as Tebonin. Clinical research has shown that Tebonin achieves vasodilation and improved blood flow, especially in deeper-seated medium and small arteries. The flow rate in capillary vessels and end arteries is increased. In elderly subjects, Tebonin alleviated dizziness and loss of memory. Ginkgo has proven to be a particularly **valuable geriatric drug**.

Mild memory loss continues to be one of humankind's tragedies and one of medicine's greatest challenges. Interestingly, ginkgolides and a bilobalide possess a structure that is unique in the vegetable kingdom. A double-blind, placebo controlled study shows yet another powerful benefit from this ancient Chinese herbal medicine.

Thirty-one patients showing mild to moderate memory impairment were followed for six months while taking a standardized extract of *Ginkgo biloba* extract (GBE). (All were over the age of 50.) The extract contained 24% flavonoid glycosides and 6% terpenes. The results show that GBE "has a beneficial effect on **mental efficiency in elderly patients** showing mild to moderate memory impairment of organic origin."

Sixty patients suffering from **arterial erectile dysfunction** received a daily treatment with 60 mg. of an extract of *Ginkgo biloba*. After 6 months, 50% of the subjects once again were **able to achieve penile erections**. Upwards of 45% of the remaining subjects showed some improvement.

Another study found that *Ginkgo biloba* extract (GBE) might prevent radical **mediated human kidney and liver damage caused by Cyclosporin A, an immunosuppressive drug used in transplants.** This herbal product was found to as be as effective as vitamin E and glutathione in protecting against such damage, adding to our understanding of the value of incorporating nutritional and herbal supplements in modern medicine. The protective effects of GBE were diminished in the presence of iron, owing to the limits imposed by this powerful oxidant.

Ginkgo's effect as an **anti-allergic, anti-asthmatic** agent has also been demonstrated. The platelet activating factor (PAF) has been implicated in pathophysilogical states including allergic inflammation, anaphylactic shock, and asthma. One study concluded that Gingkolide B is the most active PAF antagonist found in this class of gingkolides. It appears that Ginkgo **relieves bronchoconstriction** due to its PAF antagonist activity. A randomized, double-blind, placebo-controlled crossover study in 8 atopic **asthmatic patients showed that Ginkgo achieved significant inhibition of the bronchial allergen challenge compared to placebo.**

GINSENG, AMERICAN

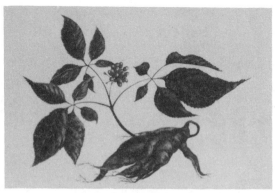

American Ginseng

SCIENTIFIC NAME: *Panax quinquefolius*
PARTS USED: Root, leaf

DOSAGE:

Powder: 1/2 teaspoon of powder to 1 cup of hot water. Drink in the morning, at lunch, at bedtime (add Lemongrass if you find the flavor wanting).

Root: Chew as desired.

Extract: 5 milliliters in 1 cup of any liquid after meals.

AMERICAN GINSENG: *Preliminary studies indicate that this North American species is quite similar in its effects to the more widely known Asian variety of this famous herb.*

Traditional Usages

A number of North American Indian tribes used Ginseng as an ingredient in love potions, reinforcing its international reputation as an **aphrodisiac**. The Meskwakis prepared a love potion consisting of Ginseng root, mica, gelatin, and snake meat. In the words of one Meskwaki, it is "a bagging agent women . . . use when they get a husband." The Pawnee made a powerful love charm by combining Ginseng with three other plants (wild columbine, cardinal flower, and carrot-leaved parsley). According to anthropologist M.R. Gilmore, when the suitor added hairs "obtained by stealth through the friendly offices of an amiably disposed third person from the head of the woman who was desired, she was unable to resist the attraction and soon yielded to the one who possessed the charm."

Many tribes used Ginseng as a normal remedy, not ascribing it the magical powers believed inherent in the plant by the Chinese, French, and English. Some Chinese viewed the plant as a panacea. The root's shape was especially important; one small piece resembling a man might bring a higher price than an entire bale. The Ginseng trade was especially brisk during the 16th century; sometimes entire Indian villages engaged in foraging for the root. In the 1790s the root sold for as high as one dollar a pound. By 1900, the commercial price was five dollars a pound. Before World War I, Ginseng was one of the chief money-making crops in America, exports in 1906 amounting to 160,949 pounds, which was then valued at $1,175,844.

A second species found is Red American "Ginseng" (*Rumex hymenosepalus*, family Polygonaceae). Native to the southwestern United States but introduced in other parts of the country, the root of this plant has been sold recently under the name of Red American Ginseng. Indeed, it has also been used as an adulterant for Ginseng. Originally utilized by the Hopi and Papago Indians to treat **colds** and **sore throats**, the plant soon found its way into early American medicine, primarily in Texas. It was employed as an **astringent for colds, loose teeth, sore throats**, and to **heal sores**.

Recent Scientific Findings

There are two species of *Panax* normally found growing in North America, only one of which is found in relative abundance, *Panax quinquefolius* (also family Araliaceae). Until recently, 90-95 percent of all *Panax quinquefolius* collected from wild-growing plants, or cultivated in the United States and Canada, was exported to the Orient. Undoubtedly, "American Ginseng" sold in the Orient was simply sold as "Ginseng," resulting in a great deal of confusion. Much of the scientific research in support of certain effects of "Ginseng" was carried out in the Orient. The evidence needed to substantiate which species was used in these experiments was never given in the scientific reports. Hence, prior to about 1965, we really cannot say whether "Ginseng" scientific studies were conducted with extracts of *Panax ginseng* (see *Ginseng, Korean White*) or *Panax quinquefolius*.

As the situation exists today, there is not a single definite report existing in the scientific literature concerning the pharmacologic testing of authentic *Panax quinquefolius*. Only preliminary studies have been carried out to identify American

Ginseng's chemical constituents, yet they seem to be quite similar to those in *Panax ginseng.* Several of the ginsenosides are common to both species. Thus, at this point, and until further studies are reported, we can only presume that the biological effect of *Panax quinquefolius* is similar to that of *Panax ginseng.*

Recent purveyors of Red American Ginseng allege effects similar to those of *Panax ginseng,* especially its supposed **aphrodisiac** properties. Needless to say, there is no evidence for any Ginseng-like activity for Red American Ginseng. The roots contain anthraquinone derivatives that would predictably result in a **laxative** effect if ingested. If you purchase a Ginseng product and the use results in loose bowel movements, it can be suspected that the product did not contain Ginseng, but rather *Rumex hymenosepalus.*

GINSENG, KOREAN

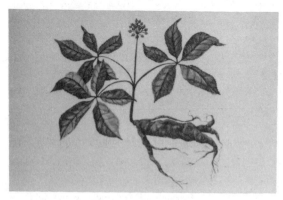

Korean Ginseng

SCIENTIFIC NAME: *Panax ginseng*
PARTS USED: Root

DOSAGE:

Powder: 1/2 teaspoon of powder to 1 cup of hot water. Drink in the morning, at lunch, at bedtime (add Lemongrass if you find the flavor wanting).

Root: Chew as desired.

Extract: 5 milliliters in 1 cup of any liquid after meals.

KOREAN GINSENG: *Long considered one of our most effective "tonics" or "adaptogens," this popular herb is now also receiving a great deal of attention as a means to enhance endurance.*

Traditional Usages

The genus name, *Panax*, is derived from the Greek goddess who "heals all," Panacea. In the Orient, Ginseng has been long revered as a tonic. It was first mentioned as a superior herb in an ancient Chinese herbal dating from 25 A.D. Chinese herb practitioners use tonics to increase overall physical strength and promote the proper functioning of the body organs. Along with being prescribed for general energy deficiency, Ginseng is used for specific ailments such as hypertension and diabetes. Ginseng is viewed as a herb that heals the spirit as well as the body.

Recent Scientific Findings

Currently, there are three major types of Ginseng available in North America. Since the names of these are often confusing, the situation needs to be clarified. Confusion results when manufacturers of Ginseng products do not clearly indicate on the label the exact Latin name for the product being sold. The name Ginseng on a bottle tells us very little about the content. One often finds labels such as Manchurian Ginseng, Swiss Ginseng, Korean Ginseng, Oriental Ginseng, and the like, with no further elaboration. Indeed, we have examined a large number of these products and find that they contain neither *Eleutherococcus senticosus,* (see *Ginseng, Siberian*) nor any of the common *Panax* species. According to a test of Ginseng products selected at random, the West German Government's State Product Test Institution reported that 25% of all Ginseng products contained little or no active ingredients.

One should presume any mention of "Ginseng" prior to about 1965, relative to human use, means *Panax ginseng* (family Araliaceae). This species is primarily found in the Orient, and it does not grow naturally in North America. Thus, "Korean Ginseng" is *Panax ginseng*, "Chinese Ginseng" is *Panax ginseng,* and so on.

The biological effects of *Panax ginseng* root extracts are fairly well defined, as are the chemical constituents responsible for most of these effects. The chemical substances that Ginseng's main active principles are complex glycosides known as "ginsenosides." These are classified as triterpene saponins and consist of about 20 identified structures. Ginsenosides of the R_b grouping are "slightly sedative" while those of the R_g grouping are more stimulating. Both types of ginsenosides show some anti-fatigue activity.

All of the Ginsengs are used primarily as adaptogens, or substances which produce nonspecific resistance in the body. By definition, an adaptogen usually exerts no specific biological effects, but it tends to **normalize adverse conditions** of the body; at least this is the claim of Russian scientists, who have contributed immensely to this field of research. Thus, a person with mild high blood pressure, after taking an adaptogen, will usually have normal blood pressure. Conversely, a person with low blood pressure, will also have normal blood pressure.

A great deal of evidence from animal studies, as well as data from dozens of human experiments, verifies the adaptogenic effects of *Panax ginseng*. However, the major use for *Panax ginseng* seems to be as a **preventive medicine** against various forms of stress, the common cold, and similar conditions. A popular belief is that *Panax ginseng* has aphrodisiac properties, but there is no evidence, in animals or humans, to verify such an action.

This herb, which has long been utilized for "tonic" or "adaptogenic" effects, is now also receiving attention for its capacity to act as an **enhancer of performance and endurance**. While not strictly a "stimulant" in the sense of being a primary CNS activator (such as caffeine and ephedrine containing plants), the various ginsengs do show some CNS stimulant activity. Ginseng is utilized for its reputed **anti-fatigue effects, improved performance and stamina**, as well as to **improve concentration and reaction times in the elderly**.

There are no reports in the scientific literature (and there have been more than 1,400 scientific papers published on this subject) that indicate any adverse effects for *Panax ginseng*. However, there are indications that regular use of this plant may cause a mild insomnia in some people. Thus, it should not be taken in the early evening or at bedtime.

Buying a *concentrated extract* of ginseng offers the consumer a far more reliable assurance that the active constituents are present at precise levels as stated on labels.

In this case, knowing that what nature provides *is there* is an improvement over nature herself.

GINSENG, SIBERIAN

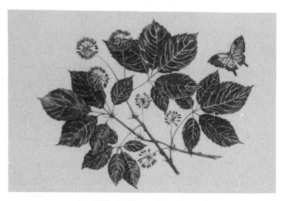

Siberian Ginseng

SCIENTIFIC NAME: *Eleutherococcus senticosus*

PARTS USED: Root

DOSAGE:

Powder: 1/2 teaspoon of powder to 1 cup of hot water. Drink in the morning, at lunch, at bedtime (add Lemongrass if you find the flavor wanting).

SIBERIAN GINSENG: *Long studied in Russia, recent research indicates that an extract stimulates cellular immunity.*

Traditional Usages

During the past decade, a new "Ginseng" has appeared in the marketplace in North America; indeed, it is being widely used throughout Europe also. This is the so-called "Siberian Ginseng," or *Eleutherococcus senticosus,* sometimes erroneously named *Acanthopanax senticosus.* Since the family Araliaceae is known popularly as the Ginseng family, many different species of this family are referred to as Ginsengs. Since the habitat for *Eleutherococcus senticosus* is primarily in Siberia, the vernacular name Siberian Ginseng was given to this plant. Indeed, because of the amazing similarity of pharmacologic effects of the *Panax* species, with comparison to *Eleutherococcus senticosus,* it seems that the name Siberian Ginseng is appropriate.

It has been used for centuries in Russian folkloric medicine as an **immune-enhancing agent.** It is also employed as an **anti-inflammatory, in cardiovascular disease, to restore concentration, memory, and cognition,** and **as a remedy for stress, depression, fatigue,** or **complete nervous breakdown.**

Recent Scientific Findings

Traditionally touted for its "aphrodisiac" effect, many people are under the impression that Ginseng is only a "male" herb. **In actuality, the Siberian Ginseng is highly valued by both sexes for its adaptogenic abilities. An adaptogen is a substance that "normalizes" adverse conditions of the body.**

Ginseng has always been perceived as a **stimulant.** In Russia a great deal of publicity comes from its **use by cosmonauts and Olympic athletes to provide energy and negate stress effects.** Most remarkably, **victims of the Chernobyl nuclear disaster were given courses of** *Eleutherococcus* **to aid them** with an anti-radiation effect. Russians prescribe Siberian Ginseng for patients undergoing chemotherapy and radiotherapy.

While the chemical constituents, "eleutherosides," differ from those of *Panax* species, the pharmacological effects of Siberian Ginseng are quite similar to those of *Panax ginseng.* This plant has been studied more rigorously by the Russians than *Panax ginseng;* they have studied both species, in fact. Extracts of Siberian Ginseng have been shown to relieve stress, lower the toxicity of some common drugs that tend to produce side effects in humans, increase mental alertness, improve resistance to colds and mild infections, and be beneficial in cases where a person is continuously in contact with environmental stresses.

A recent (1987) first-rate double-blind study demonstrated that a Siberian Ginseng extract stimulated cellular immunity. Thirty-six healthy volunteers received 10 milliliters of an alcohol extract of Siberian Ginseng three times daily for four weeks. A placebo of plain ethanol was used. A "drastic increase in the absolute number of [immune] cells," especially T lymphocytes was shown using flow cytometry. The T helper/inducer cells, as well as cytotoxic and natural killer cells were increased in number, which is clear demonstration that the human immune system can be augmented with this herb. As expected, no side effects were observed during the experiment or afterwards, a period of six months.

Flow cytometry is a highly advanced means for observing cells that permits an analysis of individual living cells. Using this method to study human immune reactions, German researchers proved that an extract of Siberian Ginseng stimulated T cell production, especially helper cells. This proof that such an "adaptogen" truly works pushes herbal science into mainstream medicine with wide application in numerous immune-related disorders.

The German scientists stated Siberian Ginseng "could be considered a nonspecific immunostimulant." This may help explain why it has been said to be of benefit or cited in "protective effects against viral infections, retardation of neoplastic growth and metastasis, or better tolerance of chemotherapy and radiation." They further speculated "about a positive effect of *eleutherococcus* in very early stages of HIV (AIDS) infection by preventing or retarding the spread of the virus, mediated by a synergistic action of elevated numbers of both helper and cytotoxic T cells."

It is not likely that any of the eleutherosides or ginsenosides will ever be used as adaptogens by themselves, since they are only present in their respective plants in small amounts. Similarly, they are too complex to expect a commercially feasible synthesis. Professor I. I. Brekhman, who has conducted numerous animal and human experiments with both *Panax ginseng* and *Eleutherococcus senticosus*, claims that the adaptogenic effect requires the total mixture of eleutherosides, in the case of Siberian Ginseng at least, and that the full effects cannot be obtained with any one of the pure eleutherosides.

Unlike *Panax ginseng, Eleutherococcus senticosus* does not seem to cause insomnia, and like *Panax ginseng,* there do not appear to be any adverse effects in humans from the use of Siberian Ginseng.

In recent years, a flood of products claiming to contain Siberian Ginseng have appeared on the market. We have found that most of these contain no *Eleutherococcus senticosus* root. The substitute products most frequently are offered for sale in capsule form. Unlike authentic Siberian Ginseng, we have found that most of the substitute products have an intense bitter taste and a characteristic "vanillan-like" odor, but it is not the typical pleasant odor of vanillin.

GOLDENSEAL

SCIENTIFIC NAME: *Hydrastis canadensis*
PARTS USED: Rhizome and root

DOSAGE:

Root: ½ teaspoon of ground, dried and powdered root, boiled in a covered container in 1 pint of water for about ½ hour, at a slow boil. Allow liquid to cool slowly in the *closed* container. Drink cold, 1 swallow or 1 tablespoon at a time, a maximum of 1 cup per day for a length of time not to exceed 1 week.

GOLDENSEAL: *Widely used by Native American healers for skin diseases, recent research has discovered potent hypotensive properties.*

Traditional Usages

Here is another Native American plant with wide usage by Amerind healers. An infusion of the roots was made into an **eye wash** for sore eyes. It was also used for **inflammation** of the mucous membrane. The Cherokees pounded the rootstock together with bear fat and smeared it on their bodies as an **insect repellent**. The root was boiled in water and the resulting liquid applied as a wash for **skin diseases** by Native Americans and later in domestic American medicine. A decoction was used as an eyewash. From 1831 to 1842, the dried rootstock was official in the *U.S. Pharmacopoeia*; it was readmitted in 1863 and remained until 1936.

Three components of the plant also

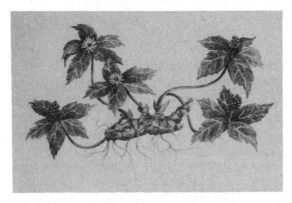

Goldenseal

were at one time official drugs; Hydrastine was entered in the *United States Pharmacopoeia* (USP) from 1905-1926, *Hydrastinine hydrochloride* in the USP from 1916-26 and the *National Formulary* (NF) from 1926-1950. All were classified as internal hemostatics. Goldenseal enjoys a tremendous reputation for its medicinal virtuosity. It has been recommended in the treatment of dozens of ailments.

Recent Scientific Findings

Recent research has corroborated Goldenseal's biological activities. The dried rhizome possesses cytotoxic activity, indicating it is useful against viruses. Since 1950, its antibacterial properties have been well-established, especially against *E. Coli* and *Staphylococcus aureus*. Not to be overlooked is goldenseal's potent hypotensive activity. In one experiment in rabbits, an extract of the root brought about a severe drop in blood pressure.

Goldenseal owes its effect primarily to the alkaloids hydrastine and hydrastinine, in addition to berberine. These alkaloids produced a strong astringent effect on mucous membranes, reduce inflammation, and have antiseptic effects.

Goldenseal can be used as an external application to the arms and legs in the treatment of disorders of the blood vessels and lymphatics. Berberine was found to have anti-convulsive effect on the intestines and uterus, and was also very effective against the bacterial *Staphylococcus aureus.*

> As a specific for uterine complaints it was given to arrest uterine hemorrhage, as well as to check excessive menstrual evacuation. In very small dosage it was advocated to cure morning sickness; however, it is critical to note that in large doses Goldenseal *may produce abortion,* and in fact has been used deliberately as an abortifacient.

Moreover, taken in too large a dose, Goldenseal can dangerously overstimulate the nervous system. **It is inadvisable to continue even limited usage for extended periods of time since the alkaloids are eliminated quite slowly from the body.**

This is a potent plant which must be utilized with care. One of its constituent alkaloids, L-Canadine, reportedly paralyzes the central nervous system and causes severe peristalsis.

GOTU KOLA or Chi-Hsing; Pai-Kuo

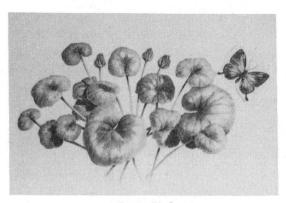

Gotu Kola

SCIENTIFIC NAME: *Centella asiatica*
PARTS USED: Whole plant

DOSAGE:

GOTU KOLA: *Long known to Fijian healers, this herb awaits discovery and possible wide adoption by the medical establishment.*

Traditional Usages

Gotu Kola is used primarily as a **sedative, diuretic, tonic,** and to **accelerate healing of wounds**. It is claimed to **strengthen** and **energize the brain**. In large doses, it is said to act as a narcotic, causing stupor, headache, and sometimes coma.

It has been employed to alleviate bowel complaints and to treat syphilis and tubercular inflammation of the cervical lymph nodes. Its ability to aid in these and urinary-tract disorders has been attributed to its demulcent properties.

Fijian healers have long known of the values of this plant; it is the most frequently utilized medicinal plant in their pharmacopoeia. It has long been known in India, and its use was probably brought to Fiji by Indian settlers.

Recent Scientific Findings

Recent pharmacological studies have shown that extracts of Gotu Kola exhibit a **sedative activity**. The mode of action appears to be mainly on the cholinergic mechanism in the central nervous system.

The major active principle in this plant is most probably the triterpene glycoside asiaticoside. Asiaticoside is well tolerated when given by mouth to mice and rabbits at a single dose of 1.0 gram. This would imply that it is a relatively safe substance. When asiaticoside is implanted under the skin, or injected subcutaneously in mice, rats, guinea pigs, or rabbits, improved blood supply of connective tissue occurs. A rapid thickening of the skin is also noted in the treated animals, as well as an accelerated growth of hair and nails.

There is some evidence in humans, because of the sum total of these effects, that asiaticoside, and hence extracts of *Centella asiatica*, **accelerate healing of wounds**. There are indications that asiaticoside are useful for infectious diseases such as **tuberculosis** and **leprosy**. The microbes that cause both of these diseases are well known to have a waxy coating that most other disease-producing organisms lack. This waxy coating prevents the body's own defense mechanisms from killing the organisms, hence it is difficult to cure both of these diseases. It is thought that asiaticoside acts to dissolve the waxy covering on the organisms, which then allows the normal defense mechanisms of the body to destroy the causative organisms of **leprosy** and/or **tuberculosis**.

It must be pointed out that the foregoing is indicated only as a reasonable explanation for part of the useful action of *C. asiatica* preparations. Further work must be carried out in animals and in humans to determine whether or not this is the case.

An extract, CATTF, has been found to be effective in promoting **wound healing** in vivo. Following up on this research, a 1991 study involving patients with post-phlebitic syndrome (PPS) confirmed that Gotu-Kola has a regulatory effects on vascular tissue. Another study of patients with varicose veins also substantiated this effect.

Two other **extracts**, TTFCA and TECA, have also proven effective in treating **venous hypertension**. In one study involving 62 patients, after four weeks of treatment those receiving TTFCA showed significant improvement while the placebo group showed no change. In another study, 94 patients suffering from edema in the lower limbs were given two different doses of TECA or a placebo. The patients given the TECA exhibited a significant difference in comparison to the placebo group.

It has also been shown that asiaticoside-pretreated rats (12.5

mg/kg/day/3 days, subcutaneously), who were subjected to cold conditions, did not develop gastric ulcers. Control animals in the experiment did develop gastric ulcers under these conditions.

Recent pharmacological studies have shown that extracts of Gotu Kola exhibit a **sedative activity** similar to that of meprobamate and chlorpromazine.

Because of the pronounced effect of asiaticoside on skin, a study was carried out to determine if repeated applications would produce cancer. A 0.10 percent solution of asiaticoside was applied to the back of hairless mice twice weekly for the lifetime of the animals (about 18 months). It was found that sarcomas (cancers) were produced on the skin of 2.5 percent of the treated mice. These findings probably have little significance, since the test is not specific, and is recognized as invalid for weak carcinogens. The results of the experiment described above would indicate that in that test, asiaticoside would be classified as a weak carcinogen. Despite these minor pharmacological problems, Gotu Kola awaits discovery and possible wide adoption by the medical establishment.

Caution: **Overdose may cause narcotic stupor.**

GREEN TEA

SCIENTIFIC NAME: Various spp.
PARTS USED: Leaves

DOSAGE:

Leaves: Approximately 1 ounce of leaves to 1 pint of water. Boil water separately and pour over the plant material and steep for 5 to 20 minutes, depending on the desired effect. Drink hot or warm, 1 to 2 cups per day, at bedtime and upon awakening.

Traditional Usages

For centuries tea has been the most commonly consumed beverage in the world, except for water. Since antiquity, Green Tea has been thought to provide various pharmacological benefits, such as combating mental fatigue as well as colds and flu. Many 19th century chemists and medical scientists believed that tea produced healthful effects on the digestive and nervous systems, facilitated cardiovascular function, and decreased blood pressure.

Recent Scientific Findings

Modern scientists are discovering new healthful benefits from the consumption of Green Tea. According to Hirota Fujiki, a chemist at the National Cancer Center Research Institute in Tokyo, "This Green Tea cannot prevent every cancer, but it's the cheapest and most practical method for cancer prevention available to the general public."

The majority of teas produced worldwide can be classified into two types: black tea, which is most common in Western nations, and Green Tea, which predominates in the Far East, especially China and Japan. When consumed, Green Tea provides more healthful advantages than black tea because it contains larger amounts of such important substances as vitamins, including twice as much vitamin C as black tea. Green Tea contains more than twice the catechins of black tea; tea's "tannins" consist mostly of these catechins. Though the content of vitamin P in other foods is very low, tea catechins have been found to have high vitamin P activity. In fact, the regular consumption of catechin-rich tea may meet the human requirements for vitamin P, according to some researchers.

While tea's favorable effect was once attributed to its caffeine content, biochemical studies have shown that tea's catechins may play an even greater role. It has been demonstrated that peculiar features of the chemical composition of tea are responsible for its important pharmacological and physiological properties. Tea's beneficial effects that were first discovered empirically over many generations have been corroborated by present-day scientific investigations.

The catechins in tea are formed by polyphenic compounds. Many researchers have found that phenolic compounds, including tea catechins, delay the development of arteriosclerosis. Clinical investigations ascertained that consumption of Green Tea had a therapeutic effect on infectious diseases, particularly dysentery. Incorporating Green Tea in the treatment of rheumatism had a favorable effect on both the general condition and capillary resistance of their patients. The researchers concluded that Green Tea exerts a favorable regulatory effect on every vital component of human metabolism.

Green Tea polyphols, which comprise from 17-30% of the dry weight of Green Tea leaves, are now known to explain the panacea-like properties of the world's most popular beverage. Found recently to account for the **anti-viral, antioxidant** effects in Green Tea, these unique polyphenols also enhance immunity and destroy bacteria. Epidemiological surveys suggest that Green Tea consumption is associated with a reduced incidence of pancreatic and stomach cancers.

In recent years there has been a growing interest in identifying the antimutagenic and anticarcinogenic constituents of the human diet. Here again, researchers are discovering that Green Tea provides healthful benefits. From a series of mouse experiments Wang and his colleagues concluded, "These results, in conjunction with our prior publications, suggest that **consumption of Green Tea may reduce the risk of some forms of human cancer** induced by both physical and chemical environmental carcinogens."

At the Fourth Chemical Congress of North America, Japanese and U.S. researchers reported that Green Tea helps shield mice against tumors of the liver, lung, skin, and digestive tract and may do the same for humans. In 1987, epigallocatechin gallate (EGCG) was found to be the key protective ingredient. EBCG seems to possess the broadest spectrum and level of activity of the Green Tea polyphenols and makes up more than 50% of the total GTP content. Researchers speculated that this **antioxidant may protect against tumor development by destroying free radicals** (highly reactive atoms or molecules) that could otherwise attack DNA and disrupt normal cell processes. In mice given a carcinogen that affects the digestive tract, 20 percent of the animals treated with EGCG developed intestinal cancer compared with 63% that did not get EGCG.

At the same time, EGCG may prevent the activation of certain carcinogens so that free radicals never form. Researchers at Rutgers University reported similar findings regarding skin cancer. The incidence of skin cancer is steadily increasing and the disease represents a major health and economic problem in the modern industrialized world. Mice that drank Green Tea instead of plain water for 10 days before and during exposure to ultraviolet light proved less susceptible to skin damage. "These broad effects of the Green Tea are quite interesting. There aren't that many things that have as broad a spectrum," mused study director Allan H. Conney. Much research remains to be done in this area, however. "The results are encouraging, but I think it would be premature to extrapolate these studies to humans," said Conney. It is not yet known how well the mouse data may apply to humans.

Currently, the speculation of Green Tea's cancer inhibiting effects in humans is based on demographic extrapolations. **It has been surmised that Green Tea may explain why Japanese cigarette smokers have a lower rate of lung cancer than smokers in the United States.** People residing in Shizuoka, Japan's tea-growing region, use tea leaves only once instead of as in other areas of Japan where the same leaves are used several times. Therefore, the people of Shizuoka consume greater quantities of the tea's chemicals. In Shizuoka the death rate from cancer, especially stomach cancer, is markedly lower than in the rest of Japan. Significant differences for habitual Green Tea consumption between Nakakawane City and Osuka City were observed. In Osuka, people drink less tea and have a high mortality rate due to stomach cancer. In Nakakawane, people drink more tea and have a low rate of stomach cancer.

Green Tea also stabilizes blood lipids, and may therefore be of value in an overall cardiac-care regimen. According to a 1991 study on mice, Green Tea extract prevented an increase in serum cholesterol even when the animals were fed an atherogenic (i.e., artery-damaging) diet. Serum lipid peroxides were also diminished, while the destruction of lecithin was reduced.

An antioxidant fraction of Green Tea Extract has been shown to efficiently scavenge the pro-oxidants hydrogen peroxide and superoxide anion radical, and to protect against the cytotoxicity of paraquat, a biocide that exhibits cellular toxicity via a pro-oxidant intermediate. Studies evaluating the ability of various polyphenols and condensed tannins (procyanidins linked to gallic acid) to scavenge the various pro-oxidants revealed that EGCG was the most potent; EGCG was also most effective at inhibiting lipid peroxidation in brain tissues from animals, exhibiting over 200 times greater activity than vitamin E (alpha-tocopherol). These investigators postulated that the galloyl groups may lend themselves to increasing antioxidant effectiveness.

EGCG and Epicatechin Gallate have recently been shown to selectively inhibit reverse transcriptase in Human Immunodeficiency Virus (HIV-RT), whereas the constituent building blocks of these compounds had no inhibitory activity. The most attractive feature of these results rests upon the observation that inhibition of HIV-RT was observed at gallocatechin concentrations over 5 times less than that which inhibited "normal" cellular DNA polymerases. This is a promising finding in that the side effects of many currently employed anti-retrovirals are due to inhibition of host cellular DNA polymerases. This means that Green Tea polyphenols inhibit viral replication at low concentrations, low enough to avoid destroying normal cells, which suggests that side-effects from EGCG would be minimal.

As can be seen, Green Tea possesses unique and broad effects. While much research must yet be done to see if all these conclusions will apply to humans, we can safely assume that the wisdom of the ages is not to be ignored. In the future, having a cup of tea might mean more than just enjoying a pleasant beverage.

GRINDELIA

SCIENTIFIC NAME: *Grindelia* spp.
PARTS USED: Leaves and flowering tops
DOSAGE:

Leaves and Flowering Tops: Approximately 1/2 ounce of leaves or flowering tops to 1 pint of water. Boil water separately and pour over the plant material and steep for 5 to 20 minutes, depending on the desired effect. Drink hot or warm, 1 to 2 cups per day, at bedtime and upon wakening.

For poison ivy or poison oak boil 1 oz. of plant material in a pint of water for about 10 minutes. Let cool, strain, and apply cold to affected parts on saturated cloth.

GRINDELIA: *Also known as Gum Plant, this has a long history of use as an expectorant.*

Traditional Usages

The principle use of Grindelia (or Gum Plant) in traditional medicine was for the treatment of bronchial catarrh, or inflammation of the bronchial mucous membranes, particularly in cases of asthma. Grindelia was thought to act as a stimulating expectorant and antispasmodic.

When combined with Stramonium, Grindelia was used in "asthma powders," which were also given for whooping cough and hayfever.

Recent Scientific Findings

The herb contains an essential oil, over 20 percent resin, grindelol, saponin, tannin, and robustic acid. In one study, a fluid extract of the aerial parts of *Grindelia squarrosa* was tested in guinea pigs, rabbits, and cats for expectorant activity. The fluidextract was administered orally. Expectorant effects were shown in the cat experiments, but not in the rabbit and guinea pig experiments. Species variation in drug testing is not uncommon and so the results are inconclusive but promising in verifying Grindelia's expectorant properties.

In the form of topical poultices and solutions, Grindelia has been reported to be **useful in treating burns, vaginitis, and genitourinary membrane infections and inflammation**. *G. squarosa* (Curly Cup) has been found to be beneficial in the treatment of **poison ivy** and other skin irritations and rashes.

GROUNDSEL

SCIENTIFIC NAME: *Senecio vulgaris*
PARTS USED: Herb

DOSAGE:

    Leaves and Flowering tops: Approximately 1/2 ounce of leaves or flowering tops to 1 pint of water. Boil water separately and pour over the plant material and steep for 5 to 20 minutes, depending on the desired effect. Drink hot or warm, 1 to 2 cups per day.

GROUNDSEL: *Both European and Native American practitoners used this in place of Ergot.*

Traditional Usages

Groundsel was used to **stimulate menstruation** and to **ease painful menstruation**, both by European and American domestic practitioners. Native Americans used the plant to **speed childbirth**. All these functions recall the applications of Ergot, and Groundsel was employed at various times as a substitute for that fungus, for example, in controlling pulmonary hemorrhage. In general, the plant has been utilized as a diaphoretic, diuretic, and tonic. **In dentistry, the herb is employed for bleeding gums.**

GUARANÁ

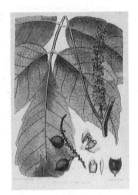

Guaraná

SCIENTIFIC NAME: *Paullinia cupana*

PARTS USED: Seeds

DOSAGE:

Seeds: The beverage, which is also used medicinally, is prepared from 1 teaspoon of Guaraná to a glass or cup of sweetened water.

GUARANÁ: This traditional Brazilian beverage alleviates migraine headaches.

Traditional Usages

A traditional beverage of the Brazilian Indians found in the native marketplaces, Guaraná is prepared from the dried seeds which are powdered, sometimes mixed with cassava flour, then kneaded into dough and formed into cylindrical or globular masses. It may also be mixed with chocolate. Besides having refreshing and nutritive value, Guaraná has been used medicinally by natives in Brazil for **bowel complaints**, both as a curative and as a preventive.

The plant was introduced into France by a physician who had been working in Brazil. It came to be employed in the treatment of **migraine and nervous headaches, neuralgia, paralysis, urinary-tract irritation**, and other ailments, as well as continuing to be administered for **chronic diarrhea**.

Recent Scientific Findings

The medicinal virtues of the plants are probably largely due to its **caffeine content**, which is higher than in any other plant source and 2$\frac{1}{2}$ times that of coffee. **The caffeine explains the efficacy of Guaraná in alleviating the pain of migraine headaches. The tannins undoubtedly act as an astringent to alleviate diarrhea.**

Aqueous extracts of Guaraná has shown positive results in a study of platelet aggregation. In both humans and rabbits, the Guaraná extracts **inhibited platelet aggregation** following either oral or intravenous administration. Guaraná has also exhibited **CNS stimulant activity** in adult humans.

GUAR GUM

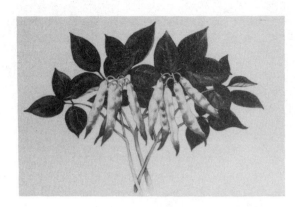

Guar Gum

SCIENTIFIC NAME: *Cyanopsis tetragonoloba*

PARTS USED: Ground endosperm of seeds

DOSAGE:

GUAR GUM: *At one time a popular laxative in southern Asia, preparations have decreased serum cholesterol.*

Traditional Usages

Guar Gum is the ground endosperm of the seeds of *Cyanopsis tetragonoloba*, a plant native to India and Pakistan. When mixed with water, it rapidly forms high viscous colloidal solutions.

Traditionally, Guar gum was most commonly used as a bulk laxative. It was also employed as an appetite suppressant and as a treatment for diabetes

Guar Gum served as a base in cosmetic preparations such as hand lotions and washable creams.

Recent Scientific Findings

Along with Psyllium, Guar Gum preparations have been found to **decrease serum cholesterol**, especially LDL cholesterol. Researchers have discovered that patients given Guar Gum preparations exhibit anywhere from a 5% to a 17% reduction of serum cholesterol.

Guar gum **stabilizes the blood sugar level** due to its delaying action on the absorption of carbohydrates in the gut. In both rabbit and human models, Guar Gum exhibited an anti-hyperglycemic effect. Anti-hyperlipemic activity has been observed in animal models.

GUGGAL

SCIENTIFIC NAME: *Commiphora mukul*
PARTS USED: Gum resin

DOSAGE:
Follow label directions of commercial preparations.

GUGGAL: A doctoral student's curiosity led to the rediscovery of this gum resin's cholesterol-lowering properties first recommended 2,500 years ago.

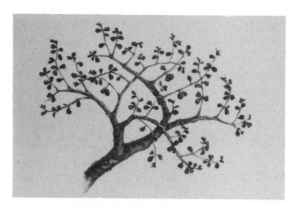

Guggal

Traditional Usages

The 2500 year old Ayurveda treatise, *Shushruta Samhita* recommends gum guggal as a treatment for obesity as well as "coating and obstruction of channels." Guggal is derived from the resin of *Commiphora mukul*, a small thorny tree 4 to 6 feet tall, which grows in the semi-arid regions of Rajasthan, Gujarat, and Karnataka in India. The tree exudes a yellowish gum resin with a balsamic odor. When tapped during winter, the average tree yields 700-900 grams of resin. Guggal oleo-resin contains a complex mixture of diterpenes, esters, and higher alcohols. The active components for **lowering cholesterol** are believed to be two steroids, Guggalsterones Z and E.

Recent Scientific Findings

In the mid-1960s, doctoral student G. V. Satyavati's curiosity was piqued by *Shushruta Samhita's* description of Guggal's uses with the ancient concept of *medoroga* (obesity) and contemporary knowledge of atherosclerosis (believed to be the principal cause of coronary heart disease). Might this mean, mused the student, that Guggal lowers cholesterol and excess fat? Satyavati's initial findings published in 1966 supported her conjecture. Since this pioneering doctoral work, more than 20 clinical studies have been published on the lipid-lowering effects of Guggal. The results clearly show that Guggal **can lower blood cholesterol**, lower blood triglycerides, lower blood VLDL (the "bad" cholesterol fraction) and raise blood HDL (the "good" cholesterol fraction).

While there currently does not appear to be support in scientific literature for the anti-inflammatory properties described in ancient Ayurvedic texts, Guggal demonstrates a cholesterol-lowering ability rivaling any natural substance—total blood cholesterol reduction of over 20% has been achieved by the use of Guggal alone without dietary modifications.

The connection between cholesterol and heart disease has been well documented both in medical journals and the popular press. Cholesterol is manufactured to provide building materials for the body, including hormones and cell membranes. However, an excessive level of cholesterol in blood vessels leads to hyperlipidemia, that is, excess lipids in the blood stream. Lipids are fat-like materials consisting of phospholipids and cholesterol and may be the prime cause of atherosclerosis, or narrowing of the arteries, and therefore, heart disease. The American Heart Association estimates that at least 60 percent of Americans have cholesterol levels that place them in the high-risk category for heart disease. If Guggal lowers cholesterol, then this gum resin may significantly reduce that risk.

Detailed pharmacological studies on Guggal have been conducted on animals and humans. Several animal studies showed a lowering of serum cholesterol by 34% to 40%, and a lowering of serum triglycerides by 26 to 30%. In human clinical studies, reductions in cholesterol and triglyceride levels of 15 to 21.5% have been achieved. The lipid-lowering effect has no correlation to age, sex or body weight, and no side effects were found. The authors of one study stated, "From these studies we conclude that gugulipid is a safe and effective lipid-lowering agent comparable in its efficacy to clofibrate but with better compliance and fewer side effects."

Clofibrate is a standard lipid-lowering drug. Comparison studies showed that Guggal was equal to or better than clofibrate regarding normalizing blood lipid profile. Other preliminary studies have demonstrated that Guggal decreases platelet adhesiveness and increases the blood's fibrinolytic (fibrin-breaking) activity. Both of these actions are extremely beneficial in protecting against thrombosis (heart attack and stroke). If further research confirms these findings, this would be an important breakthrough because few nutrients both normalize blood lipids and protect against thrombosis.

Twenty years after her initial doctoral research, Satyavati writes, "In conclusion, the saga of gum guggal serves as a highly fascinating and inspiring account of how an 'ancient insight' can lead to a significant 'modern discovery,' provided modern scientists with an open mind (i.e., those without any prejudice against the traditional systems of medicine) care to undertake a serious study of ancient Ayurvedic texts and then carry out carefully planned scientific studies to test some of the rich fundamental concepts and hypotheses available in time-honored ancient systems of medicine."

HAWTHORN

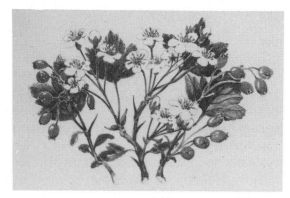

Hawthorn

SCIENTIFIC NAME: *Crataegus oxycantha*
PARTS USED: Flowers, leaves, and berries

DOSAGE:

Flowers: 1 teaspoon flowers per 1 pint of boiling water, poured over the flowers and steep for 5 to 20 minutes, depending on the desired effect. 1 to 2 cups per day, a mouthful at a time.

Fruit: For the fruit, place 1 teaspoon crushed fruit in 1/2 cup cold water. Let stand for several hours (7 to 8), then boil and strain. 1 to 2 cups per day, a mouthful at a time.

HAWTHORNE: *In Europe, this is often prescribed as a substitute for digitalis.*

Traditional Usages

Hawthorn leaves and berries were used for digestive and urinary ailments. Parkinson recommended the berries or seeds as a remedy for kidney stones and dropsy.

Hawthorn has a history of use for various heart conditions dating from the 17th century. However, its use as a heart medicine was not widespread until the late 19th century, when an Irish doctor became well known for his **secret remedy for heart disease.** After his death in 1894, the doctor's daughter disclosed that the remedy was a Hawthorn berry tincture. Hawthorn then became a **popular remedy for heart and cardiovascular ailments.** It was believed to strengthen the heart muscle and, taken over a long period of time, to **lower blood pressure.**

Other uses for Hawthorn include as a **diuretic and astringent.** A tea was drunk as a nerve tonic.

In traditional Chinese medicine, Hawthorn has a history of use for a thousand years. It was given as a treatment for **dyspepsia** as well as to improve digestion of both children and adults.

Recent Scientific Findings

Since the turn of the century, Hawthorn has been a widely used **heart remedy.** Hawthorn exhibits **vasodilatory action** and **lowers peripheral resistance to blood flow.** The mode of action and active principles are still being investigated, though it is known that Hawthorn is not a digitalis-like substance. Hawthorn is rich in flavonoids, which in general are known to have cardiotonic attributes. Because the flowers and leaves contain different amounts of Hawthorn's flavonoids, preparations commonly combine the parts.

In Europe, where Hawthorn is more

widely prescribed than in the United States, it is often given in conjunction with digitalis or in place of digitalis when the latter's side effects need to be avoided. In Hawthorn's nearly 100 years of clinical use, there has yet to be a reported case of a toxic reaction. In animals studies where even high doses of Hawthorn has been administered, there have not been toxic reactions.

The specific cardiac symptoms for which Hawthorn is most commonly prescribed include myocardism, geriatric or stressed heart, hypertension, and dysrhythmia. **In combination with digitalis, Hawthorn is given for cardiac disturbances such as palpitations, anginal complaints, and tachycardia (rapid heart action).** It is recommended that treatment be long-term, at least several months.

A 1981 double-blind placebo study was conducted with 120 patients suffering from loss of cardiac output. The researchers found that in comparison to the placebo group, the Hawthorn group exhibited improvement both in subjective symptoms, especially **palpitations** and **shortness of breath**, and in cardiac function.

A 1990 experiment found that a mixture of Hawthorn and Motherwort might prove an effective preventive and/or treatment for atherosclerosis. Also, dried Hawthorn flowers were tested pharmacologically and found to have a **positive inotropic effect.**

HELLEBORE, AMERICAN

SCIENTIFIC NAME: *Veratrum viride*
PARTS USED: Rhizome

DOSAGE:

Root: *Extreme Caution:* When prescribed as a tincture, 0.8 ounces of the dried root to 16 ounces of diluted 0.835 alcohol is macerated for 2 weeks, then expressed and filtered. Tincture: Dose is 0.6-1.8 milliliters. Fluidextract: 0.065-0.13 grams.

AMERICAN HELLEBORE: *The alkaloids are utilized to treat high blood pressure.*

Traditional Usages

Known also by the names of Indian Poke, Poke Root, Swamp Hellebore, and Itch Weed, like its European cousin the Black Hellebore, the American Hellebore is **highly toxic.**

A 17th century account asserts that Hellebore was employed by one tribe as part of an ordeal. "He whose stomach withstood its action longest was decided to be the strongest of the party, and entitled to command the rest." In the 18th century it was used to **treat gout.**

In standard medicine, Hellebore was employed for its **irritant and sedative action** in a wide range of complaints, including pneumonia, gout, rheumatism, typhoid and rheumatic fevers, and local inflammations.

A related species, *V. californicum*, or False Hellebore, is a famous contraceptive plant of Nevada tribes and surrounding regions. Shoshones and other Native Americans employ a root decoction daily for the three weeks to insure sterility. The plant is called by its Shoshone name, *div-h-savva*, meaning "sterile."

Recent Scientific Findings

Producing distressing nausea and extreme depression of the circulation and the nervous system, **American Hellebore's use in generalized herbal practice as a home remedy is to be avoided.**

American Hellebore preparations are well known to contain a complex mixture of steroid alkaloids (including jervine, pseudojervine, and meratroidine) that are still used by the medical profession to treat severe cases of high blood pressure and related cardiovascular conditions. It must be pointed out, however, that **this is one of our most potent drug plants**. It is effective only in selected types of high blood pressure, and has many side effects if used over a long period of time.

As with many other toxic herbs, **minute doses of Hellebore are an important remedy in the homeopathic discipline of medicine;** the homeopathic preparations are utilized as nervines and especially for their sedative action on the circulation. Homeopaths report that in suitable doses, it can be relied upon to bring the pulse down from 150 beat per minutes to 40 beats per minutes or even as low as 30 beats per minute. **However, even the homeopaths warn of the dangers of overdosing and prescribe as an antidote in case of accidental poisoning morphine or laudanum in a little brandy or ginger.**

HELLEBORE, BLACK

SCIENTIFIC NAME: *Helleborus niger*
PARTS USED: Rhizome

DOSAGE:
   Caution: Toxic

BLACK HELLEBORE: *Once cruelly used to treat insanity, this plant contains a potent cardiac drug.*

Traditional Usages

This perennial plant is **quite toxic** and its usage in herbal medicine was restricted by physicians, who were fully aware of its poisonous properties. Used properly by a knowledgeable herbalist or physician, Hellebore has been given as a **purgative**, to **excite sneezing**, to **provoke menstrual evacuation**, and, externally applied, to cause blistering and inflammation of the skin. Perhaps it is most famous for its use in dropsy.

There is a peculiar story regarding Black Hellebore. In 1806 a group of French prisoners were suffering from hemeralopia (blindness from sunset to sunrise). After attempting a variety of treatments, a powdered snuff of Black Hellebore was given to them; they recovered in a few days. At the same time they reported a welcome side-effect—relief from dyspeptic symptoms!

The root has also been used throughout history, dating from the ancients, as a remedy for insanity. The

Greek myth of Melampus describes this healer curing the mad daughters of the King of Argos with Black Hellebore. Its reputed efficacy in such psychiatric disorders was attributed to its drastic purgative property of expelling the "black bile" from which such maladies were thought to originate. One can only presume that the doctors believed the patient, brought to the doors of death with this violent purgative, would be literally shocked back to reality, the fear of further treatment being more than sufficient incentive to quit irrational behavior. The brutal treatment of the mentally ill by continual application of violent drugs remains one of the most tragic chapters in medical history, a chapter not yet finished.

Recent Scientific Findings

Black Hellebore contains the cardiac glycoside hellebrin, as well as many related chemical substances which would explain the claimed beneficial effects for this plant in dropsy.

Caution: Not for general "at home" herbal use.

HEMLOCK

SCIENTIFIC NAME: *Conium maculatum*
PARTS USED: Entire plant, except root

DOSAGE:

Dangerous. Avoid. Hemlock contains the poisonous alkaloid coniine in all parts of the plant. However, the high toxic risk of using even dilute extracts of Hemlock, for any human condition, cannot be discounted.

HEMLOCK: *Used in ancient Athens as a means of capital punishment, this highly toxic plant should not be used medicinally.*

Traditional Usages

Sedative and antispasmodic when used medicinally, Hemlock is a **deadly poison**, which in sufficient doses paralyzes the motor centers. It appears to be well established by scientists and historians that the poison administered as a mode of execution in Athens was principally, if not wholly, composed of the juice of the leaves and the green seeds of this plant.

Conium was first mentioned as a medicinal by Dioscorides, who reported the use of an **external plaster** in the treatment of **herpes** and other skin eruptions. From that time on we find a veritable explosion of diseases this plant was reputed to cure, ranging from cancer of the breast to syphilis, epilepsy, ulcers, and jaundice, to mention only a few.

However, when we read the following account of the death of Socrates, we can only wonder at the herbalists who used

Hemlock successfully, and without incurring charges of homicide:

> But Socrates, after walking about, now told us that his legs were beginning to grow heavy, and immediately lay down, for so he had been ordered. At the same time the man who had given him the poison examined his feet and legs, touching them at intervals. At length he pressed violently upon his foot, and asked if he felt it. To which Socrates replied that he did not. The man then pressed his legs and so on, showing us that he was becoming cold and stiff. And Socrates, feeling it himself, assured us that when the effects had ascended to his heart, he should be gone. And now the middle of his body growing cold, he threw aside his clothes, and spoke for the last time: "Crito, we owe the sacrifice of a cock to Aesculapius. Discharge this, and neglect it not." "It shall be done," said Crito; "have you anything else to say?" He made no reply, but a moment after moved, and his eyes became fixed. And Crito, seeing this, closed his eyelids and mouth.
>
> — Charles F. Millspaugh, *American Medicinal Plants,* pp. 268-269

Recent Scientific Findings

Hemlock contains the poisonous alkaloid coniine in all pasts of the plant. Very small amounts of Hemlock will produce effects that explain the medicinal uses of this plant. However, the high toxic risk of using even dilute extracts of Hemlock, for any human condition, cannot be discounted.

HENBANE

SCIENTIFIC NAME: *Hyoscyamus niger*
PARTS USED: Seeds, leaves, and root

DOSAGE:
   Caution! Avoid.

HENBANE: *The effects of this plant are quite similar to Belladonna.*

Traditional Usages

Related to Belladonna, Henbane is a poisonous plant, extremely dangerous in overdose. Dioscorides declined to use Henbane because he believed it was too poisonous. Administered properly and in correct doses, Henbane is a valuable folk remedy, and has been employed in traditional medicine as a **sedative, anodyne, calmative,** and **antispasmodic.** It is similar to atropine in its ability to dilate the pupil of the eye. The dried leaves have been **smoked for toothache.**

Recent Scientific Findings

Henbane's action is similar to that of Belladonna, but its effects on the cerebrum and motor centers are more pronounced, while its stimulant action on the sympathetic nervous system is less. Overdose can produce headache, nausea, vertigo, extreme thirst, dry burning skin, dilated pupils, loss of sight and voluntary ocular motions, and in extreme cases, mania, convulsions, and death. **Use by the amateur herbalist is obviously quite risky, since the toxic effects can be swift and fatal.**

HENNA

SCIENTIFIC NAME: *Lawsonia alba*
PARTS USED: Leaves and fruit

DOSAGE:
Recommended for external use only. **Do not use internally.**

HENNA: *Since antiquity, the leaves have been used as a hair dye.*

Traditional Usages

Henna has been applied as a **hair dye** since antiquity. Henna leaves were used by the people of ancient civilizations to dye the manes and tails of their horses. The Arabs have employed the leaves for centuries to dye their beards, nails, palms, and soles. Henna imparts a reddish tint to the hair. Mixed with Indigo, it imparts a fine blue-black gloss to beard and hair.

Interestingly, the mummies of ancient Egypt were found wrapped in henna-dyed cloth. In Africa the flowers are used to give a fine scent to pomades and oils.

The fruits have been thought to **stimulate the menstrual function.** In powdered form, the leaves have been utilized both internally and externally to treat various skin diseases, including **leprosy.** In Arabic medicine the powder was employed in the treatment of jaundice, most likely on the basis of coloration (as implied by the Doctrine of Signatures); it is unlikely that Henna benefitted the patient at all and perhaps it only turned him more yellow. In India the leaves were made into an **astringent gargle.**

Recent Scientific Findings

Extracts of Henna leaves have been shown to act in a manner similar to Ergot with respect to **inducing uterine contractions.** It is therefore quite possible that extracts of this plant could induce menstruation and be effective emmanagogues. In test tube experiments, extracts of the leaves of Henna have shown good **antibacterial activity,** although not specifically against the leprosy bacillus, which is not possible to test against since it does not grow in non-living tissues. The active principle for these effects most likely is the coloring principle, lawsone.

The topical application of two chemical components of this shrub, lawsone and dihydroxyacetone, has been reported useful as a protective filter against ultraviolet light for people with chlorpromazine-induced light sensitivity. Experimentally, a water extract of the leaves inhibited gram-positive and gram-negative bacteria. **Antitumor** activity in experiments with mice tends to support folkloric uses of Henna as an anticancer agent.

Henna has experienced a renewed popularity as a hair dye.

HOLLY

SCIENTIFIC NAME: *Ilex aquifolium* (European Holly), *I. opaca* (American Holly)

PARTS USED: Leaves and berries

DOSAGE:

Leaves: To reduce the effects of intermittent fevers, an infusion of the powdered leaves was taken 2 hours *before* the paroxysm in the dose of 3.9 grams.

Berries: 10 or 12 berries are the emetic dose.

HOLLY: *Both the European and American varieties were at one time employed for a variety of uses.*

Traditional Usages

The leaves of the European Holly were employed medicinally for their ability to increase perspiration. In infusions they were also utilized to treat **inflammations** of the mucous membranes, **pleurisy**, **gout**, and **smallpox**.

The leaves also enjoyed a brief reputation in France as a cure for intermittent fevers. The berries were said to have purgative, emetic, and diuretic properties, and the juice of the berries has been used in the treatment of jaundice.

American Holly was used for essentially the same purposes. Two species growing in the southern United States, *I. vomitoria* and *I. dahoon*, were utilized by North Carolina tribes in ritual as well as medicine.

A decoction made from the toasted leaves, known as Black Drink or Yaupon, had emetic properties.

Recent Scientific Findings

Holly leaves are known to contain theobromine, which explains the **diaphoretic** and **febrifuge** effects attributed to herbal teas prepared from them. No studies have been reported on the berries of this plant.

HOLY THISTLE

SCIENTIFIC NAME: *Cnicus benedictus*
PARTS USED: Leaves and flowering tops

DOSAGE:

Leaves: Approximately ½ ounce of leaves and flowering tops to 1 pint of water. Boil water separately and pour over the plant material and steep for 5 to 20 minutes, depending on the desired effect. Drink hot or warm, 1 to 2 cupfuls per day.

HOLY THISTLE: *Used as a medicinal for 2,000 years, the leaves contain cnicin, which stimulates gastric juices.*

Traditional Usages

The Holy Thistle has been recorded as a medicinal since the first century A.D. Credited with the medical virtues of a **diuretic, diaphoretic, febrifuge,** and **cholagogue,** it has been used to treat a variety of ailments. It is a **bitter tonic** and a **good appetite stimulant;** it is still used today to **treat indigestion.** At one time this herb was ascribed the nearly supernatural qualities of a "cure all," but current knowledge yields no evidence to support such a belief.

Recent Scientific Findings

While there is no direct experimental evidence that preparations of Holy Thistle leaves will give the emetic effect claimed by some writers, if given in large enough quantity most any plant would produce emesis due to the presence of low concentrations of irritant principles.

On the other hand, the use of leaf decoctions as a bitter tonic is well founded. The bitter principle in this plant is known to be cnicin, and human experiments have shown that **extracts of Holy Thistle stimulate the production of gastric juices.**

Although widely used as a herbal tea for the treatment of **amenorrhea** (absence of menses), there is no experimental evidence that Holy Thistle seeds have this effect.

HOPS

SCIENTIFIC NAME: *Humulus lupulus*
PARTS USED: Strobiles

DOSAGE:

An infusion prepared with ½ ounce of Hops and a pint of boiling water was given in the dose of 4 fluid ounces. As a fluidextract the usual dose was 2.0-5.8 grams. In making Hop pillows, the dried herb should be moistened with water diluted with a trace of glycerin to prevent rustling of the dried strobiles, which might upset the insomniac more than offering a calming influence.

HOPS: *This well-known ingredient in beer contains a complex mixture of substances with proven sedative action.*

Traditional Usages

Best known as a flavoring and preservative ingredient in the brewing of beer, the Hop plant has also been utilized traditionally in the treatment of **hysteria, restlessness,** and **insomnia.** In Gerarde's herbal of 1633, he wrote "The buds or first sprouts which come forth in the spring are used to be eaten in sallads; yet are they, as Pliny saith, more toothsome than nourishing, for they yield but very small nourishment." Only the young shoots are tasty, the older ones being so bitter and tough that they are softened by bleaching with sulphuric oxide. King Henry VIII feared that he would be poisoned by this violent bleaching agent; he passed an

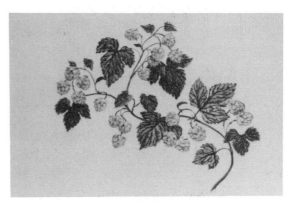

Hops

edict that forbade the addition of hops to ale brewed in his household. In 1787, when King George III was seriously ill, the court physicians filled his pillow with hops instead of opiates to calm his nerves and to promote sleep.

The ancient Hebrews relied on Hops to ward off the plague. Hops contain effective **antibacterial** principles, and were in fact valuable against the infectious agent *Yersinia pestis,* the plague bacillus.

In North America, Native Americans discovered Hop's value independent of Europeans. The Mohegans prepared a **sedative medicine** from the conelike strobiles and sometimes heated these blossoms and applied them for toothache. One Meskwaki practitioner **cured insomnia** with Hops. The Dakotas prepared a tea of the steeped strobiles to **relieve digestive pains.**

At the end of the 19th century, hops were widely used in American medicine for their **tonic, diuretic,** and **sedative** properties. Hops were believed to exert calming effects on the heart and nervous system. The side effects described were colic and constipation.

Recent Scientific Findings

The dried strobiles of Hops contain a complex mixture of substances known as "hop acids" (although not all of them are acids), which are all very bitter substances. Some of these hop acids are **very effective sedatives**, as determined from animal experiments. However, it is most likely that an essential oil in Hops also contributes to the sedative effects, although the active principle(s) in the oil has not yet been identified.

Pillows stuffed with hops have been used to produce sleep in nervous disorders. To prevent rustling of the contents, it is advisable to moisten them with water and glycerin or spirits before placing them under the head of the patient.

A 1966 experiment validated Hops sedative action. One recent study showed that Hops was truly sedative and not merely a muscle relaxant. Other experiments have found anti-hyperglycemic activity in human adult model and antibacterial activity in vitro against *Staphylococcus aureus*.

HOREHOUND

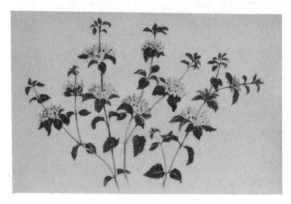

Horehound

SCIENTIFIC NAME: *Marrubium vulgare*
PARTS USED: Leaves and flowering tops

DOSAGE:

    Leaves: 1 teaspoon of leaves and/or flowering tops per cup of boiling water. Drink when cold; 1 tablespoon at a time, 1 cup per day.

HOREHOUND: *This popular folk remedy for respiratory problems contains high concentrations of mucilage.*

Traditional Usages

A very popular folk remedy, Horehound is **mainly tonic and laxative in its action**, but has also been considered valuable for removing obstructions in the system. It was used to treat chronic hepatitis, and a wide range of ill health due to malignancies, advanced pulmonary tuberculosis, leukemia, malaria, and hysteria.

In domestic use, however, it is more often employed in respiratory complaints, such as the treatment of sore throats, to promote the expectoration of phlegm in bronchitis, for asthma, pulmonary consumption, and for obstinate cough.

Recent Scientific Findings

White Horehound has a high concentration of mucilage, which would be expected to **ease the irritation accompanying sore throats**.

HORSE CHESTNUT

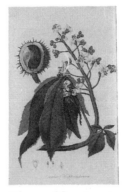

Horse Chestnut

SCIENTIFIC NAME: *Aesculus hippocastanum*

PARTS USED: Bark, leaves, nut (kernel and oil)

DOSAGE:

Bark: A decoction of the bark, when used for fevers, was given in the dose of 16 trams (1/2 ounce) of the bark in 24 hours.

Leaves: A leaf decoction was made from 1 teaspoon of the plant material, boiled in a covered container with 1 pint of water for about 1/2 hour, at a slow boil. The liquid is allowed to cool slowly in the *closed* container. Drink cold, 1 swallow or 1 tablespoon at a time, 1 to 2 cups per day.

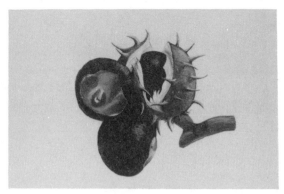

Horse Chestnut

HORSE CHESTNUT: *The seeds of this beautiful tree contain escin, a widely used anti-inflammatory agent.*

Traditional Usages

This easily recognized, stately tree migrated originally from the north of Asia, by Constantinople, about the middle of the sixteenth century. It is not known in what year, but Matthiolus is the first botanist to mention Horse Chestnut. Parkinson states in his *Paradisus* that he cultivated it in his orchard as a fruit tree, esteeming the nuts superior to the ordinary sort.

The powdered kernel of the nut causes sneezing and the oil extracted with ether from the kernels has been used in France as a **topical remedy for rheumatism**. A decoction of the leaves was formerly employed in the United States as a treatment for whooping cough, while the seed oil has been considered useful against sunburn. California tribes combined bear fat with the nut kernel as a paste for hemorrhoids. Dr. Millspaugh described the nuts of the Horse Chestnut as **narcotic** and states that "10 grains are equal to 3 grams of Opium."

Recent Scientific Findings

The active principle of Horse Chestnut seeds is the complex triterpene glycoside *escin*. Escin is not absorbed in the stomach when taken in its natural form. However, when converted to an amorphous form, a derivative (which is sold as Reparil) can be taken orally. Escin is widely utilized in Europe as an **anti-inflammatory** agent for a variety of conditions, in addition to being used for **vascular problems**. There is ample evidence supporting the folkloric usage of Horse Chestnut to treat **varicose veins** and **inflammatory disorders of the legs**. Ointments and gels are applied externally in conjunction with the internal preparation.

Many animal experiments have repeatedly confirmed the **anti-inflammatory** and **anti-edema** actions of escin. One group of researchers studied the process of inflammation in detail and learned that escin inhibits the movement of inflammatory cells, especially macrophages, without lessening their activity or phagocytic properties.

This remarkable glycoside also has potent powers to reduce edema. It achieves this by normalizing the permeability of blood vessel walls. In human therapy, Italian researchers found this compound to be "well tolerated throughout treatments lasting 50 consecutive days."

The leaves *A. glabra*, the Ohio Buckeye, are felt to be quite efficacious in the treatment of chest congestions. Buckeye seeds contain constituents similar to those in *A. hippocastanum* seeds, and thus would be expected to have beneficial effect in the treatment of portal congestion.

When next you gaze at these thickly armored fruits consider the sweet healing balm contained therein.

HORSETAIL (SHAVEGRASS)

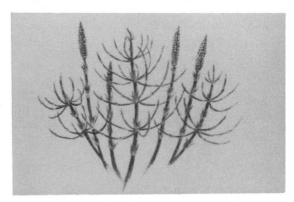

Horsetail

SCIENTIFIC NAME: *Equisetum arvense,*
E. hiemale
PARTS USED: Whole plant

DOSAGE:
   1 teaspoon of plant per cup of boiling water. Drink cold, 1 to 2 cups per day, 1 tablespoon at a time. (Do not continue usage longer than 3 days.)

HORSETAIL: *Used by Native Americans to help wounds to heal, this plant's high silica content makes it ideal for sitz baths.*

Traditional Usages

Also known as Shavegrass, Native Americans used Horsetail as a poultice to promote wound healing. The Thompson tribe in British Columbia applied the ashes of Horsetail fern stems to burns. A mild diuretic, Horsetail was administered to promote urination in dropsical complaints and kidney dysfunctions. Because the **diuretic action** of Horsetail grass is quite weak, it is likely to have been utilized in cases of very sensitive or weakened patients, or for pregnant women, as there were no deleterious side effects.

The cuticle of the stems contains abrasives which made the plant useful in scouring metal culinary articles; it was widely used by artisans for polishing wood, ivory, brass, and objects of similar materials.

Recent Scientific Findings

Although diuretic effects are attributed to extracts of *Equisetum hyemale* very frequently in literature, very few experiments have been carried out to verify this effect. At best, the experiments show a low level of diuretic activity, which is almost entirely attributable to the irritant action of silica that is present in the plant in high concentrations. It is highly questionable whether diuresis should be induced on the basis of a purely irritant effect on the kidneys, in that long-term ramifications of this continuous irritation could be detrimental.

Horsetail's silica content makes it useful in sitz baths, which aid in treating peripheral vascular disorders, chilblains, post-thrombotic swelling, as well as treating ligaments and tendons after ankle sprains and fractures. **The silica Horsetail contains is highly absorbable and is utilized to promote bone growth and collagen formation, two very important functions for menopausal women.** Horsetail has a high content of minerals in general, such as calcium, which promote the rebuilding of body tissue.

Current pharmacology indicates a reduction of edema in some cases of **arthritis** and swelling of legs, and tuberculostatic activity. A Horsetail tea has been recommended for **stomach ulcers**.

Caution: Long-term use could be detrimental to kidney function.

IPECAC

SCIENTIFIC NAME: *Cephaelis ipecacuanha, Euphorbia ipecacuanha*

PARTS USED: Root

DOSAGE:

Caution: Do *not* use the fluid-extract, unless advised by a physician. The syrup is far less dangerous.

IPECAC: *The aborigines of Brazil first discovered the properties of this popular emetic.*

Traditional Usages

The name *Ipecacuanha,* from the language of the Brazilian aborigines, has been applied to various **emetic** roots of South America. The Portuguese learned of this Indian remedy for **bowel problems** when they settled Brazil, and the root was introduced to Europe around 1672 as a remedy for **dysentery**.

Originally sold in Paris as a secret cure, the plant showed such value in bowel affections that no less a personage than Louis XIV eventually bestowed a large sum of money and public honors on the physician who popularized its use, on the condition that he make it public.

Like many other similar drugs, **Ipecac is emetic only in large doses**. In intermediate doses it is a nauseant, diaphoretic, and expectorant; **in small doses it is a mild stomach stimulant**, increasing the appetite and aiding digestion. Very small doses have also been used to treat the vomiting of pregnancy. When used as a nauseant, Ipecac was also observed to exert a **sedative effect** on the vascular system; hence it came to be employed for hemorrhages, particularly of the uterus.

Recent Scientific Findings

After it was introduced in Europe, Ipecac appeared to work extremely well in some cases of dysentery while it did nothing in others. Later evidence showed that the drug has no value against bacteria. Since there are two types of dysentery, one due to a specific amoeba and one due to a bacillus, Ipecac is useless against the bacillary form, while its amebecidal properties account for its being considered **probably the most efficacious remedy available against the amoebic type of dysentery**.

The major active constituents of Ipecac root are the alkaloids emetine and cephaeline. These potent drugs can cause adverse effects on the heart, but in proper dosage, they are not appreciably absorbed from the stomach or intestinal tract, and thus the bad effects are rarely encountered.

Perhaps the major use for Ipecac is in the form of *syrup* of Ipecac, which is widely publicized as a useful vomitive (emetic) to administer when people (especially children) have accidentally swallowed a poisonous substance and it is desired to remove the poison by using an emetic agent. If the proper amount is administered, emesis will take place within 15-20 minutes, and no adverse effects are noted.

Unfortunately, there have been a large number of cases in which *fluidextract* of Ipecac has been *erroneously* used for this purpose, and several deaths have been recorded due to such mistakes. *Fluidextract* of Ipecac is about twenty times more potent than *syrup* of Ipecac. When utilized as an expectorant, very small doses of Ipecac are required.

Recently, physicians have been recommending and research supports the use of activated charcoal instead of Ipecac in pediatric medicine.

IVY

SCIENTIFIC NAME: *Hedera helix*
PARTS USED: Leaves, berries, and exudate

DOSAGE:

No recommended dosages for internal use.

Resin: For external application, an infusion may be prepared using approximately 1 ounce of resin to 1 pint of water. Boil water separately and pour over the resin and steep for 5 to 20 minutes, depending on the desired strength.

Leaves: The leaves for external use are applied fresh, after being bruised and/or macerated.

IVY: *The leaves, berries, and gum exudate were each used for a variety of external and internal ailments.*

Traditional Usages

The resinous substance, which exudes through incisions in the bark, was used in medicine under the name Ivy Gum as a **stimulant** and an **emmenagogue** (stimulating the menstrual function). When placed in cavities of teeth, Ivy gum relieved **toothache**. Externally the resin has been used to **heal sores, ulcers**, etc.

Fresh Ivy leaves have been utilized as a dressing for wounds and sores that exude pus, and in decoction the leaves have been used to treat skin ulcers and various eruptions. The leaves were also employed as an **insecticide**.

The berries have been used as a purgative and emetic as well as to induce perspiration; in smaller doses they have been recommended as a cathartic.

Recent Scientific Findings

Recently, Ivy's saponins have been reported to be effective against internal **parasites**. Antimutagenic activity has also been observed.

The young twigs are a good source of a yellow and brown dye.

JALAP

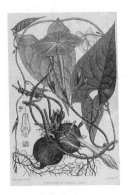

Jalap

SCIENTIFIC NAME: *Ipomoea purga*
(*Exogonium jalapa*)

PARTS USED: Root

DOSAGE:
Caution: Do not use.

JALAP: *The root resin is a very powerful cathartic.*

Traditional Usages

Jalap is a powerful cathartic. It was used widely during the seventeenth century in Europe as a purgative and to reduce fluid retention of tissues and organs in dropsical complaints.

At one time in the United States, Jalap root was administered in cases of complaints due to liver congestion, including constipation, headache, loss of appetite, and fever accompanied with vomiting of bile.

Recent Scientific Findings

Jalap root resin is well known to act as a **powerful hydragogue cathartic**, resulting in profuse watery stools when preparations of this plant are taken orally by humans. The action is due to a complex resin mixture which contains long chain fatty acids linked to glycerin.

> The cathartic action of Jalap is so harsh, powerful, and unpleasant that it is doubtful whether it should be used for any purpose.

We have been unable to verify any diuretic effect for this plant as reported in the scientific literature, nor any useful property that would allay the symptoms of dropsy.

JASMINE, YELLOW

SCIENTIFIC NAME: *Gelsemium sempervirens*

PARTS USED: Root

DOSAGE:

Caution: Not recommended for amateur use. A very potent drug. Overdose can cause death: 35 drops of bark tincture have caused death in 1½ hours, while 0.7 milliliter proved fatal to a 3-year-old boy.

When *prescribed*, the dose is usually 0.6 milliliter of the tincture or 0.12 milliliter of the fluidextract.

YELLOW JASMINE: *The roots contain gelsemine, a potent analgesic.*

Traditional Usages

Yellow, or Carolina, Jasmine was formerly employed as an arterial sedative and as an agent to reduce high fevers. According to Dr. Millspaugh, the herb's powers were discovered by accident when Jasmine was mistaken for another herb yet cured the patient's fever.

During the latter half of the nineteenth century, Jasmine was given to treat spasmodic diseases such as asthma and whooping cough. Due to recognized dangers of *Gelsemium* poisoning, use of the plant declined by World War I.

Recent Scientific Findings

The rhizomes and root contain a complex mixture of alkaloids, the major and most important one being gelsemine. Gelsemine has **very potent analgesic** effects of a specific type that has led to its valuable use in the relief of pain due to *tic douloureux* (trigeminal neuralgia), which is a condition relating to nerve pain in the cheek. The use of Yellow Jasmine to treat this condition is not without risk, however, since gelsemine does have a high order of toxicity.

Resembling Hemlock in its action, Yellow **Jasmine may lead to death by asphyxia.**

JIMSON WEED

SCIENTIFIC NAME: *Datura stramonium*
PARTS USED: Leaves

DOSAGE:
   Caution: Very potent drug.

JIMSON WEED: *The narcotic-like leaves are similar to Belladonna in their medicinal action.*

Traditional Usages

Tribes in California, southwestern United States, Mexico, and Central and South America took the varieties of this genus for a **narcotic effect.** Most commonly, Jimson Weed was used for divination. The leaves, stems, and roots were pounded and soaked in water for several hours. The solution was strained and then drunk. California tribes drank Jimson Weed as part of male puberty rites. California tribes and the Zuni also used it as an **anesthetic** when treating injuries such as broken bones. Many other tribes, including the Mohaves and Paiutes utilized the plant for similar purposes.

The name Jimson Weed originated in colonial Virginia. According to Robert Beverly's *History of Virginia*, soldiers sent to Jamestown to put down Bacon's Rebellion in 1676 gathered young shoots of Jimson Weed and cooked them as a vegetable.

   . . . the Effect of which was a very pleasant Comedy; for they turn'd natural Fools upon it for Several Days; One would blow up a Feather in the Air; another would dart Straws at it with much Fury; and another stark naked was sitting up in a Corner, like a Monkey, grinning and making Mows at them; a Fourth would fondly kiss, and paw his Companions, and smear in their Faces, with a Countenance more antick, than any in a *Dutch* Droll. In this frantick Condition they were confined, lest they should in their Folly destroy themselves; though it was observed, that all their Actions were full of Innocence and good Nature. Indeed, they were not very cleanly; for they would have wallow'd in their own Excrements, if they had not been prevented. A Thousand such simple Tricks they play'd, and after Eleven Days, return'd themselves again, not remembering any thing that had pass'd.

In 37 and 38 B.C. Anthony's legion consumed Jimson Weed with equally comic results.

Dr. Millspaugh describes the plant being employed as a cure for rabies. In the early 1900s, leaves of Jimson Weed were made into cigarettes and smoked for **asthma.** Interestingly, the violent mania and other mental symptoms produced by the plant led to its use in treating insanity and epilepsy, with some reported success.

Homeopathic doses were administered to treat skin eruptions, hemorrhoids, hysteria, and neuralgias. In spasmodic asthma, the leaves, smoked in cigarettes, or their steam, inhaled from an infusion, reportedly provided great tem-

porary relief and facilitated expectoration, but extreme caution was advised in any such use of the plant.

Recent Scientific Findings

All parts of the plant contain Belladonna-like alkaloids that render it both **medicinal and toxic.** Jimson Weed is very similar to Belladonna in its action in both large and small doses, and in its toxicity and therapeutic action. The two plants were used interchangeably to check secretions, stimulate circulation, stimulate respiration, overcome spasms of the involuntary muscles, and externally as a local anodyne. Atropine poisoning may follow external as well as internal application.

While Jimson Weed is employed for about the same purposes as Belladonna, **Jimson Weed usually contains higher concentrations of scopolamine than does Belladonna.** Because of this, Jimson Weed has been used to some extent as a recreational hallucinogenic drug, either by taking extracts orally, or by smoking the plant parts. There are a large number of published medical reports that confirm this effect in humans.

Jimson Weed is also very effective in relieving the symptoms of asthma by either burning the leaves and inhaling the smoke, or by inhaling the smoke from *stramonium* cigarettes. The active alkaloids are volatile and pass with the smoke into the lungs. They then exert their effect by relaxing the smooth muscle of that organ, which is constricted during an asthmatic attack, thereby allowing the person to breathe more freely.

As with Belladonna, similar precautions in use must be observed because of the powerful action of this plant.

JUNIPER BERRY

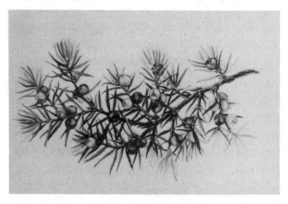

Juniper Berry

SCIENTIFIC NAME: *Juniperus communis*
PARTS USED: Berry

DOSAGE:

Berries: 3 ounces of the berries to 1 pint of boiling water, poured over the berries and steep for 5 to 20 minutes, depending on the desired effect. Drink hot or warm, 1 cup every 4 to 5 hours, to which may be added extract of Dandelion, or cream of tartar.

JUNIPER BERRIES: *Long used as a gentle diuretic, preliminary studies indicate this may also be a valuable arthritis treatment.*

Traditional Usages

Juniper berries are a **gentle stimulant and diuretic,** imparting an odor of violets to the urine. Taken in large quantities, they occasionally produce irritation of the urinary passages. Their principal use was as an adjuvant to more powerful diuretics in problems of fluid retention. The berries were also used as carminatives, stomachics, antiseptics, and stimulants. The volatile oil distilled from the berries was used as a carminative to aid the expulsion of intestinal flatulence, and also as a diuretic. For a period of time, the *U.S. Pharmacopoeia* recommended them to **promote menstruation**. The aromatic berries have been employed in folk medicine to **lower serum cholesterol** and as an **anticancer remedy**.

Juniper berries make an excellent survival food because they are edible and available through part of the winter. The tree's inner bark is also edible and was eaten by many Native Americans to fight off starvation. Some tribes dried the berries and baked the ground fruits into cakes or mush. Roasted juniper berries were ground and substituted for coffee. In British Columbia, the stems and leaves were boiled to make an astringent tea. Juniper berries are also the primary source of flavoring for gin.

Recent Scientific Findings

Though the USFDA considers this plant an "unsafe herb," there is no known data to substantiate this conclusion. Experimentally, **antitumor activity** has been shown in animals, along with strong cytotoxic activity in cell culture against HELA cancer cells. Studies have also found **antiviral activity** in cell culture against influenza virus A2 and herpes simplex virus I and II, as well as antibacterial activity in vitro against several human pathogens.

The primary use, however, has been as a **diuretic**, and this effect has been substantiated in animal studies. The active diuretic principle has been shown to be a simple terpene, terpinene-4-ol.

Although there is no direct experimental evidence that Juniper berries would be effective in the treatment of **gout**, studies have been conducted in humans that indicate a value in treating **arthritis**. Both gout and arthritis are acute inflammatory conditions, and drugs effective for one of these conditions are usually found useful in the other.

The mildly stimulant effect attributed to Juniper berries is due to the action of constituents in the essential oil.

Caution: May irritate kidneys. Do not use more than six consecutive weeks. Juniper may stimulate uterine contractions and cause abortion.

KAVA KAVA

SCIENTIFIC NAME: *Piper methysticum*
PARTS USED: Root

DOSAGE:

Root: The Fiji Islanders take one large handful of the dried, powdered root and wrap it in a cheesecloth. In one quart of cold water they knead the Kava-Kava until the liquid is a *dark* chalky gray. They stir and drink at once, several cupfuls, unsweetened. They then add water, reknead the root, and drink as desired until sedation is felt.

KAVA KAVA: *This drink has been a part of Polynesian religious and social life since antiquity.*

Traditional Usages

Kava is native to the Pacific Islands. In early times it was distributed eastward through tropical islands by migrating people, who valued the root both as a drink and medicine. In Hawaii more than 15 varieties were known. In many islands of the Pacific, Kava has long played an important part in the life of the people, being used in ceremonies, festivals, and as a sign of good will.

The root is used to prepare the ceremonial drink of many inhabitants of Melanesian and Polynesia. This drink is reputedly **sedative, aphrodisiac, tonic, stimulant, diuretic,** and **diaphoretic.** While both men and women drink Kava nowadays, in former times tribal custom forbade women to partake. Young virgins would masticate the root to prepare the beverage for the men's ceremonial purposes. The root has a faint but characteristic odor, an aromatic, bitter, pungent taste, with a slight local anesthesia resulting.

Recent Scientific Findings

A number of compounds referred to as "Kava pyrones" (for example, kawain, dihydrokawain, methysticin, and dihydromethysticin) are claimed to have mild **sedative** and **tranquilizing** effects. Kawain is marketed in Europe as a mild sedative for the elderly. Extracts of Kava, and most of the Kava pyrones have been shown to have **antiseptic** properties in test tube experiments.

Animal studies clearly point out a marked ability of extracts of Kava to calm enraged animals. **Anticonvulsant** activity has been observed in adult human and animal models. The principle responsible for this effect has not yet been discovered.

Regular and prolonged use of Kava extracts results in the production of a skin rash, which is pigmented yellow. This condition, among Kava users in the South Pacific, is known as "Kawaism." The condition subsides following restriction of the Kava beverage, with no ill effects. It is important to remember that this plant has been utilized for it calming effects in Oceania since antiquity. While the introduction of alcohol has created many social problems, those groups still using this plant in its traditional way enjoy a mild insulation from life's vicissitudes.

KINO

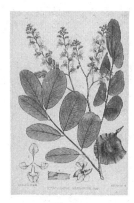

Kino

SCIENTIFIC NAME: *Pterocarpus marsupium,*
P. indicus,
P. echinatus

PARTS USED: Exudate (juice from incisions in trunk of tree)

DOSAGE:

Exudate: For internal use—
.05-2.0 grams of powdered exudate, dissolved in 1 cup of boiling water, taken 1 cup per day, 1 tablespoon at a time. For external use, powdered exudate is applied directly to the affected area.

KINO: *The juice is a powerful astringent.*

Traditional Usages

Kino is the name given to the juice that exudes from incisions in the trunk of the tree *Pterocarpus marsupium.* It was deemed a powerful astringent and as such was used externally to check discharges from wounds, scrapes, and skin ulcers. In combination with Opium or chalk mixtures, it was administered to treat **non-inflammatory diarrheas.** Kino was never given in the presence of fever.

It has also been used to treat passive hemorrhages of the intestines and uterus, diabetes, and as a gargle to relax the throat. Aromatic substances were often added to the Kino to make it more palatable.

A related species, from Africa, *P. angloensis* (Bloodwood), used as substitute for Indian teak, is famed as an aphrodisiac.

The roots were employed for this activity in the Congo, Angola, Tanzania, Mozambique, and the Transvaal.

Recent Scientific Findings

Kino's **astringent action** is primarily due to the presence of a tannin-like substance, kinotannic acid, which also gives it application in the treatment of leucorrhea by injection.

LADY SLIPPER,
Domesticated

SCIENTIFIC NAME: *Cypripedium
parviflorum*

PARTS USED: Root

DOSAGE:

.05 to 2.0 grams of pow-
dered root, dissolved in 2 cups
of boiling water. Drink 1 tablespoon at a time during the entire day.

LADY SLIPPER: *This beautiful flower
deserves further research as a mild nerve
medicine.*

Traditional Usages

Several North American tribes used
the Lady Slipper as a **nerve medicine**. It
later became an accepted cure for
insomnia in domestic American
medicine. A medical botanist of the first
half of the 19th century, Rafinesque,
introduced Lady Slipper to medical
circles.

Of this beautiful genus, all the species
are equally medical; they have been long
known to the Indians . . . They produce
beneficial effects in all nervous diseases
and hysterical affections, by allaying
pain, quieting the nerves and promoting
sleep.

The roots were official in the *U.S.*
Pharmacopoeia from 1863 to 1916. They
were primarily used as an **antispasmodic**
and a **nerve medicine**. Dr. Millspaugh
wrote that "This is one of our drugs that
has not been sufficiently thought of by
provers . It merits a full proving . . ." And
it still does!

Recent Scientific Findings

Lady Slipper is another drug plant
that was once popularly prescribed but
has been superseded by synthetic agents.
Lady Slipper may act similarly to
Valerian, in milder form, to **lessen
anxiety and restlessness.**

LAVENDER

SCIENTIFIC NAME: *Lavandula officinalis*
(*L. vera* and *L. spica*)

PARTS USED: Flowers (and oil)

DOSAGE:

Flowers: 1 teaspoon of the flowers, cut small or granulated, to 1 cup of boiling water. Boil water separately and pour over the plant material and steep for 5-20 minutes, depending on the desired effect. Drink cold, a large mouthful at a time, 1 cup during the day.

LAVENDER: *The aromatic oil of the flower often is used in combination with other herbs and pharmaceuticals.*

Traditional Usages

The flowers, as well as the oil, are employed chiefly in perfumery, but their fragrance also led to their use to disguise nasty-smelling herbal and other pharmaceutical preparations. Bunches of the dried flowers are used to make sachets and for imparting a gentle scent to linen.

Oil distilled from Lavender flowers is utilized medicinally as an aromatic stimulant, mild carminative, tonic, and to treat nervous languor and headache. Interestingly, the oil (known as "oil of aspic") is also used in varnishes to dilute delicate colors in china paintings.

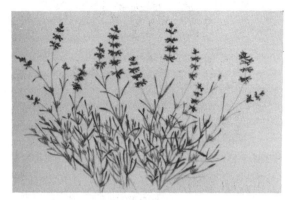

Lavender

Recent Scientific Findings

Chemically, the plant contains 1-linalyl acetate, geraniol, and linalol. Lavender flowers contain large amounts of a highly aromatic oil, and have definite **spasmolytic**, **antiseptic**, and **carminative** activity. These activities are all attributed to the essential oil, and its aromatic principles.

LEMONGRASS

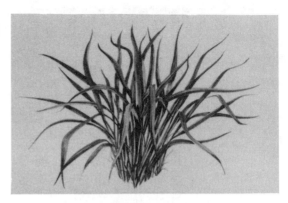

Lemongrass

SCIENTIFIC NAME: *Cymbopogon citratus*
PARTS USED: Oil

DOSAGE:

LEMONGRASS: *The tasty tea has long been a mild sedative due to myrcene, an analgesic that may also reduce cholesterol.*

Traditional Usages

Lemongrass tea has long been used as a before bed drink to promote sleep. In traditional Brazilian medicine, Lemongrass has been widely used as an analgesic and as a sedative.

Lemongrass oil is found in all citrus fruits. It is a common food flavoring and ingredient in cosmetics and perfumes. The oil is a source of ionone, which is made into a synthetic violet.

Recent Scientific Findings

Lemongrass's essential oil contains the monoterpene myrcene, an **analgesic**, thus confirming Lemongrass tea's traditional use as a **mild sedative**. One team of researchers concluded that "Terpenes such as myrcene may constitute a lead for the development of new peripheral analgesics with a profile of action different from that of the aspirin-like drugs."

Myrcene was also found to reduce the toxic and mutagenic effect of cyclophosphamide in in vitro experiments. In other words, myrcene may possess **antimutagenic** properties.

Lemongrass oil has also been reported to possess strong **antibacterial** activity in vitro against several human pathogens. For instance, a 1988 study found an appreciable increase in activity against *Escherichia coli* and *Staphylococcus aureus.*

Lemongrass oil is also rich in geraniol and citral, both of which may contribute to **lowering serum cholesterol levels**. In one study involving 22 hypercholesterolemic patients, cholesterol levels were lowered.

However, to date there is no laboratory evidence to support Lemongrass' reputed folkloric ability to relieve anxiety.

LETTUCE, WILD

SCIENTIFIC NAME: *Lactuca elongata*
PARTS USED: Latex

DOSAGE:

Latex: When used for its sedative effects, the latex of Wild Lettuce was taken in a dose of 3.0 to 12 grams every 24 hours.

WILD LETTUCE: *Since ancient times, the milk latex has been an effective mild sedative.*

Traditional Usages

Wild Lettuce has been used in use as a **painkiller** and **relaxant** since ancient times. It is mentioned by the Greeks Dioscorides, Galen, and Theophrastus, among others.

In North America, Meskwaki women imbibed a lettuce leaf tea to promote the **secretion of milk after childbirth**, as did the Flambeau Ojibwas. The Menominees applied the milky juice to **poison ivy** rash.

The medicinal effects depend upon the milky juice that exudes when the stem or the flower stalks are lacerated. In color, taste, and odor, this juice strongly resembles Opium. The medicinal preparation consists of the juice in hardened, evaporated form and is known as lactucarium. As a sedative and diuretic, it was official in the *U.S. Pharmacopoeia* from 1820 to 1926. More recently, it has been revived to some extent among the drug culture in the form of a commercial preparation known as "**Lettuce Opium.**"

Recent Scientific Findings

Lactucarium, found in this and other species of Lettuce, is obtained by wounding the plants in the flowering season when their vessels are filled with juice and so irritable that they often spontaneously burst or are ruptured by very slight accidental injuries.

This fresh milky latex contains a sedative principle known as lactupicrin. The best way to collect this juice is by placing successive small pieces of cotton on the cut stem and throwing them into a little water. After a quantity has accumulated, the water holding in solution the contents of the pieces of cotton is evaporated, and an extract thus procured. An easier way to collect the latex is by macerating the stems and leaves in water, just after the seeds have matured and before the plant decays. The maceration is to be continued for 24 hours, then the liquid is boiled for 2 hours, and finally evaporated in shallow basins.

Lactucarium has very mild pain allaying and calmative effects, somewhat **like a weak dose of opium**. It may best be employed as a **mild sedative**. It was also used as a draught in constipation, intestinal disorders such as engorgements, and for other gastric upsets.

LICORICE

SCIENTIFIC NAME: *Glycyrrhiza glabra*
PARTS USED: Root

DOSAGE:

Root: 1 teaspoon of the root or subterranean stem, boiled in a covered container with 1½ pints of water for about ½ hour, at a slow boil. Allow liquid to cool slowly in the *closed* container. Drink cold, 1 swallow or 1 tablespoon at a time, 1 to 2 cups per day.

LICORICE: *The roots contain glycyrrhizin, which is about 50 times sweeter than sugar and exhibits a powerful cortisone-like effect.*

Traditional Usages

Among the ancient Greeks, Licorice root had a reputation for quenching thirst, and was used in this connection to treat dropsy. It is an excellent **demulcent** and is soothing to the mucus membrane, hence was given to treat irritated urinary, bowel, and respiratory passages. It was often given in combination with Senega and Mezereon, when these drugs were used on persons with irritated or inflamed eliminatory organs. The root also reportedly had expectorant and **laxative** properties.

The Blackfoot steeped the leaves in water and used this liquid for **earaches.** The edible roots of American licorice were boiled and the tea drunk by the early white settlers, who either learned of this remedy from Native Americans or adapted a European remedy.

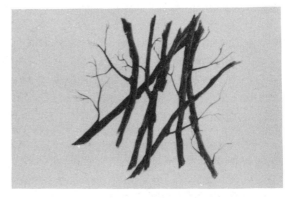

Licorice

In China, Licorice root became a major tonic to combat fevers and as a remedy for infections. For centuries, it has one of the most commonly employed herbs in Chinese medicine; most prescriptions include Licorice as a component.

Children suck on Licorice sticks both as candies and as a remedy for coughs. Licorice is a valuable flavoring adjunct to medicines with unpleasant tastes. The powered root was utilized in the preparation of pills, both to give them more substance and to coat the surfaces to prevent their sticking together.

In the 1940s, Dutch physicians tested Licorce's reputation as an aid for indigestion. Their research resulted in the

the drug carbenoxolone, which was used to aid peptic ulcer patients. Though the drug proved effective, it also resulted in the adverse side effect of excessive swelling of the limbs and face.

Recent Scientific Findings

The multitude of pharmacological effects of Licorice rhizomes and roots are practically all attributed to the presence of a triterpene saponin called *glycyrrhizin,* which is about fifty times sweeter than sugar, and has a powerful cortisone-like effect. Several cases have been reported in medical literature in which humans ingesting 6-8 ounces (a very large amount) of licorice candy daily for a period of several weeks are "poisoned" due to the cortisone-like effects of licorice extract in the candy. Proper treatment restores patients to normal. The above amount of this compound is very large compared with the relatively small amount found in supplements.

In addition, Licorice rhizomes and roots have a high mucilage content. When mixed with water, the resulting preparation has a very pleasant odor and taste, and acts as an effective demulcent on irritated mucous membranes, such as accompany a **sore throat**. One study found that glycyrrhizin was as effective a **cough suppressant** as codeine. A 1991 experiment with mice found that glycyrrhizin protected against skin cancer. The authors speculated that it might prove useful in protecting against some forms of **human cancer** as well.

It is not surprising that Licorice and glycyrrhizin have such wide applications. It should be noted that this chemical constitutes only 7 to 10% of the total root (on a dry weight basis). Glycyrrhetic acid (G.A.) is obtained when acid hydrolysis is applied to the main component of licorice. This compound is extensively used in Europe for its **anti-inflammatory** properties, especially in **Addison's disease** and **peptic ulcer**. Some European researchers concluded that G.A. may be preferred to cortisone because it is safer, especially when prolonged treatment is required.

A recent study (1990) demonstrated that G.A. exerts its activity *not* as a *direct effect* but by reducing the conversion of cortisol to cortisone, its biologically inactive product. The authors concluded that hydrocortisone, a "weak anti-inflammatory agent," can be greatly potentiated (i.e., made more powerful) by the addition of 2% GA. To lessen the toxic effects of corticosteroids, the authors suggested that patients use hydrocortisone *together* with GA. Here is another example of the growing marriage between prescription pharmaceuticals and herbal preparations.

Glycyrrhizin has also exhibited **antiviral** activity. A 1979 study demonstrated that **glycyrrhizin inhibited Epstein-Barr Virus (EBV), cytomegalovirus (CMV),** and hepatitis B virus. In Japan, glycyrrhizin has long been successfully used to treat **chronic hepatitis B**. This has led to speculation that glycyrrhizin holds promise in the treatment of HIV.

A note of caution: Side effects from the ingestion of large amounts of Licorice have been reported. Glycyrrhizin in very large amounts can promote hypokalemia and hypertension. For these reasons people with heart problems and high blood pressure are advised to avoid consuming large quantities of Licorice or its components.

LILY-OF-THE-VALLEY

SCIENTIFIC NAME: *Convallaria majalis*
PARTS USED: Root, fruit, flowers

DOSAGE:

Flowers or Root: Of either the flowers or the root, as a cardiotonic, 0.32-0.65 gram.

Caution: This plant has a powerful digitalis-like effect.

LILY-OF-THE-VALLEY: *This lovely flower contains glycosides that make a powerful cardiotonic that is currently popular in Europe.*

Traditional Usages

The major traditional use for Lily-of-the-Valley seems to be as a cardiotonic. It has long been used as a popular remedy for dropsy. It was also employed to expel worms from the intestinal tract.

The flowers were believed to stimulate the secretions of the mucous membranes of the nose. They also were employed in the treatment of apoplexy, epilepsy, coma, and vertigo. Spirits distilled from the flowers were applied externally on sprains and to treat rheumatism.

The root was employed for the same maladies as the flowers. Also an extract of the root was used for its gentle stimulant and laxative properties.

Recent Scientific Findings

Lily-of-the-Valley's effective use as a cardiotonic is explained on the basis of the presence of cardiac glycosides similar in structure and effect to the *Digitalis* glycosides. The major cardiac glycoside in Lily-of-the-Valley is convallatoxin.

Since there are no advantages of *Convallaria* as a cardiotonic over the effect of *Digitalis purpurea* (Foxglove), it is not commonly used in the United States. However, it is employed extensively in Europe at the present time.

LINDEN

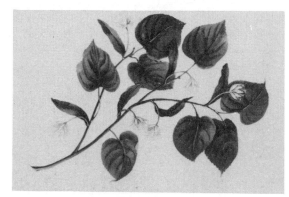

Linden

SCIENTIFIC NAME: *Tilia cordata,*
Tilia europaea
PARTS USED: Flowers and leaves

DOSAGE:

Leaves: Approximately 1 ounce of leaves to 1 pint of water. Boil water separately and pour over the plant material and steep for 5 to 20 minutes, depending on the desired effect. Drink hot or warm, 1 to 2 cups per day, at bedtime and upon awakening.

LINDEN: *Once a popular home remedy in Europe and North America, little recent research has been conducted to confirm or deny folkloric claims.*

Traditional Usages

The flowers of many of the different species of this tree were used in both Europe and North America as a **home remedy for colds, sore throats, coughs,** and flu. The leaves were also sometimes used in North America for the same afflictions. The flowers were also an **antispasmodic** and **nervine.**

Externally, the inner bark's mucilage was applied for various skin conditions, such as sores, burns, and wounds. The burned wood was also used as a wound application.

Recent Scientific Findings

Linden contains flavonoids. However, no medical use has been found for Linden, though it does make a pleasing tea.

LOBELIA

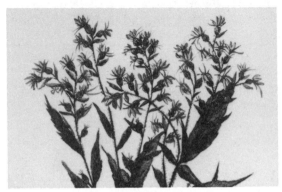

Lobelia

SCIENTIFIC NAME: *Lobelia inflata*
PARTS USED: Leaves and seeds

DOSAGE:

Tincture: When used in asthma was given in doses of 0.9 millimeter every hour(!).

Fluidextract: When used as an antispasmodic, was given in doses of 0.13-0.5 gram.

LOBELIA: *This controversial herb was at the center of the Thomsonian system of herbal medicine; current evidence suggests that Lobelia may aid smokers to quit.*

Traditional Usages

Sometimes called "Indian Tobacco," this species of Lobelia is a very common weed, growing throughout the United States. The Meskwaki tribe finely ground the roots of red and blue lobelias and secretly put it into the food eaten by a quarreling couple. This tribe felt this preparation "averts divorce and makes the pair love each other again." The Iroquois used a root decoction of Lobelia to treat syphilis. In the early 1800s, English physicians adapted this cure. Dr. Millspaugh theorizes why the plant failed to effect a cure when employed in Europe:

> The natives of North America are said to have held this plant a secret in the cure of syphilis, until it was purchased from them . . . and introduced . . . as a drug of great repute in that disease. Euro-pean physicians, however, failed to cure with it, and finally cast it aside, though Linnaeus, thinking it justified its Indian reputation, gave the species its distinctive name, *syphilitica*. The cause of failure may be the fact that the aborigines did not trust to the plant alone, but always used it in combination with May-apple roots (*Poldophyllum peltatum*), the bark of the Wild Cherry (*Prunus Virginica*), and dusted the ulcers with the powdered bark of New Jersey tea (*Ceanothus Americanus*). Another chance of failure lay in the votality of its active principle, as the dried herb was used.

This controversial herb was the mainstay of the system of herbal medicine introduced by Samuel Thomson, who wrote in the third edition of his *Botanic Family Physician* (Boston, 1831): "In consequence of their [accredited doctors] thus forming an erroneous opinion of this herb, which they had no knowledge of, they undertook to represent it as a deadly poison; and in order to destroy my practice, they raised a hue and cry about my killing my patients by administering it to them." Thomson's book is largely given over to passionate protestations toward the medical establishment, which he felt was persecuting him.

Lobelia was reported useful in treating bronchitis, laryngitis, asthma, and convulsive and inflammatory disorders such as epilepsy, tetanus, diphtheria, and tonsillitis.

As a **muscle relaxant**, Lobelia was employed in midwifery to alleviate rigidity of the pelvic musculature during childbirth, according to the recommendations of one of Thomson's followers. Use externally in a poultice with Slippery Elm and a little soap, Lobelia was helpful in bringing abscesses and boils to a head.

Recent Scientific Findings

The precautions about the poisonous potential of the plant are always mentioned by herbalists other than those practicing the Thomsonian system. Lobelia, along with twenty-six other plants, has been declared an "unsafe herb" by the U.S. Food and Drug Administration, which describes it was "a poisonous plant which contains the alkaloid lobelia, plus a number of other pyridine alkaloids. Overdoses of the plant or extracts of the leaves or fruits produce vomiting, sweating, pain, paralysis, depressed temperatures, rapid but feeble pulse, collapse, coma and death in the human being." The effects of excessive doses, classified by herbalists as "acro-narcotic," are similar to those of tobacco; hence its popular name, Indian Tobacco.

Lobelia leaves and flowering tops do contain the alkaloid lobeline, which is know to relax smooth muscle and thus would give rise to an **antispasmodic** effect. Extracts of the leaves have been shown experimentally to have expectorant properties, most likely due to the lobeline content.

Lobeline is used to stimulate respiration in newborn infant. It is a popular smoking deterrent when taken orally in small doses. Human experimental evidence attest to its value in aiding smokers to drop the habit, contradicting the possibly excessive cautions of the USFDA.

MADDER

SCIENTIFIC NAME: *Rubia tinctorum*
PARTS USED: Root

DOSAGE:

   Root: 1 teaspoon of the root, boiled in a covered container of 1½ pints of water for about ½ hour, at a slow boil. Allow liquid to cool slowly in the *closed* container. Drink cold, 1 swallow or 1 tablespoon at a time, 1 to 2 cups per day.

MADDER: *The ancient Greeks thought the roots treated a number of complaints, but in modern times Madder fell largely into disuse except as a facial to remove freckles.*

Traditional Usages

   The principal use of the Madder root has been as the source of a red dye for fabrics. Madder seemingly became popular as a medicinal only because of its very unusual ability to impart a red color to the urine and bones when taken internally, especially in young animals. It does not dye the surrounding tissues and seems to concentrate on the bones nearest the heart.

   Madder enjoyed a striking reputation among the ancient Greek physicians for its reported ability to promote the flow of urine and menstruation, cure dysentery and jaundice, and aid in childbirth. Its use to promote menstruation and its inclusion in remedies for dropsical complaints, as well as its employment to treat internal wounds and bruises, may have been traceable to the early physicians' belief that a plant that could dye urine and bones, as well as the beaks and feet of birds that fed upon it, must be good for the blood and bones. More recently Madder roots and rhizomes have been used for their tonic and astringent properties.

Recent Scientific Findings

   Dyers' Madder has become virtually obsolete in medicine in more recent times. However, **Madder roots are known to cause contractions of uterine muscle in certain types of laboratory experiments.** In some cases, contraction of uterine muscle can result in the induction of menstruation, and thus would have beneficial effects in women suffering from amenorrhea. A Madder extract, Lucidin, have proven genotoxic in laboratory tests.

   We have been unable to locate experimental evidence that would substantiate the use of Madder in treating dropsy. **Nevertheless, the bruised roots and leaves have attained some reputation as a facial for the removal of freckles!**

MAGNOLIA

SCIENTIFIC NAME: *Magnolia glauca* and other *Magnolia* species

PARTS USED: Bark and root bark

DOSAGE:

Bark: For medicinal applications, 1 teaspoon of the bark, cut small or granulated, is boiled in a covered container with 1½ pints of water for about ½ hour at a slow boil. Allow liquid to cool slowly in the *closed* container. Drink cold, 1 swallow or 1 tablespoon at a time, 1 to 2 cups per day.

MAGNOLIA: *The bark of this beautiful tree mitigates malaria and future research may confirm preliminary antitumor findings.*

Traditional Usages

Various Native American tribes employed Magnolia as a remedy for **rheumatism**, to expel **worms**, and for cramps. Colonial settlers employed the bark by putting it into brandy or boiling it any other liquor. They used it to ease pectoral diseases, as well as internal pains and fever, and dysentery.

Owing to their diaphoretic properties, the barks of various Magnolias were taken to **mitigate the ravages of malarial as well as other intermittent fevers.** Used in place of Cinchona (Quinine), Magnolia could be administered for longer periods of time with no side effects.

There is some record of the Magnolia bark's usefulness as a substitute for tobacco and as an aid for breaking the habit of chewing tobacco. Official in the *U.S. Pharmacopoeia* from 1820 to 1894, the dried bark of three magnolia species (*M. virginiana, M. acuminata,* and *M. tripetala*) was recommended in doses of 2.0 to 3.9 grams.

M. officinalis is prized in Chinese herbalism as a tonic, and is considered aphrodisiac. In Mexico, *M. Schiedeana* in a flower decoction applied topically is used to treat scorpion stings. Perhaps most interesting of all medicinal properties of Magnolias is reported of a species found in Brazil (*M. pubescent*). The stems, leaves, and seeds contain saponins capable of stupefying fish and are employed for this purpose by fishermen wanting an easier catch.

Recent Scientific Findings

Only recently have the various Magnolias begun to be subjected to the scrutiny of the laboratory. One team of researchers isolated three neolignans from Magnolia bark. They found that these extracts exhibited **"remarkable inhibitory effects" on tumors in mice and in vivo.**

One of these three extracts, Magnolol, possessed the qualities of an **antiplatelet agent** in a preliminary study.

MAIDENHAIR FERN

SCIENTIFIC NAME: *Adiantum pedatum,*
A. capillus-veneris

PARTS USED: Herb

DOSAGE:

Herb: For medicinal use, one teaspoon of the herb is added to 1 cup of boiling water. Drink cold, 1 tablespoon at a time, up to a total of 1 to 2 cups per day.

MAIDENHAIR FERN: *This herb was commonly used for coughs and congestion.*

Traditional Usages

Maidenhair Fern was most commonly employed to **relieve coughs of colds and nasal congestion**. It was believed to relieve thirst and fever, as well as stimulate secretions of the bronchopulmonary mucous membranes. In this latter expectorant function, it was used for asthma and other pulmonary congestive disorders.

A **dandruff remedy** employing Maidenhair Fern was reported by some herbalists. The ashes of this fern were combined with vinegar and olive oil, and applied to the scalp.

Recent Scientific Findings

Extracts of a related fern, *Adiantum caudatum,* have been studied in animals. These experiments indicate that extracts of the fern are capable of relaxing smooth muscle, a finding that is in support of the use of *A. pedatum* and *A. capillusveneris* for **asthma**. Further work is obviously necessary before one can validate the effectiveness of these herbal remedies.

MALE FERN

SCIENTIFIC NAME: *Dryopteris filix-mas*
(Aspidium filix-mas)
PARTS USED: Rhizome

DOSAGE:
See below.

MALE FERN: *Since the ancient Greeks, this plant has been employed to relieve intestinal worms.*

Traditional Usages

The ancient Greeks Theophrastus, Dioscorides, and Pliny all recommended Male Fern for use in expelling **tapeworms** and other **parasitic worms** from the intestines; they advised combining the fern with wine and barley meal. A certain Madame Nouffer sold her secret remedy to Louis XVI for 18,000 francs, which led to widespread use of Male Fern in the 19th century. It was often taken on an empty stomach, followed in two hours by a dose of castor oil or other mild purgative. **Excessive doses can be poisonous, so this fern was always used very carefully.**

Recent Scientific Findings

The oleoresin from the rhizomes of Male Fern is a **well-known anthelmintic**, owing its activity to a complex mixture of substances known collectively as "filicin." Male Fern oleoresin is almost exclusively employed to remove tapeworms from the intestinal tract. When used properly it is quite safe, but if used improperly it can be more toxic to the person taking it than to the tapeworm.

Thus, before using Asidium oleoresin, a person should maintain a fat-free diet for 24 hours. A saline cathartic such as citrate of magnesia should then be taken, but not oily cathartics. The reasons for this is that the filicin is very poisonous if it is absorbed into the body from the intestine. It will only do this if there is fat or oil present. The cathartic will not remove the tapeworm since it has "hooks" on its head (scolex) that attach to the intestine wall. When a single dose of Aspidium oleoresin is taken, the filicin numbs and/or paralyzes the tapeworm and it releases its hold on the intestinal wall. After a short period of time another dose of the saline (not oily) cathartic is taken and the tapeworm is flushed out of the body.

It is important that the feces be examined to see if the head (scolex) of the tapeworm has been removed. Tapeworms can be up to 15 or more feet in length, and practically all of the worm could be flushed out of the body, but if the scolex remains, it will continue to reproduce and form another full-size parasite.

MANDRAKE

SCIENTIFIC NAME: *Podophyllum peltatus*
(American),
Mandragora offici-narium (European)

PARTS USED: Root

DOSAGE:
Caution: Safer purgatives than the American Mandrake exist.

MANDRAKE: *At one time the subject of horrific superstitions, extracts of this plant recently have proven effective for rheumatoid arthritis.*

Traditional Usages

The fantastic myths and legends surrounding the Mandrakes result from the root's uncanny likeness to a human body with its appendages. The more closely it resembles the human figure, the more highly is the root's value in folkloric medicine. It was such a prized commodity at one time that collectors invented dire horror stories surrounding inappropriate methods of collection, predicting horrible consequences, to discourage entrepreneurs from trading.

European Mandrake's shape gained it a reputation as an aphrodisiac, probably based on the "doctrine of signatures." The Greeks associated the plant with Aphrodite. During the Middle Ages, superstitions abounded concerning Mandrake.

The American Mandrake, or May Apple, was used by Native Americans for its cathartic effects long before its "rediscovery" for American medicine.

American Mandrake has been employed in cases of **chronic constipation** for its cathartic effect, as well as in problems arising from liver congestion, and also as a remedy for ridding people of **worms**. The resin derived form the root was considered a safe and reliable substitute in all cases where mercury was indicated, earning this plant its nicknames, "Vegetable Mercury" and "Vegetable Calomel."

While the drug is characterized as a "drastic purgative," an early visitor to North America reported than an Indian woman had used the root to commit suicide. An 1890 medical journal described a case of a 60-year-old woman's death after ingesting five grams of the resin.

It was widely employed by the ancients for its **narcotic value** and as an anesthetic prior to surgery. "Morion," or "Death Wine," said to have been administered previous to the torture, was made from it.

Recent Scientific Findings

European Mandrake is related to *Atropa* species and contains tropane alkaloids similar in structure and biological effects to those in *A. belladonna*. Hence the **anodyne, sedative,** and **poisonous** effects attributed to the use of this plant have a sound basic in fact. The plant is on the March 1977, USFDA unsafe herb list. For side effects and contraindications to the use of European Mandrake, the reader should refer to Belladonna.

The rhizomes and roots of American Mandrake contain the toxic and irritant principles podophyllotoxin, alpha-pelatin, and beta-peltatin. They are responsible for the well established purgative effect of this plant. Podophyllotoxin is a safe and effective application for external **genital warts.**

Another podophyllum extract, CPH 82, has been shown to be effective against **rheumatoid arthritis.** A double-blind placebo-controlled study was conducted over a 12-week period. The placebo patients showed no improvement. However, the patients treated with CPH 82 showed significant improvement.

There is no scientific evidence that this plant has sedative, anodyne, or aphrodisiac effects as has been claimed by some folkloric practitioners.

MANNA

SCIENTIFIC NAME: *Fraxinus ornus*
PARTS USED: Dried exudate from bark

DOSAGE:

Exudate: Approximately ½ ounce of the dried exudate, powdered to pint of water. Boil water separately and pour over the plant material and steep for 5-20 minutes, depending on the desired effect. Drink hot or warm, 1 to 2 cups per day.

MANNA: *Not the "manna from heaven," however, the bark is a safe laxative for children.*

Traditional Usages

This is not the manna of the Bible. Most botanists agree the Scriptural manna was probably the lichen *Lecanora esculenta,* from which bread may be produced; others say it was from the shrub *Tamarix mannifera.*

Rather Manna is the name given to the dried saccharine exudate of the "Manna-Ash" tree. The Manna exudes spontaneously from the bark, but for commercial purposes, when it is cultivated as a crop, incisions are made in the trunk to produce a larger yield.

Recent Scientific Findings

In combination with Senna or Rhubarb, whose taste is concealed by the aromatic Manna, the effect is **purgative.** Taken alone, Manna is a **gentle laxative,** which may occasionally produce the side effect of stomach gas and some cramping pains. Generally, however, it is considered safe for children. The principal constituent is mannite, or Manna sugar, which possesses similar laxative properties to the exudate, and is often employed in Italy for that purpose.

Manna contains a high concentration of sugar alcohols, primarily mannitol. These sugar alcohols, when taken orally, cause fluids surrounding the intestinal tract to be drawn inside of the intestine. This results in an increased volume of fluid within the lower bowel, which causes a laxative effect.

MARIGOLD

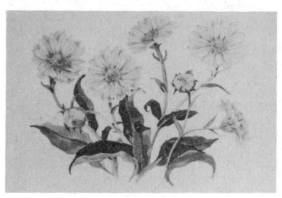

Marigold

SCIENTIFIC NAME: *Calendula officinalis*
PARTS USED: Flowers

DOSAGE:

> **Flowers:** The medicinal dose is 1 to 4 grams of granulated flowers per cup of boiling water, 1 cup per day.

MARIGOLD: *Considered a natural antiseptic, an Austrian patent was issued for the flowers as an emollient.*

Traditional Usages

Applied locally as a tincture, oil, or lotion, **Marigold is considered a "natural antiseptic" by homeopaths.** The crushed petals may be combined with olive oil to form an ointment for external application to **cuts, bruises, sores, and burns.**

The infusion was used to soothe watery, irritated eyes, and for relief in bronchial complaints. The Marigold was frequently used as a home remedy in liver disorders. It was also thought to induce perspiration in fever.

Recent Scientific Findings

The flowers contain an essential oil, an amorphous bitter compound and calendulin. **Experimentally, Marigold flower extracts have been shown to lower blood pressure and to have sedative effects in several animals species**, and it thus seems that the use of Marigold tea would have a beneficial effect on these conditions as well. Marigold is a common adulterant to Saffron.

An Austrian patent was issued in 1955 for the use of extracts of Marigold flowers as an emollient in the treatment of burns in humans.

MARIJUANA

SCIENTIFIC NAME: *Cannabis sativa*
PARTS USED: Flowering tops

DOSAGE:
As required.

MARIJUANA: *This illegal weed has proven to be an effective treatment for glaucoma and an aid for cancer patients undergoing chemotherapy.*

Traditional Usages

Currently an illegal drug in almost every country of the world, Cannabis has enjoyed a long and respectable history as a medicinal agent. As early as 2737 B.C. the plant was included in the pharmacopoeia of the Chinese Emperor Shen Nung. The ancient Scythians used it in their funeral rites, and seeds have been found in funerary urns dating back to the 5th century B.C.

Cannabis was formerly utilized in medicine to treat insomnia, allay pain, and soothe restlessness. The herbalist Culpepper recommended Cannabis in the treatment of colic, bloody noses, and jaundice. Cannabis has been given in the treatment of neuralgias, spasmodic coughs as in pertussis and asthma, as well as in tetanus and hydrophobia and other painful spasmodic diseases.

Inhalation of Cannabis smoke produces great exhilaration and can cause muscle fatigue to temporarily disappear. These psychic effects of the drug have made it useful as a nervine and stimulant for raising the spirits. Held to be narcotic and antispasmodic, it was recognized in the 1918 *U.S. Dispensatory* as a general nerve sedative for use in hysteria, mental depression, and neurasthenia.

Besides its medicinal applications, Hemp is an important fiber crop; it has been observed that plants grown in colder climates yield better fiber while those from warmer climates have more pronounced intoxicant and medicinal properties, owing to a higher content of the resin which contains the active principles.

The fruits, known as Hemp seeds, are a popular ingredient in bird seed. At one time they were employed medicinally in the treatment of mucous membrane inflammations.

Recent Scientific Findings

Currently, it is estimated that one in seven Americans twelve years of age or older has used Marijuana, and its number seems to have stabilized over the past few years. Although many refer to Marijuana as a "narcotic" or "hallucinogen," in a strict scientific sense neither term is applicable. Marijuana is not "addicting," nor does it produce true hallucinations, except in extremely high doses. Its anodyne and soporific action resembles that of Opium, but without the undesirable aftereffects of constipation and appetite loss.

Pharmacologists have been unable to place Marijuana into a neat "category" for purposes of explaining its effects; it is a drug in a class by itself. However, it is safe to say that currently the most popular use for Marijuana is as a recreational euphoriant.

The major active euphoric principle in Marijuana is a substance known as ê-9-tetrahydrocannabinol (ê9-THC). It is an extremely unstable substance in its pure form, but in the living or dead plant it is quite stable. It is amazing to learn that there is only one plant—*Cannabis sativa*—known to contain ê-9-THC, or compounds related to this principle. Although some botanists, with reasonable arguments, claim three major species of Marijuana exist, i.e., *Cannabis sativa* (most common), *Cannabis indica,* and *Cannabis ruderalis,* most chemical and pharmacological evidence seems to support the existence of only one species, i.e. *Cannabis sativa.*

Recent clinical experience demonstrates that Cannabis has a wide range of useful applications in medicine. **Certain types of glaucoma that are resistant to conventional types of treatment can be controlled by smoking Marijuana. Administration of THC to cancer patients who experience nausea and vomiting as a common side effect of chemotherapy produces relief of these symptoms.** Marijuana or its constituents, however, do not have anticancer properties.

Based on results of human studies, other remarkable effects of THC are to relieve pain, control seizures of epilepsy, relieve symptoms of asthma, and to act as a sedative. It is now well established that the use of Marijuana in the treatment of pain, to induce sleep, and for other maladies, has been fully justified on the basis of solid scientific evidence. Indeed, if it were not for the undesirable mind-altering side effects, Marijuana would probably be widely used in the practice of medicine.

MARSH-MALLOW

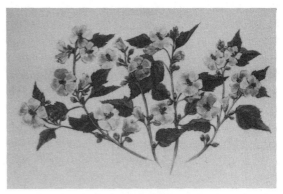

Marshmallow

SCIENTIFIC NAME: *Althaea officinalis*
PARTS USED: Root, leaves, and flowers

DOSAGE:

Root: ¹/₂ teaspoon of the crushed root, boil for ¹/₂ hour, strain, and mix well with honey. Drink cold, 1 to 2 tablespoonfuls at a time, 1 to 2 cups per day.

MARSHMALLOW: *Considered a cure-all by the ancient Greeks, the roots' mucilage content make this plant an excellent emollient.*

Traditional Usages

The ancient Greeks praised the virtues of Marshmallow and seemed to consider it a medicinal that would help cure any ailment. Hippocrates especially felt it was an immense aid in the treatment of wounds.

During the Renaissance, herbalists used marshmallow to treat **sore throat, stomach problems, gonorrhea, leucorrhea, toothache**, and **mouth infections.**

Marshmallow root is an excellent **demulcent** and **emollient.** The decoction is taken internally to relieve irritation and inflammation of the mucous membranes. The crushed leaves and flowers are boiled and applied externally in poultice form as a soothing dressing for **scrapes, chafing,** and other irritated skin conditions.

Recent Scientific Findings

Marshmallow root is well known to have a very high mucilage content. When the mucilage comes into contact with water it swells and forms a very soft, soothing, and **protective gel.** Thus, the external application of water extracts of this plant will have a demulcent and emollient effect on mucous membranes, or on the skin, or will have lubricant effect. If a water extract of Marshmallow was applied to a burn or skin abrasion, its **emollient** effect would reduce the amount of pain from the burn or abrasions, and in this context, it would have pain relieving properties.

MATÉ

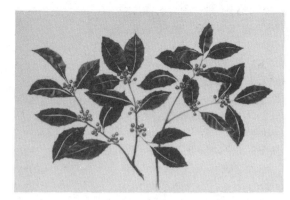

Maté

SCIENTIFIC NAME: *Ilex paraguensis*
PARTS USED: Leaves

DOSAGE: 1 teaspoon of the leaves, steeped in 1 cup of freshly boiled water for 2 minutes. Drink warm, 1 to 2 cups per day.

MATÉ: *In South America this is a popular drink due to its high caffeine content.*

Traditional Usages

Just as millions of people drink coffee and tea in other parts of the world, millions in South America enjoy Maté. The characteristic aromatic flavor and the stimulant caffeine are extracted by pouring water, either hot or cold, over dried leaves. As with tea, the most expensive grade of Maté is composed of the youngest leaves, while cheaper grades contain twigs, stems and older leaves. Botanically, Maté is a species of holly. It is cultivated and is also found growing wild.

Recent Scientific Findings

Maté is a rich source of caffeine. At the Sixth International Caffeine Workshop in Hong Kong, researchers concluded that the consumption of "normal levels" of caffeine posed "no significant health hazards."

The recurring concern of the putative link between cancer and caffeine was specifically dispelled; there being no association for esophageal, stomach or liver cancer; a slight relationship for pancreatic cancer; and a protective effect against colorectal cancer.

Pregnant women who consumed the substance were studied over a 7 year period with no effect seen on newborns, infants, and 4 to 7 year old children.

As noted earlier, the *method* of brewing coffee *does* have some effect on serum cholesterol levels (boiling coffee is the worst as far as cholesterol-watchers are concerned).

Coffee and tea drinkers no longer need be overly fearful of their "daily cup" so long as they follow a "moderate" intake (2-3 cups per day). What remains to be studied, in the editor's opinion, is the relationship between styrofoam containers and cancer of the pancreas as well as the health effects of *highly sweetened* caffeinated beverages.

It will not surprise inveterate coffee drinkers to learn that **caffeine promotes the burning of fat.** A series of recent studies, most notably that of Astrup and colleagues, confirms what coffee and tea "addicts" have long known, that these beverages promote slimming in humans.

It has been discovered that caffeine stimulates the expenditure of energy and the burning of fats.

Astrup's was a placebo-controlled, double-blind, dose-response study. (In other words, it met all the requirements of mainstream science.) Caffeine was tested in dosages of 100, 200, and 400 mg and compared against three different doses of ephedrine, and two placebos.

Six healthy subjects were recruited from the University of Copenhagen Medical School. Excluded were people habituated to caffeine from other sources—coffee, tea, colas, chocolate, and cocoa. The test subjects were put on a weight-controlling diet, consisting of about 250 grams of carbohydrate and a fixed amount of sodium. Their body fat content was measured before and after taking the placebo (lactose) or caffeine (100, 200, or 400 mg.) in gelatin capsules. Through a series of wonderful experimental analyses, the authors discovered that caffeine has a *thermogenic* effect (i.e, raises body heat) when taken in *moderate* doses on a daily basis. "A significant thermogenic effect was found even after the *lowest* dose of caffeine (100 mg.)..." Interestingly, even this relatively small intake of caffeine was found to produce a lasting effect on energy expenditure. **When caffeine was taken together with physical activity the thermogenic effect was enhanced.**

The *mechanism* by which caffeine exerts this fat-burning effect is thought to be associated with the thermogenic cori cycle. This is where glycogen and glucose are converted to *lactate* in fat and muscle tissue. Lactate then triggers thermogenic processes in the liver.

MATHAKÉ (TROPICAL ALMOND)

SCIENTIFIC NAME: *Terminalia catappa*
PARTS USED: Leaves and bark

DOSAGE:

MATHAKÉ: *Commonly used in the South Pacific, tropical almond is one of the most effective anti-fungal plants.*

Traditional Usages

This species, widely distributed in the tropics, is one of the most effective anti-fungal plants yet is not widely known.

Recent Scientific Findings

In 1984, I introduced the tropical almond to several physicians who report strong activity against *Candida albicans* in trials with patients. My decision to bring this plant into western medicine was based on first-hand observations of its **powerful anti-fungal activity** when used in Fijian folk-medicine.

Subsequent literature analysis indicated that a decoction of the leaves (mixed with other plants) is used to induce abortion in New Guinea. However, Mathaké by itself is perfectly safe; it is being used as a tonic in Mexico and the nuts have been eaten by children since antiquity. The compounds found within the leaves, kill *staphylococci*, which may explain its folkloric use as a tonic.

A related species, *T. arjuna*, has been shown to reduce total cholesterol and triglycerides while raising HDLs in experiments with rabbits. This study was based on an Ayurvedic prescription for the treatment of Hrid-Roga, the cardiovascular disorders.

Robert F. Cathcart, III, M.D., of Los Altos, California, reports that Mathaké should be utilized as an alternative to Pau D'Arco.

At this time we do not know if Mathaké acts directly to kill yeast or if any of its compounds enhances the immune system. Owing to its clinical effectiveness in initial trials and its long history of usage, this plant is worth utilizing as part of an overall immune-enhancing program.

The following was written about Mathaké by Richard W. Noble, M.D., a physician familiar with herbal medicine.

It would be difficult to overstate the usefulness of the medicinal herb, Mathaké, in my medical practice. I am particularly grateful for your effort to make this material available for use in this country . . . I was looking for alternatives to oral Nystatin, particularly in children with Candidiasis. In the intervening years Mathaké has become the first treatment of choice in patients with Chronic Candiasis related illness

The wide variety of agents, both prescription and non-prescription, that are available to treat yeast infections is well known. As a medical doctor experienced in the use of botanical medicine I have used through the years a variety of these agents including medicine Garlic, Pau d'Arco, Grapefruit Seed Extract, and Caprylic acid.

All of these materials may be helpful in certain cases but none of them provide the ease of use, the economy, and the low side effects I have experienced in patients using Mathaké. It will be readily verified by any physician who has attempted to treat this puzzling problem that continued therapy measured in months, not days or weeks is the usual case. It is for this reason prolonged use of prescription medications are not advised. . . .

Mathaké can be used for up to three months at a time. It has the advantage of being an easily prepared medication: All that is necessary is boiling water to produce a pleasant tasting cup of tea. Children, particularly, accept this method. Adults find the ease of use and the low toxicity very appealing.

Thank you again for your efforts in bringing this valuable herb to the continent. Please keep me advised of your research with Mathaké.

MEADOW SAFFRON

SCIENTIFIC NAME: *Colchicum autumnale*
PARTS USED: Corn (bulb), seeds

DOSAGE:

Caution: Not for home use. When used in medicine, the alcohol extract was given in a dose of 0.016-0.065 gram. The fluidextract was given in a dose of 0.12-0.5 milliliter; the tincture was given in a dose of 0.3-0.9 milliliter, while Cochicum wine was given in a dose of 0.6-2.5 milliliters.

"Wine of Colchicum seed is made by mixing together 10 milliliters of fluidextract of Colchicum seed, 15 milliliters of alcohol, and 75 milliliters of sherry wine. In gout this wine is frequently given in connection with magnesium sulphate." (U.S.D.) As little as 9.3 milliliters of the wine have caused death!

MEADOW SAFFRON: *This strikingly beautiful flower is the source of the potent drug colchicine.*

Traditional Usages

This beautiful plant has long been known for its potent medicinal properties. The generic name is derived from Colchis, a town in Natolia (near the Black Sea), which abounded in this and other medicinal plants. It perhaps gave

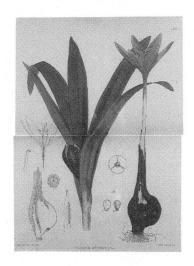

Meadow Saffron

rise to some of the myths concerning Medea, who was sometimes called Colchis after her birthplace.

Colchicum has been used in home remedies to treat **gout, rheumatism**, and **dropsy**, but owing to varying times of collection of the corns with varying degrees of success. Climate and soil influence the potency, but the season of collection is most important. In spring, when the corns are most potent they are often eaten by animals, with fatal results.

The old French name, *Tue-chien,* intimates that dogs are especially vulnerable to the poison. Country people in 19th century England called the flowers "Naked Ladies" because they come up without any leaves or cover.

Recent Scientific Findings

All parts of the Meadow Saffron plant contain the alkaloid colchicine, which has a specific action in **relieving the pain and inflammation associated with gout**. However, only a very small amount of colchicine will produce this effect, and if larger than necessary quantities are taken, severe toxic effects will occur.

Instances are recorded where death ensued within a day after about 4 grams of the wine of Colchicum had been taken for dropsy. (The seeds possess the same properties as the bulbs and are used for the same purposes.)

The toxic alkaloid colchicine is so potent as to be used in experimental genetics to induce "new permanent characteristics in plants and animals."

MEZEREON

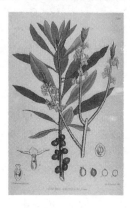

Mezereon

SCIENTIFIC NAME: *Daphne mezereum*
PARTS USED: Bark, berries

DOSAGE:
　　Not for home use.

MEZEREON: *The bark of this plant contains mezerein, a substance that could be a co-carcinogen.*

Traditional Usages

While the berries and bark of Mezereon have reportedly been useful in European folk medicine (to cure paralysis of the mouth), the plant is a strong *internal* poison. However, an ointment made of the berries gained a folkloric reputation in northern Europe as a treatment for **cancer, canker sores**, and **ulcerous lesions**.

Linnaeus stated that the Swedes applied the bark to parts bitten by poisonous reptiles and rabid animals.

Recent Scientific Findings

Mezereon contains an extremely irritant substance, known as mezerein, that is toxic to cells. **In animal experiments, mezerein, as well as extracts of Mezereon, inhibit experimental tumors.** These properties explain most of the effects claimed for this plant.

It must be pointed out that mezerein is a chemical substance closely related to other substances classified as co-carcinogens. This means that by itself the substance cannot cause cancer. However, it will increase the cancer-causing effects of other chemical substances when they are put together. **Thus, it is possible that the use of Mezereon by a tobacco user will increase the risk of cancer, due to this additive effect.** Other environmental cancer-causing agents, which we are all exposed to continuously, could possibly react with mezerein and enhance the production of cancer cells in humans who are expose to both types of agents.

For these reasons, one must understand the risk potential in using Mezereon for any purpose.

MILK THISTLE

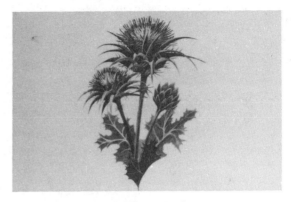

Milk Thistle

SCIENTIFIC NAME: *Silybum marianum*
PARTS USED: Seeds

DOSAGE:
    Seeds: 1 teaspoon seeds steeped in ½ cup water; 1 to 1½ cupfuls per day, 1 tablespoon or mouthful at a time.

MILK THISTLE: *The seeds contain silymarin, a flavonoid that is effective for liver disorders.*

Traditional Usages

For centuries, Milk Thistle has been used in folkloric medicine. The seeds were believed to act most directly to protect the **liver.**

Recent Scientific Findings

One active component extracted from milk thistle seeds, silymarin, is a flavonoid long recognized for its ability to benefit people with **liver disorders** and as a protective compound against liver-damaging agents as diverse as mushroom toxins, carbon tetrachloride, and other chemicals. This flavonoid demonstrates **good antioxidant** properties, both *in vivo* and *in vitro*.

Chilean scientists found that silymarin also increases the content of liver glutathione (GSH), an effect *not* known with other closely related flavonoids such as (+)- cyanidanol-3 (cathequin). These experiments also showed an increase of glutathione content and antioxidant activity in the intestine and stomach. The effects selectively occur only in the digestive tract, and not in the kidney, lung, and spleen.

A double blind, prospective, randomized study performed on 170 patients with cirrhosis of the liver supported the fact that **silymarin protects the liver.** All patients received the same treatment with a mean observation period of 41 months. The 4-year survival rate was significantly higher in silymarin-treated patients than those in the placebo group. No side effects of drug treatment were observed.

Another study found that Milk Thistle may offer us some protection against the toxic side-effects of the common pain-reliving drug acetaminophen, which is a widely used analgesic and fever medication. In overdosage severe hepatotoxicity may result, characterized by glutathione (GSH) depletion, suppression of GSH biosynthesis, and liver damage. GSH is considered the most important biomolecule against chemically-induced cytotoxicity.

Silybin, a soluble form of silymarin, is thought to exert a membrane-stabilizing action which inhibits or prevents lipid peroxidation. Silybin and silymarin may be useful in protecting the liver in many cases besides acetaminophen overdosage. Alcohol also depletes GSH and these flavonoids offer protection for those who continue to drink. Interestingly, silybin dihemisuccinate remains medicine's most important antidote to poisoning by the mushroom toxins a-amantin and phalloidin.

MISTLETOE

SCIENTIFIC NAME: *Viscum album* (European), *Phoradendron flavescens* (American)

PARTS USED: Berries, leaves, and wood

DOSAGE:

Leaves and Wood: Because of the confusion surrounding this herb, there is no recommended dose of Mistletoe for domestic use. However, when used in medicine the leaves and wood were given in the dose of 3.9 grams. To lower blood pressure, a water extract of 0.2 gram daily was prescribed.

MISTLETOE: *Sacred to the Druids, this plant has been used in medicine since ancient times, yet modern research is discovering new medicinal properties.*

Traditional Usages

This parasitic plant was sacred to the Druids, and was supposedly used therapeutically by that mysterious ancient people as a cure for sterility and epilepsy, and as an antidote to poisons. Its medicinal use is recorded over centuries. Hippocrates, Dioscorides, and Galen highly extolled the virtues of the glutinous extract of Mistletoe as an external remedy. However, only Hippocrates recommends it internally, in disorders of the spleen.

Mistletoe is considered briskly purgative and emetic. Through the early part of this century it was thought to have beneficial effects on nervous conditions, but by 1917 it was already out of vogue as a nervine. The glutinous substance viscin is obtained by boiling the bark in alcohol; this material was felt to be beneficial as an external application for irritated and chafed skin.

American Mistletoe, Phoradendron flavescens, is a plant that is parasitic on a number of different woody species. The leaves and branches are diuretic and the drug obtained from them was thought to aid asthma and whooping cough. It was used to arrest postpartum and other uterine hemorrhage. In Mendocino County in California, Native Americans made a tea from the leaves of American Mistletoe. If taken in large quantities, **it was reputed to cause abortion or prevent conception.**

Extracts have been employed by the medical profession to prevent postpartum hemorrhage and to aid in the induction of labor at term in pregnancy. It was used most frequently in the mid-1800s in the United States, and was claimed at that time to be superior over Ergot preparations (see article on Ergot for additional details).

Recent Scientific Findings

Accounts on the use and safety of "Mistletoe" preparations in the scientific literature are at best confusing. In most cases, the conclusions drawn are erroneous because most people consider "Mistletoe" to be a single plant. The situation is not so simple. A large number of Mistletoes grow naturally in the United States and Canada, but Viscum album does not. All of the North American Mistletoes are classified in the related group of plants, *Phoradendron*. The European Mistletoe is correctly referred to as *Viscum album*; the American Mistletoe can be any one of a number of species, but most commonly *Phoradendron flavescens*.

Several reports can be found that suggest ingestion of "Mistletoe" or "Mistletoe berries" results in adverse effects and even death (in animals and small children). In carefully checking into each of these reports, there is good reason to believe that they are incorrect. It was found that either there was no evidence by a qualified person that the plant material ingested was really a "Mistletoe," or there was no evidence that the plant material was even ingested. When one considers that up until about 1968, "Mistletoe" (*Viscum album*) preparations were official in the pharmacopoeia of several European countries as a means of treating high blood pressure, it is difficult to believe that such a plant results in the toxic effects described by some.

On the other hand, there is both animal and human test evidence available that *Viscum album* preparations do have sedative (nervine) properties. However, we have not been able to find good evidence that an emetic effect will result from use of such preparations.

A point of caution to the use of *Viscum album* preparations is that one should make absolutely sure that he or she is not taking at the same time any prescription medicine that contains a monoamineoxidase inhibitor, since the mixture will cause very serious side effects. Tyramine is a well established constituent of *Viscum album*. Tyramine will not have any appreciable effects in humans when taken by mouth, unless a monoamineoxidase inhibitor is taken at the same time. In this case, a serious drop in blood pressure will result. This should not be cause for alarm, since many foods, as well as Chianti wine, contain large amounts of tyramine, and the same caution holds true for them as with *Viscum album* preparations.

There is no evidence that American Mistletoe, if taken before sexual relations, will prevent conception. However, **it is quite possible that taken a short time after fertilization has occurred, menstruation might be induced.** In that case it would be acting as an early abortifacient.

A Mistletoe extract, iscador, has been found to have immuno-modulatory properties. Preliminary evidence reports that iscador enhances the activities of Natural Killer (NK) cells and cytotoxic T lymphocytes (CTL).

American Mistletoe has similar effects as those of *Viscum album* (European Mistletoe). American Mistletoe also contains tyramine, and the same precautions should be observed as for European Mistletoe.

MORNING GLORY

SCIENTIFIC NAME: *Ipomoea purpurea* and other *Ipomoea* species

PARTS USED: Seeds

DOSAGE:
   Caution: See text.

MORNING GLORY: *Of the more than 175 varieties of this flower, only seven have been found to contain hallucinogenic components.*

Traditional Usages

A great deal of confusion revolves around the use of Morning Glory as an herbal remedy. This is due to more than one plant species being widely used. A great deal of difference in effect occurs, depending on whether the seeds or the roots are used.

The most common cultivated garden ornamental Morning Glory is *Ipomoea purpurea*. No part of this species is capable of producing hallucinogenic effects. However, the roots contain a complex mixture of fatty acid-like substances that produce a rather harsh purgative effect.

In recent years, the seeds of *Ipomoea violacea (Ipomoea tricolor)* have been widely employed as a hallucinogen in North America. Ironically, this use was known in Mexico for centuries for a plant known as Badoh Negra, and it was only about two decades ago that Badoh Negra was botanically authenticated as *Ipomoea violacea.*

Recent Scientific Findings

The **hallucinogenic** effect of this plant is due to chemical substances very closely related to lysergic acid diethylamide (LSD). The active compounds are found in trace amounts in all parts of the plant, highest concentrations being found in the seeds. More than 175 horticultural variants of *Ipomoea violacea* are known, but the lysergic acid-like substances have only been found in seven of these.

Early controversy arose as to whether or not Morning Glory seeds were, in fact, hallucinogenic. Some persons taking the seeds claimed this effect while others failed to experience the effect. This variance in experience is explained by the fact that the seeds are very hard and if boiled in water, the active constituents will probably not be extracted. Similarly, when the whole seeds have been taken by mouth, most people who have used them have found that the seeds were not digested and thus that little or no effect was experienced. It has been estimated that about 350 seeds are required to produce hallucinations in most humans.

MOTHERWORT

SCIENTIFIC NAME: *Leonurus cardiaca*
PARTS USED: Tops and leaves

DOSAGE:

Tops and Leaves: 1 teaspoon of leaves and tops to 1 cup of boiling water. Taken cold, 1 mouthful at a time, to 1 or 2 cups per day.

MOTHERWORT: *For centuries this herb was given for menstrual problems; modern research reveals it may also aid the heart.*

Traditional Usages

In Chinese legend, Motherwort prolonged life. The herb's name comes from the fact that the fruit, stem, and leaf are always thick and abundant. Motherwort was commonly prescribed for **menstrual disorders**, during childbirth to aid the placenta, and for general abdominal pains.

In Western medicine Motherwort was recommended as a treatment for **vaginitis** when employed as a douche. The plant has been utilized to provoke menstruation and to aid the continuation of the flow of the lochia following childbirth. Reportedly it was used to **calm epileptics** during the 17th century, and more recently it has been employed as a **nerve tonic** and **sedative**, especially for administration after childbirth.

Recent Scientific Findings

While most uses of this aromatic perennial herb, as evidenced by the common name, have been directed toward the female anatomy, **recent evidence has confirmed its utility in heart problems.** Experimentally, Motherwort extracts have been reported to have cardiotonic effects based on experiments involving application of extracts of the plant on isolated animal hearts. The action was confirmed in whole animals. Hot-water extracts also show **sedative** and **anti-epileptic effects** in animals. These experiments tend to confirm the accuracy of the species epithet (*cardiaca*).

A 1990 experiment found that a mixture of Hawthorn and Motherwort might prove an effective preventive and/or treatment for **atherosclerosis.** Animals experiments have produced interesting results that warrant further investigation in regards to Motherwort's effect on **breast cancer.** A methanol extract of Motherwort was added to the drinking water of mice. The extract stimulated the excretion of carcinogenic factors and suppressed the development of one type of mammary cancer. Yet, it also enhanced the development of a different type of mammary cancer.

After flowering the herb is richest in its drug component, consisting of various glycosides, resins, tannins, saponins, and organic acids.

MUGWORT

SCIENTIFIC NAME: *Artemisia vulgaris*

PARTS USED: Leaves and flowering tops

DOSAGE:

Leaves or Flowering tops: Approximately ½ ounce of leaves or flowering tops to 1 pint of water. Boil water separately and pour over the plant material and steep for 5-20 minutes, depending on the desired effect. Drink hot or warm, 1 to 2 cups per day, at bedtime and upon awakening.

MUGWORT: *This plant has been used by cultures throughout the world to assist and promote menstruation.*

Traditional Usages

The leaves of the common Mugwort were used to make "moxas." The term *moxa* designates a small mass of combustible matter, which by being burnt slowly in contact with the skin, produces an eschar, a slough or scab produced from cauterization. As a treatment for disease, cauterization by fire has been commonly practiced from the earliest periods of history both by primitive tribes and advanced civilizations. The ancient Egyptians and Greeks were acquainted with the use of moxa, as were the ancients in China, Japan, and other Asian countries.

The early Portuguese navigators brought the practice from Asia to Europe. In the 1830s moxas were a popular remedy in France for amaurosis, loss of taste, deafness, paralytic affections of the muscles, asthma, chronic catarrh and pleurisy, phthisis, chronic engorgement of the liver and spleen, rachitis, diseased spine, coxalgia, and other forms of scrofulous and rheumatic inflammation of the joints. The *British Flora Medica* has this to say:

The dried leaves, bruised in mortar, and rubbed between the hands until the downy part is separated from the woody fibre, and rolled into little cones, is a good substitute for Chinese moxa. The part is first moistened and then a cone of the moxa is applied, which is set on fire at the apex and gradually burns down to the skin, producing a dark-coloured spot; by repeating this painful process an eschar is formed, and this on separation leaves an ulcer which may be kept open or healed as circumstances may require.

Hippocrates recommended Mugwort taken internally to aid in the delivery of the placenta; Dioscorides utilized it to expedite labor and delivery. It has been used as a tonic and as a cure for intermittent fever.

Recent Scientific Findings

Mugwort is one of the most commonly employed herbal preparations for the treatment of amenorrhea, i.e., used to assist and promote menstruation. We have records showing that it is used in the Philippines, Vietnam, India, Korea, China, Portugal, Europe, and in the United States for this purpose. There is evidence that water extracts of Mugwort will cause a stimulation of uterine muscle in the test tube; thus, on a theoretical basis, it could act as an emmenagogue in humans. There is no really effective means to establish whether or not a substance has an emmenagogue effect in animals or in humans, and thus it is difficult to use evidence such as this in support of this effect. However, when a plant is used for the same purpose in as many geographically separated areas as is Mugwort, this adds credibility to the alleged effect.

Certain of its extracts injected into laboratory animals give rise to a **sedative** effect. Thus, it is possible that this sedative effect could be beneficial in a person with epilepsy, an illness in which Mugwort has been employed.

MULLEIN

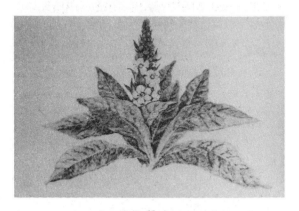

Mullein

SCIENTIFIC NAME: *Verbascum thapsus*
PARTS USED: Leaves and flowers

DOSAGE:

Leaves: The medicinal preparation consists of 1 teaspoon of leaves, steeped in 1 cup of boiling water. Drink cold, 1 to 2 cups per day, 1 tablespoon at a time.

MULLEIN: *This plant has long been used as a treatment for respiratory problems.*

Traditional Usages

Mullein was introduced from Europe into North America. In all probability Native Americans learned from early settlers to treat **respiratory problems** with Mullein. The Menominees smoked the pulverized, dried root for respiratory complaints. The Potawatomis, Mohegans, and Penobscots smoked the dried leaves to relieve **asthma**. The Mohegans steeped the leaves in molasses to make "an excellent **cough remedy**." Catawbas prepared a sweetened syrup from the boiled root as a **cough medicine** for their children.

During the Civil War, the Confederate army used Mullein to treat respiratory problems. Dr. Millspaugh noted that Mullein was principally employed around 1887 to relieve painful, phlegmy coughs. He also described a "cure" for **hemorrhoids** consisting of a fatty oil that resulted after the bottled flowers were allowed to set in the sun.

By 1913, Mullein had become extremely popular in America as a treatment for coughs and inflamed mucous membrane lining the throat. The corolla of the golden yellow flowers brought a wholesale price of 70 to 80 cents a pound. The steam was often inhaled to relieve cold symptoms such as **nasal congestion** and **throat irritation**.

Recent Scientific Findings

Mullein leaves have high concentrations of mucilage, which is responsible for the emollient and demulcent effects of water extracts of this plant. In its application as an external emollient, a fomentation of Mullein leaves in hot vinegar and water makes an agreeable application to **piles** and **itching** complaints. Boiled with lard, it makes an ointment for dressing wounds. Fomentations or poultices of the leaves or flowers beaten up with Linseed meal have been applied to **burns**, **scalds**, and **boils**.

Internally **demulcent**, Mullein soothes the **throat** and **lungs**. It is also **diuretic**, **allays pain**, and is **antispasmodic**. It does not have a very pleasant taste, so the addition of an aromatic, together with boiling the herb in milk, is advised.

MUSTARD

SCIENTIFIC NAME: *Sinapis alba,*
S. nigra

PARTS USED: Seeds

DOSAGE:

Caution: Mustard plasters can rarely be taken for more than 10 or 15 minutes. As an emetic (especially used in narcotic poisoning), mustard powder was given in the quantity of 3.9-7.7 grams.

MUSTARD: *Mustard plasters continue to be a common remedy.*

Traditional Usages

Powdered Mustard seeds are a common condiment; they promote the appetite and stimulate the gastric mucous membrane, with some effect on pancreatic secretions, thereby aiding digestion. By virtue of these effects they can sometimes relieve **obstinate hiccough**.

Mustard is also a valuable **emetic**, when it is desired to empty the stomach without accompanying depression of the system, as in cases of narcotic poisoning. Taken whole, the seeds are **laxative** and can aid in upset stomach due to acid indigestion.

An important use of mustard has been externally, as a rubefacient (reddening the skin, producing local congestion, the vessels becoming dilated and the supply of blood increased); with longer applications vesication, or blister formation, occurs, drawing deeper fluids to the surface. Mustard poultices may be mixed with alcohol, almond oil, or olive oil. The poultice should be carefully attended, as too long an application can result in pain and tissue damage.

Recent Scientific Findings

Black and White Mustard seeds both contain highly irritating so-called "mustard-oil" glycosides, typified by "mustard oil," or allyl isothiocyanate. The irritant effect is mild in water extracts, but in concentrated extracts, the irritation can actually induce blistering. A combination of mild irritation due to the mustard-oil glycosides, in addition to a high fat content, causes the laxative effect of Mustard seeds. In larger doses, the irritant action of the mustard-oil glycosides causes emesis.

Mustard plasters are still widely used, and their effective utility requires special handling. The mustard plaster is simply a thin layer of deflated Mustard seeds, applied to a piece of paper with a suitable glue. Prior to use, the mustard plaster is dipped into lukewarm (never hot) water. This contact with water sets off a chemical reaction in which the end-product is "mustard oil." The plaster is then applied for a short period of time. While the plaster is in contact with the skin, the blood rushes to the area of application. The additional blood supply serves to produce an anti-inflammatory response, relax muscles, and in general provide relief from muscle strains and similar ailments. It must be pointed out that the mustard plaster should not be allowed to remain in contact with the skin for any prolonged period of time, or it will result in the formation of blisters. The blisters are very painful and there is always a

possibility that infection will result. However, mustard plasters, applied externally for periods up to 15 minutes, will usually not result in blistering, and are quite safe and effective for those whose skin is of normal sensitivity.

Mustard oil itself is used in many proprietary ointments intended for external application for the relief of minor aches and pains, much the same as mustard plaster.

MYRRH

SCIENTIFIC NAME: *Commiphora myrrha*
PARTS USED: Oleo gum-resin from stem

DOSAGE:

Gum-resin: For internal complains, an infusion is prepared with approximately 1/2 ounce of myrrh to 1 pint of water. Boil water separately and pour over the plant material and steep for 5 to 20 minutes, depending on the desired effect. Drink hot or warm, 1 to 2 cups per day.

An external plaster of Myrrh is made by rubbing together powdered Myrrh, Camphor, and Balsam of Peru, 1 1/2 oz. each, adding to 32 oz. of lead plaster previously melted, and stirring well until the plaster thickens on cooling.

MYRRH: *This ancient aromatic resin is an excellent decongestant.*

Traditional Usages

Myrrh is a gummy substance exuding from a small tree of eastern Africa and Arabia. In Greek mythology, Myrrha, the daughter of the king of Syria, was punished by Aphrodite, who caused her to disguise herself and commit incest with her father. When her father discovered her identity, he attempted to kill her, but the gods intervened, turning Myrrha into a myrrh tree. The gum resin is said to be her tears. The gum's name comes from the Arabic word meaning "bitter."

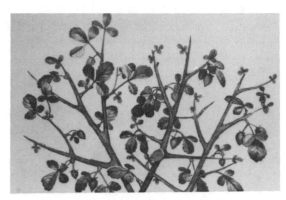

Myrrh

Myrrh has been used for thousands of years as an ingredient in incense and perfumes. The gum-resin was used by the ancients for embalming. Its use is mentioned in an Egyptian papyrus from about 2000 BC. There are numerous Biblical references to myrrh, including the *Song of Solomon* in which "A bundle of myrrh *is* my wellbeloved unto me; he shall lie all night betwixt my breasts." The Chasidic prayer book contains a formula for a holy incense containing myrrh that was prepared by the ancient Hebrews. Myrrh was also one of the wise men's gifts to the baby Jesus.

As a medicinal, Myrrh is a stimulant tonic and expectorant, and was most commonly administered to patients suffering from chest problems in order to stimulate mucous secretions and promote their drainage.

A second major area of usage concerned the female reproductive organs. Myrrh was taken to stimulate the menstrual flow or to bring it on, even when the patient had never menstruated. In this connection it was often combined with aloes for the laxative properties contributed by the latter. Myrrh was also applied to spongy gums and mouth ulcers. For centuries myrrh has been used by the Chinese to treat menstrual difficulties, and hemorrhoids

A gentle rubefacient in external application, Myrrh was employed to make a plaster where it was desirable to produce blisters slowly and with a minimum of pain.

Recent Scientific Findings

Myrrh gum contains several volatile oils, rendering this herb an excellent promoter of **free breathing** during congestive colds. Myrrh acts on the mucous membranes of the respiratory tract.

NETTLE

SCIENTIFIC NAME: *Urtica dioica*

PARTS USED: Roots, leaves, and seeds

DOSAGE:

Leaves or Root: For medicinal use one teaspoon of the granulated leaves or root per 1 cup of boiling water. Drink cold, one tablespoon at a time, 1 cup per day.

NETTLE: *Ironically, this stinging plant is sometimes used in cosmetics as a facial.*

Traditional Usages

The Nettle has been used medicinally either to excite the skin locally or to affect the nervous system generally. The poisonous stinging hairs of the fresh Nettle will produce intense itching and stringing. However, both Pliny and homeopathic physicians applied the juice to cure its own sting! The leaves will stimulate, irritate, and cause blisters, so they are used where a rubefacient is desired, such as to heal wounds and burns.

In the 2nd and 3rd centuries B.C. several practitioners made reference to the medicinal properties of Nettles. It was used as an antidote for Hemlock, a counterpoison for Henbane, and as a cure for snakebite and scorpion sting. It was reputedly an aid for gout, asthma, and tuberculosis. Other recorded applications of the plant are as a diuretic and to arrest uterine hemorrhages. Nettle juice at one time formed the main component (93 percent) of a preparation known as Brandol, which was commercially marketed. Nettle seeds are sometimes used in home remedies for hair troubles, coughs, and shortness of breath.

The tops of the plants, boiled, are eaten as greens by many people in soups. It is recommended as an emergency food plant and has been suggested as a possible source of chlorophyll, for commercial purposes.

Recent Scientific Findings

Extracts of Nettle have been tested in animals and show **anti-inflammatory** effects, and also lower the amount of sugar in the blood. Nettle is sometimes used in hair products and facials.

NIGHTSHADE, BLACK

SCIENTIFIC NAME: *Solanum nigrum*
PARTS USED: Leaves

DOSAGE:
> **Leaves:** For external use only, as a leaf poultice.

BLACK NIGHTSHADE: *Since the ancient Greeks, a poultice of crushed leaves has been applied externally.*

Traditional Usages

Used to produce vomiting, and purging, Black Nightshade was felt to purify the blood of toxins. In North America the Comanches, Houmas, and Rappahannock employed the plant internally as a treatment for tuberculosis, to expel worms, and induce sleep.

The external application of the leaves in skin problems has been recorded since the ancient Greek Dioscorides. Arabic physicians utilized the bruised leaves as an application for burns. A poultice of freshly crushed leaves or a compress soaked in concentrated decoction was applied as an analgesic in cases of itching, hemorrhoids, and arthritis.

Recent Scientific Findings

The leaves and berries are **poisonous**, especially in the unripe state. The berries are often involved in the poisoning of children, who find them attractive to eat. As the fruit ripens, the solanine (active principle) content gradually decreases to nontoxic levels. The ripe berries have sometimes been used to make preserves and pies. Boiling apparently also destroys the toxic principles.

OAK, WHITE

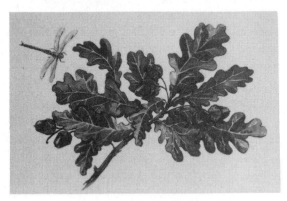
White Oak

SCIENTIFIC NAME: *Quercus alba*
PARTS USED: Bark

DOSAGE:

>**Acorns:** Decoct ½ to 1 ounce in 1½ pints of boiling water, allow to simmer, at breakfast.

WHITE OAK: *There is renewed interest in the inner bark of this stately tree due to its high tannin content.*

Traditional Usages

Of the more than fifty species of oak found in the United States, the White Oak has been the most important medicinal, both to Native Americans and whites. The acorns formed the staple of the diet of many tribes, especially in California. After leaching the bitter tannins, the nuts were ground into a meal that was made into bread.

The Menominees treated **piles** by squirting an infusion of the scraped inner bark into the rectum with a syringe made from an animal bladder and the hollow bone of a bird. This type of syringe was reputedly made by many tribes. The Iroquois and Penobscots also boiled White Oak bark and drank the liquid to treat diarrhea.

In my antique copy of *The Dispensatory of the United States* (1834) White Oak bark is accorded all the respect that a major pharmaceutical would receive in a current textbook of pharmacology. The inner bark was listed in the *U.S. Pharmacopoeia* from 1820 to 1916. Oak bark was taken in the form of a powder, extract, or decoction, primarily for its high tannin content. It was not used internally to a great extent, but a **decoction of the bark has been found useful in treating chronic diarrhea, advanced dysentery, and other conditions.** The bark's principal use has been for external application, as an astringent wash, especially for flabby ulcers, as a gargle, and internally via injection for leucorrhea and **hemorrhoids.**

Recent Scientific Findings

The inner bark of White Oak is known to contain about 10 percent of a tannin complex, often referred to as quercitannic acid. As with all tannins, it predictably exerts an **astringent** and **mild antiseptic action**, the latter effect being due primarily to the phenolic nature of the tannin complex. Thus, as reported in folklore accounts, decoctions or infusions of *Quercus alba* bark, when applied locally, would have an astringent effect that tends to **shrink hemorrhoids** and accelerate the healing of flabby ulcers.

It is not known whether tannins kill **parasites** directly or if they act to protect an invaded intestinal wall by the above-described mechanism. That they do work is attested to by the fact tannins are going through a revival owing to their medicinal properties. With the proliferation of intestinal parasites this class of plant-derived substances is receiving the respect once seen in older books on pharmacognosy and botanical medicine. Tannins precipitate proteins from solution, and act to protect injured tissues by precipitating their proteins to form an antiseptic, protective coat under which the regeneration of new tissues may take place. They are utilized in medicine as astringents in the G.I. tract, on **burns**, on skin abrasions, for bleeding or infected **mouth sores**, as a local application for **hemorrhoids**, and as a douche for vaginal and cervical discharges.

It should be noted, however, that tannins should *not* be taken for prolonged periods. An increased incidence of cancer of the esophagus and buccal cavity has been noted among habitual betel-nut chewers (*Areca catechu*) in India and South Africa. This is linked to the high content of condensed catechin tannin found in the nuts, which are chewed for their stimulant drug content.

OAT STRAW

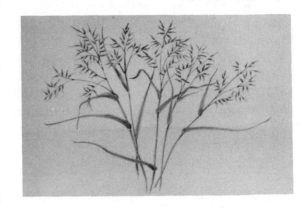

Oat Straw

SCIENTIFIC NAME: *Avena sativa*
PARTS USED: Straw

DOSAGE:
 1 to 2 teaspoons, once per day
in beverage or food.

OAT STRAW: *This popular grain has been shown to lower cholesterol.*

Traditional Usages

This annual grass has been cultivated as a primary food source for centuries. It is a rich nutritive addition to the diet and that has been its primary used. Oats are thought to promote healthy skin, hair, nails, and teeth.

Oat baths have long been popular in Europe for rheumatism as well as kidney and bladder problems.

Recent Scientific Findings

Rich in the element silicon. Silicon is necessary to build the outer layer of skin, hair, the fingernails.

Workers in the United States and in Israel have shown oats to have both estrogenic and anti-estrogenic effects in rats and mice.

Oat bran has been shown to lower cholesterol, reducing cholesterol levels in the blood by about 20%. It has also been found to reduce fecal pH, which may be a risk factor for colorectal cancer.

OPIUM

SCIENTIFIC NAME: *Papaver sominferum*
PARTS USED: Seed capsules

DOSAGE:
Only to taken under medical supervision.

OPIUM: *This has been called the most important and valuable medicine in the whole materia medica.*

Traditional Usages

Although we consider this the mother of medicinal plants, the Latin name *Papaver* is thought to be derived from the Celtic *papa* (whence "pap," the soft food given to children), a food in which the Opium seeds were formerly boiled to induce sleep.

The use of Opium as a medicine can be traced back to the time of Hippocrates. It has been called the most important and valuable medicine of the whole materia medica, and "the source, by its judicious employment, of more happiness, and by its abuse, of more misery, than any other drug employed by mankind." (Pereira)

Laudanum (tincture of Opium) was regularly given to infants and small children to treat colic during the 19th century.

The following formula for camphorated tincture of Opium (paregoric) was once a standard in medical practice.

4 grams powdered opium
4 grams benzoic acid
4 grams camphor
4 milliliters oil of anise

Macerate mixed drugs in stoppered container, with 40 milliliters of glycerin and 950 milliliters of diluted alcohol. Continue maceration with frequent agitation during 3 days, transfer mixture to a filter and, when the liquid has drained off completely, gradually wash the residue on the filter with enough alcohol to make one thousand milliliters of finished tincture.

Recent Scientific Findings

The gummy latex of this annual herb contains many alkaloids, including morphine, codeine, narcotine, laudenine, and papaverine. Various medicines made from Opium alkaloids are used for their sedative, hypnotic, narcotic, antispasmodic, and analgesic effects. The highly addicting *synthetic* heroin is made by modifying morphine.

There is no substitute for the narcotic abilities of Opium. Many terminally ill cancer patients in this country whose major concerns is dying with dignity, drug addiction not being a problem of any concern whatever, are denied this most efficacious painkiller, to suffer out their last weeks and months in needless agony for themselves—and for their families, who must stand by helplessly.

It is the author's fervent hope that Opium and its derivatives will once again be made available in this country to ease the suffering of the terminally ill, and with proper controls, for use in place of the synthetic tranquilizers. Ultimately, we would like to see this plant regain its status as the valued natural drug it is.

ORCHID, WILD

SCIENTIFIC NAME: *Orchis* spp.
PARTS USED: Tubers

DOSAGE:

Tubers: First macerate the tubers in cold water until they soften and then rapidly dry them. Take 1 to 2 ounces per day.

WILD ORCHID: *These tubers of these beautiful flowers are the source for salep.*

Traditional Usages

Orchids have enjoyed a widespread reputation as restoratives, rejuvenants, and aphrodisiacs, seemingly more because of the splendid and opulent flowers than from any specific excitant or stimulant properties.

A product known as salep is prepared from the tubers of various *Orchis* species. The tubers are strung on strings, scalded to destroy their vitality, then dried to a hard consistency; after maceration in water they regain their original form and volume. These strings of dried tubers, or salep, are highly prized in India, Persia, and Turkey for restoring the strength of debilitated or aged persons, and especially as an aphrodisiac. One writer has speculated that it is the odor and appearance of the salep, and the tubers from which it is derived, that suggested its application as an aphrodisiac, on the basis of the "doctrine of signatures."

Recent Scientific Findings

Fundamentally, the tubers are nutritive and compare favorably with tapioca and sago in the convalescent's diet. Salep has also been used to treat **diarrhea, dysentery,** and **nervous fevers.**

OREGON GRAPE

SCIENTIFIC NAME: *Berberis aquifolium*
PARTS USED: Root

DOSAGE:

Root: The traditional medicinal preparation consists of 1 teaspoon of granulated root per 1½ pints of boiling water, steeped for ½ hour and strained. Take 1 tablespoon 3 to 6 times per day.

OREGON GRAPE: *At one time, the roots were a major trade item; they are rich in berberine.*

Traditional Usages

Oregon Grape is the state flower or Oregon. The Kwakuitls made a bark tea to offset the digestive disorder characterized by an excess of bile. In California, many tribes boiled the roots to make a tea they drank as an aperitif.

Soon adopted for domestic uses, the roots became a major trade item such that at the beginning of this century the species was almost exterminated around larger towns and cities. The roots, which contain berberine, were official in the *U.S. Pharmacopoeia* from 1905 to 1916.

Oregon Grape has also been used to treat **jaundice, chronic hepatitis, syphilis**, and **scrofula**. It was believed to have specific action on the spleen and was administered in cases of malaria where the spleen was dangerously enlarged; this was a risky procedure, however, since the ability to produce contraction was so strong that there was a possibility of rupture and fatal hemorrhage if the herb was taken by a person whose spleen was dangerously softened.

The plant was also been considered diuretic, mildly tonic, and gently laxative. It has been applied topically for various minor skin irritations.

Recent Scientific Findings

All *Berberis* species are quite similar in chemical composition, and hence would give rise to similar pharmacological effects. See remarks in article on Barberry (*Berberis vulgaris*) for further details.

ORRIS

SCIENTIFIC NAME: *Iris germanica* and other *Iris* species

PARTS USED: Rhizome

DOSAGE:

Rhizome: 1 teaspoon of rhizome, boiled in a covered container with 1½ pints of water for about ½ hour at a slow boil. Allow liquid to cool slowly in the *closed* container. Drink cold, 1 swallow or 1 tablespoon at a time, 1 to 2 cups per day.

ORRIS: *No longer used as a medicinal, the root and oil are common ingredients in cosmetics.*

Traditional Usages

Orris root is prepared by stripping away the outer layer of the rhizome and the roots. The remainder of the root is distilled to yield a solid oil. This oil (one part diluted with 3-4 parts alcohol) has a scent resembling the smell of violets. Consequently, it is valued in the perfume and cosmetics businesses.

Medicinally Orris is reputedly cathartic and diuretic, and in stronger doses it has been reported to be emetic. **It was felt to be useful in treating dropsical conditions** (water retention of tissues and/or organs). The root was also chewed as a coverup for **bad breath**.

Blue Flag (*Iris versicolor*), another herbaceous perennial found in the eastern United States, was once used for its emetic, diuretic, and cathartic effects.

This rhizome contains an acrid resin and essential oil.

Recent Scientific Findings

At this time, Orris is not used for medicinal purposes. However, **Orris root is a common ingredient in talcum powders and is a contact allergen.**

PANSY, WILD

SCIENTIFIC NAME: *Viola tricolor*
PARTS USED: Herb, flowers and root

DOSAGE:

    Root: Boil 1 teaspoon of the root in a covered container with 1½ pints of water for about ½ hour at a slow boil. Allow liquid to cool slowly in the *closed* container. Drink cold, 1 swallow or 1 tablespoon at a time, 1 to 2 cups per day.

WILD PANSY: *Used both internally and externally, this lovely flower has a long history of treating certain skin conditions.*

Traditional Usages

The Pansy's use in medicine can be traced back to ancient herbalists. In the 17th century it was reported that a North American tribe treated boils and swellings with a yellow-flowered pansy. It is not clear whether the Indians learned this plant remedy from the newly arriving Europeans. By the late 1800s, Wild Pansy was being ground up for application with a variety of skin diseases such as **scabies.**

The herb, which contains mucilaginous material, functions as an **external soothing lotion** for **boils, swellings,** and **skin diseases of various kinds.** It is also a **good and gentle laxative,** also because of the mucilage. This part of the Pansy has been utilized to treat pectoral and nephritic diseases.

The flowers also have **demulcent** properties, again because of the mucilage, and are made into syrup and administered as a **laxative** for infants. The root is both emetic and cathartic.

Sweet Violet (*V. odorata*) is much used as a flavoring and in candy making, while a leaf tea is a good cough remedy. The Wonder Violet (*V. mirabilis*) is used in decoction in Ukrainian folk medicine to treat heart ailments, palpitation, and shortness of breath.

Recent Scientific Findings

Wild Pansy contains saponins. Recent reports describe a tea made from the plant as effective on certain **skin conditions.** Given both as a tea internally and as compresses externally, it has been found useful in cases of **eczema** and other skin complaints in infants.

PAPAYA

SCIENTIFIC NAME: *Carica papaya*
PARTS USED: Leaf and latex

DOSAGE:

Leaves: The leaves are wrapped directly on wounds.

Latex: Latex used as needed; avoid internal use due to presence of protein-digesting properties.

PAPAYA: *The dried latex of this delicious fruit contains an enzyme that has been experimentally successful in cases of slipped discs.*

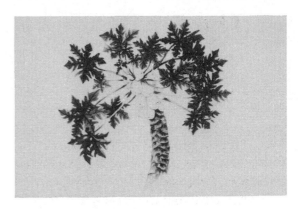

Papaya

Traditional Usages

Although the Papaya is best known for its delicious fruit, fresh Papaya leaves were used medicinally as a dressing for wounds by the aborigines indigenous to the tropical areas where the plant grows. They also wrapped meat in these leaves to make the flesh more tender.

In the Fiji Islands a filtrate of the inner bark is used to treat **toothache**, while the fresh milky white sap (latex) is applied directly on large **boils** and also utilized to **treat wounds.**

Recent Scientific Findings

The dried latex of the Papaya is marketed under the names papayotin, papain or papoid, and is given to treat **dyspepsia** and **gastric catarrh.** In powder form it is applied to treat skin diseases, including **warts** and **tubercle swellings.** Much of this medicinal product is supplied from Ceylon and the West Indies. It is still employed as a **meat tenderizer** and is **contained as an additive in one brand of beer to dissolve excess proteins, thereby making the beer more clear.**

The enzyme chymopapain, a derivative of the latex of the Papaya, has been used on an experimental basis by neurosurgeons to dissolve herniated ("slipped") intervertebral discs in patients complaining of **back pain.**

Preliminary research has also revealed **cardiac depressant** activity when given orally to human adults and **cardiotonic** activity.

PARSLEY

SCIENTIFIC NAME: *Petroselinum sativum*
PARTS USED: Leaf, root, and seeds

DOSAGE:

Leaves: Approximately 1 ounce of leaves to 1 pint of water. Boil water separately and pour over the plant material and steep for 5 to 20 minutes, depending on the desired effect. Drink hot or warm, 1 to 2 cups per day, at bedtime and upon awakening.

PARSLEY: *This popular cooking herb contains Apiol, which has been marketed in Russia to promote uterine contractions during labor.*

Traditional Usages

This popular cooking herb also has a long history of use as a medicinal. It was believed to be invigorating to the blood. Parsley was used to **regulate menstrual flow** with the oil of the seeds reputedly an **abortifacient**.

Parsley was employed for a variety of abdominal ailments, including **liver** and **spleen complaints** such as **jaundice** and **gastritis**. It was also considered a digestive aid that **promoted urination** and helped **expel gallstones**.

Recent Scientific Findings

A great deal of research has been conducted on Parsley's effect on cells and DNA. Some of the medical implications involve the enzymes that are integral to disease resistance response. In vitro studies have shown Parsley has **antibacterial** and **antifungal** effects. Unfortunately, little research has occurred to confirm or deny Parsley's folkloric claims as a remedy for liver ailments.

One of Parsley's chemical constituents, Apiol, is a **uterine stimulant**, as to a lesser extent is another constituent, myristicin. The Russian product "Supetin," comprised of 85% parsley juice, is used to stimulate uterine contractions during labor. At one time, Apiol was used in capsules as an abortifacient. Apiol and myristicin also contribute to Parsley's effectiveness as a diuretic.

Parsley is rich in nutrients, including vitamins A, B, C, and K as well as protein and potassium.

Caution: **Use of Parsley should be avoided during pregnancy.**

PASSION FLOWER

SCIENTIFIC NAME: *Passiflora incarnata*
PARTS USED: Plant and flower

DOSAGE:

Herb: For medicinal use, 1/2 to 1 teaspoon of the dried herb is used to 1 cup of boiling water. The resultant infusion may be taken every 3 to 4 hours. As a fluidextract, 3-4 drops every 4 hours.

PASSIONFLOWER: *Modern research is confirming Native American's use of this flower as a superior natural tranquilizer.*

Traditional Usages

All but about 40 species of the nearly 400 known species of *Passiflora* are natives of America; the 40 are natives of Asia, South Pacific islands, and Madagascar. Early European travelers in tropical America gave the strange flower the name Passionflower, as it suggested to them the passion of Christ: the 10 equal sepals and petals represented the crown of thorns; the 5 stamens, the five wounds; the 3 styles, the three nails; the tendrils, the cords or scourges; the leaves, the hands of the persecutors. The white color symbolizes purity; the blue, heaven.

In the Yucatan, it is an old remedy for **insomnia, hysteria,** and **convulsions in children.** Interestingly, the early Algonquins brewed this woody vine to soothe their nerves. The Houmas believed it was a systemic tonic and so added the pulverized root to their water. However, Passionflower was largely ignored in conventional North American medicine until the late-1800s. The flowering and fruiting tops were used to relieve insomnia and to soothe nerves. They were official in the *National Formulary* from 1916 to 1936.

Recent Scientific Findings

The state flower of Tennessee appears to be a useful bridge between traditional medicine and modern ills, especially anxiety states. Physicians could well recommend this plant to patients who want to wean themselves from synthetic sleeping pills and tranquilizers.

As a **sedative,** Passionflower has qualities unlike those of any other herb. It is very effective, with a pleasant taste, and yet surprisingly gentle. **It is helpful in a variety of ailments, from insomnia, dysmenorrhea, nervous tension, and fatigue, to muscle spasms.** It can be used with safety even for small children. In Italy the plant drug is used to treat **hyperactive children.**

Passiflora incarnata may be our best tranquilizer yet. The dried leaves and stems both induce a natural sleep and calm hyperactive people. It is currently being employed as a non-addictive substitute natural tranquilizer by physicians in the treatment of tranquilizer-addicted patients.

Surprisingly, one kind of Passionflower (*P. quadrangularis,* or Giant Granadilla) was recently found to contain serotonin. Low levels of this compound in the cerebrospinal fluid of patients with chronic depression have led some researchers to speculate that adding it to circulating blood would relieve states of depression. This may be confirmed by the fact that LSD-like compounds which are used to induce clinical psychoses are known to have potent anti-serotonin activity; perhaps Passionflower therefore acts as a natural calming agent by promoting the transmission of subtle nerve impulses. It appears to aid concentration, alter perception, and gently shift mood.

PATCHOULI LEAF

SCIENTIFIC NAME: *Pogostemon patchouli (P. cablin)*

PARTS USED: Herb

DOSAGE:

No recommended dose. Not medically active for folkloric usage. Ill effects, such as loss of appetite and sleep, and nervous attacks have been ascribed to the excessive employment of patchouli as a perfume.

PATCHOULI LEAF: *More known for its sexual use, the oil is a common ingredient in perfumes.*

Traditional Usages

The Arabs, Chinese, and Japanese believed that the oil of the Patchouli prevented venereal disease when applied prior to and during sexual intercourse.

It has a valuable property of fixing odors, giving it broad application in the perfumery business as an odor and scent preservative added to other fragrances.

Recent Scientific Findings

Almost all essential oils form plants have inhibitory activity against some type of microorganism. However, they rarely are tested against the organisms responsible for venereal disease, and thus it is difficult to project whether or not the use of Patchouli oil as a prophylaxis for venereal diseases is valid.

Although the author has not personally used Patchouli oil as an application to the genitalia to prevent venereal disease, I nevertheless pass on a word of caution. Virtually any essential oil, when applied undiluted to any mucous tissue, including the genitalia, produces a rush of heat to the area due to rapid evaporation and dilation of blood vessels in the area. This could produce a very uncomfortable condition if Patchouli oil was applied to the sensitive tissue of the penis and/or vagina!

PAU D'ARCO OR TAHEEBO

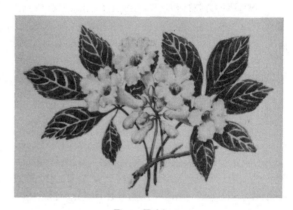

Pau D'Arco

SCIENTIFIC NAME: *Tabebuia impetiginosa* and other species

PARTS USED: Inner bark

DOSAGE:

A decoction of the bark is preferred. Steep ½ ounce or 1 teabag in 2 cups boiling water for 10-15 minutes. Cool, drink 1 tablespoon at a time, 2 to 4 cups per day.

PAU D'ARCO: *This "miracle" bark from South America may have anticancer properties.*

Traditional Usages

Traditionally, Pau D'Arco bark was used as a strengthener for increased energy and endurance.

Recent Scientific Findings

The inner bark of these stately, full leaved trees of Central and South America have received so much attention for their medicinal properties that sales of nearly $200 million have been reported. This is no doubt in part due to the keen marketing program undertaken by Brazilian and Argentinean suppliers of "taheebo." However, this marketing was based on solid reports of the bark's anticancer properties, first published in the 1960's.

The bark is rich (2-7%) in lapachol, a naphthoquinone,[72] and also contains lapachone and xyloidone, both quinoids. **Studies in the 1970's showed evidence that lapachol was active against mouse lymphocytic leukemia.**

Currently, Pau D'Arco is widely utilized for its reputed **anti-candida properties.** While no direct evidence exists to confirm or deny this activity, the anecdotal evidence is quite overwhelming. Moreover, a carefully controlled animal study published by a researcher at the prestigious Naval Medical Research Institute in Bethesda, Maryland demonstrated that **dietary intake of lapachol is protective against penetration and infection by another deadly parasite,** *Schistosoma mansoni.*

From the available evidence it appears that this **"miracle"** bark from South America, which has gained wide acceptance for its **anti-fungal** properties, will continue to gain in its applications, most notably against **intestinal parasites.**

PENNYROYAL

SCIENTIFIC NAME: *Hedeoma pulegioides* (American), *Mentha pulegium* (European)

PARTS USED: Whole plant

DOSAGE:

Whole plant: 1 teaspoon per cup of boiling water. Boil water separately and pour over the plant material and steep for 5-20 minutes, depending on the desired effect. Drink hot or warm, 1 to 2 cups. *Caution:* the essential oil has caused death.

PENNYROYAL: *The pleasant tea of this herb is an aromatic carminative.*

Traditional Usages

The Onondagas, one of the divisions of the Iroquois, steeped Pennyroyal leaves and drank the resulting tea to cure **headaches.** A related species (*H. reverchoni*) was also used by the Mescalero Apaches as a headache remedy by crushing the twigs and inhaling the mintlike odor.

Extensively employed in domestic American medicine, Pennyroyal induced sweating in the early stages of colds. It was also employed to **promote menstruation** as well as being used with brewer's yeast to induce abortion and with raw linseed oil to dress burns. In the Thomsonian system of medicine, Pennyroyal was utilized to check **nosebleed;** the patient sat with feet immersed in a tub of quite warm water while drinking a tea made from the plant.

This was thought to equalize circulation and alleviate pressure to the head. From 1831 to 1916 the dried leaves were official in the *U.S. Pharmacopoeia.*

> It is a gentle stimulant, and as an aid in relieving the common cold, a draught was often drunk at bedtime to promote perspiration, again with the feet soaking in hot water. It was also used the same way to bring on suppressed menstruation.

Recent Scientific Findings

The two species both have the medicinal properties of the official Mints, being **stimulant, aromatic, carminative,** and **stomachic.** The volatile oil has similar properties to the herb and is frequently used in domestic practice to **promote the menstrual flow.** Pennyroyal is considered inferior in its medicinal qualities to Peppermint, which largely superseded it in regular medicine, but Pennyroyal has continued to be popular in domestic practice. The alcoholic infusion has been utilized to treat fainting, asphyxia, paralysis, asthma, hysteria, atonic gout, and flatulence.

Experimentally, **extracts of Pennyroyal are known to stimulate the uterus** in test tube studies, which could account for the menses-inducing effect.

It is a very soothing tea, and produces a nice sense of comforting warmth.

> *Caution:* Large doses of this plant are known to produce nausea, vomiting, and possible toxic effects. A recent death was found to be the result of the ingestion of Pennyroyal essential oil, not an infusion of the herb.

PEPPERMINT

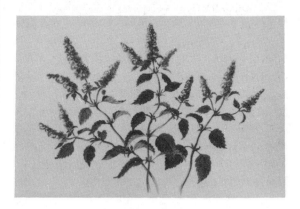

Peppermint

SCIENTIFIC NAME: *Mentha piperita*
PARTS USED: Leaves and flowering tops

DOSAGE:

> **Leaves:** Approximately ½ ounce of leaves to 1 pint of boiling water. Boil water separately and pour over the plant material and steep for 5-20 minutes, depending on the desired effect. Drink hot or warm, 1 to 2 cups or more per day.

PEPPERMINT: *This remains one of our most refreshing carminatives.*

Traditional Usages

The genus name, *Mentha*, originated in Greek mythology; the nymph Mintha was metamorphosized into this plant. It is recorded that Peppermint was cultivated by the ancient Egyptians, and its usage is documented in the Icelandic pharmacopoeia of the thirteenth century. The most agreeable and powerful of the mints, it possesses aromatic, carminative, stimulant, antispasmodic and stomachic properties.

Peppermint is frequently used to allay nausea, relieve stomach and bowel spasms and griping, and to promote the expulsion of flatus. It is often drunk after mealtime as an aid to digestion. The volatile oil, which has been similarly used in medicine, is also employed as a flavoring agent in cordials and candles, and has also been added to less palatable medicines to mask disagreeable odors and/or tastes.

Recent Scientific Findings

Peppermint tea is one of the most common herbal remedies, **used primarily as a carminative and intestinal antispasmodic**. These effects are all explained on the basis of animal experiments using the essential oil from Peppermint, or purified essential oil constituents, the results of which mimic the effects claimed in humans. This essential oil has a high menthol content. **Menthol both stimulates the flow of bile to the stomach and is an antispasmodic.**

PERIWINKLE, TROPICAL

SCIENTIFIC NAME: *Catharanthus roseus, Vinca rosea*

PARTS USED: Herb

DOSAGE:
> *Caution:* See discussion.

TROPICAL PERIWINKLE: *This lovely ornamental plant is the source of the potent anti-cancer drugs vinblastine and vincristine.*

Traditional Usages

The Tropical Periwinkle is a pantropical plant that is often cultivated in temperate climates as an ornamental. However, in the Philippines, Periwinkle has long been taken orally as a folkloric remedy for the treatment of hyperglycemia. A leaf extract was used to treat diabetes.

Recent Scientific Findings

The Tropical Periwinkle is an extremely important example of a traditional folk medicine whose use was investigated by a major pharmaceutical company, resulting in the discovery of two alkaloids with **practical application in the treatment of cancer.**

In 1953 Dr. Faustino Garcia reported at the Pacific Science Congress on Periwinkle's use in the Philippines to treat hyperglycemia. Researchers at the Lily Company, conducting a general survey of many folk remedy plants through preliminary testing in a cancer-screening program, found that the Periwinkle showed striking anticancer activity in test animals.

In the early 1960s it was discovered that extracts of the leaves of *C. roseus* would significantly prolong the life of mice in which leukemia had been clinically induced. **This finding eventually led to the discovery of two potent anticancer drugs, vincaleukoblastine (vinblastine, VLB) and leurocristine (vincristine, VCR), both of which are now available on a worldwide basis for the treatment of human cancer.** While nearly identical structurally, the these two alkaloids each effect different types of tumors.

Vincristine is one of our most important anticancer drugs, being most useful for the treatment of **childhood leukemias**. Vinblastine is of lesser importance, but is effective in treating certain types of **Hodgkin's disease**.

Since vincristine odes have neurotoxic side effects, and vinblastine can cause a marked decrease in the number of white blood cells, these must be considered as **very potent drugs**. Thus, it cannot be recommended that the Tropical Periwinkle be used as a herbal remedy, since the danger of potential life-threatening complications is very real.

The leaves have also been used most extensively as an **oral insulin substitute**. Proprietary products have been sold in Africa and the Philippines for this purpose.

At least seven or eight scientific publications are available in which investigators have reported no effect on blood sugar levels in normal, as well as diabetic animals, when aqueous extracts of Periwinkle leaves were administered orally. Other studies have been published in which hot-water extracts of the leaves of this plant were given to diabetic patients, but in every instance there was no significant benefit to the patients.

Vinca major (Greater Periwinkle) and *Vinca minor* (Lesser Periwinkle): Both of these "Periwinkles" are often confused with the Tropical Periwinkle (*Catharanthus roseus*), and although *Vinca* and *Catharanthus* are related in being members of the Dogbane (Apocynaceae) family, they are chemically and pharmacologically quite different.

Although Greater Periwinkle and Lesser Periwinkle are somewhat different in chemical makeup, they have both been used externally to stop hemorrhages, such effect most likely being due to astringent tannins present in both plants. Any effect of preventing menstrual hemorrhaging (menorrhagia) could be due to vincamine, an indole alkaloid present in both species, which has been shown to contact uterine muscle in test tube experiments. Neither of these effects has been confirmed, however, by direct experiments involving the use of extracts from these plants.

Vincamine has also been found to effect the flow of blood in the brain. A series of ECG studies and double blind trials found that vincamine improved the cerebral vascular system.

PINEAPPLE

SCIENTIFIC NAME: *Ananas comosus*
PARTS USED: Enzyme: Bromelain

DOSAGE:
No recommended dose.

PINEAPPLE: *This delicious fruits contains an enzyme that may have anticancer properties.*

Recent Scientific Findings

Pineapple contains **bromelain**, an enzyme whose exact chemical structure is currently being investigated. However, bromelain has exhibited some interesting pharmacological possibilities. It appears to interfere with the growth of malignant cells, inhibit platelet aggregation, fibrinolytic activity, anti-inflammatory action, and skin debridement properties.

These properties therapeutically might prove effective in treating tumor growth, blood coagulation, inflammatory changes, debridement (removal of unhealthy tissue) of third degree burns, enhancement of the absorption of drugs.

Animals experiments with rats indicated that **Pineapple enzymes rapidly effect debridement of skin burns.**

PINKROOT

SCIENTIFIC NAME: *Spigelia marilandica*
PARTS USED: Rhizome and roots

DOSAGE:
Not recommended. Requires expertise of a skilled herbalist to be effective yet not toxic.

PINKROOT: *Native Americans discovered the root's ability to treat intestinal worms.*

Traditional Usages

Overdose can be fatal, but use of Pinkroot has rarely been reported to produce ill effects so long as it is eliminated. For this reason it is commonly prescribed in combination with Calomel, Senna, or some other cathartic.

Pinkroot is one of the clearest examples of acceptance of a Native American remedy by the medical profession. The Cherokees prepared a **worm medicine** by boiling a large quantity of the freshly dug root in water.

In the early 1700s, two physicians from Charleston, South Carolina, learned about Pinkroot from Native Americans. Quickly spreading to the general public, Pinkroot was praised as a worm treatment, particularly roundworms, and commonly used for the next 200 years. In the early 1900s, Pinkroot fell into disuse when greedy herb dealers adulterated or substituted other plants.

The 23rd edition of the *Dispensatory of the United States* lists the prescribed adult dose of the powdered root as four or eight grams each morning and evening for several days, then to be followed by a strong laxative.

A preparation sold under the name Worm Tea contained Spigelia, Senna, Manna, and Cedar Berry. It was mixed in different strengths by the apothecary to suit individual needs.

Recent Scientific Findings

The roots contain spigeline, which resembles coniine (found in Hemlock) and nicotine, which explains its stimulant effects.

PIPSISSEWA

SCIENTIFIC NAME: *Chimaphila umbellata, C. Maculata*

PARTS USED: Leaves and herb

DOSAGE:

Leaves or Herb: Approximately ½ ounce of leaves or herb to 1 pint of water. Boil water separately and pour over the plant material and steep for 5-20 minutes, depending on the desired effect. Drink hot or warm, 1 to 2 cups per day. Still, the best method of taking the herb is in the form of fluidextract, which is readily made into a syrup: dose, 2-6 grams.

PIPSISSEWA: This Native American remedy remains a first-rate medicinal for urinary-tract infections.

Traditional Usages

Why the generic name of these plants is formed of two Greek words for "winter" and "love" remains a mystery, although their use in folk medicine is readily explained. This Native American remedy for rheumatism and **scrofula** (a type of tuberculosis) was also used by the settlers for the same purposes. Both groups also took the plant as a tea to induce sweating.

The Mohegans and the Penobscots steeped the plant in warm water and applied the liquid externally to draw out blisters. The Thompsons of British Columbia pulverized the entire fresh plant and applied the mass in the form of a wet dressing to swellings of the lower legs and feet.

At one time, Pipsissewa was a popular home remedy among the early settlers of the United States, especially the Pennsylvania Germans who used it as a tea to induce sweating. From 1820 to 1916 it was official in the *U.S. Pharmacopoeia* as an **astringent** or tissue-drying agent.

It is credited with tonic, astringent, and diuretic properties, and was administered in the treatment of cystitis and was held to be diuretic and antiseptic to the urinary tract. A decoction was applied externally for blisters and scrofulous sores and swellings, but the Pipsissewa remains a **first-rate folk remedy for miscellaneous urinary-tract infections.**

Recent Scientific Findings

The leaves of this half-shrub contain ericolin, arbutin, chimaphilin, urson, tannin, and gallic acid. Chimaphilin, as well as extracts of this plant, show **antibacterial** properties in test tube experiments. This can explain the use of this plant in scrofula, and in treating cystitis.

PLANTAIN

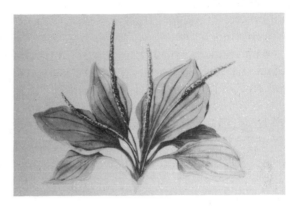

Plantain

SCIENTIFIC NAME: *Plantago major, P. lanceolata* and var. spp.

PARTS USED: Seeds, leaves

DOSAGE:

Seeds and Leaves: In 1 pint of boiling water, steep for 20 minutes, drink hot or warm, 1 to 2 cups. Infusion of ½ ounce of seeds to 1 pint of water, steep for 5-20 minutes; drink 1 tablespoon 3-6 times per day.

PLANTAIN: *Called "white man's foot" by Native Americans, the leaves are an effective treatment for poison ivy rash.*

Traditional Usages

Plantain has been used medicinally since antiquity. Formerly this common weed was utilized to relieve thirst and reduce fever, to remove obstructions within the system, and as an astringent. Later it was seldom used internally but remained a popular external stimulant application to **boils, sores,** and **wounds.** The leaves were bruised and applied whole to the affected area in poultice form. To relieve bee stings, the fresh leaves are rubbed on.

Native Americans named Plantain white man's foot due to the plant's trait of growing in the footsteps of the white man; the plant was commonly introduced wherever a settlement developed. The Shoshoni heated the leaves and applied them in a wet dressing for wounds. In early American domestic medicine, the leaves were employed as an antidote to the bites of venomous snakes and insects, while the seeds were used as a worm remedy. Boerhaave, an 18th century botanist, recommended that Plantain leaves be bound to aching feet after long hikes to relieve pain and fatigue. In Ayurvedic medicine, Plantain is used to treat ulcers.

Recent Scientific Findings

P. media, the Hoary Plantain, and *P. lanceolata,* the Narrow-Leaved Plantain (Rib Grass), possess the same properties as *P. major* and may be utilized interchangeably. A European species, *P. psyllium,* the Fleawort, has seeds which are used medicinally due to their mucilaginous nature. They are **demulcent** and **emollient** and were used for the same purposes as Flax seed (see article on Flax).

The seeds of most *Plantago* species contain high concentrations of mucilage, and thus will have a demulcent and emollient effect externally, and will act as a **laxative** if taken internally due to the swelling of the seeds.

An Italian study found that **Plantain served effectively in contributing to weight loss in conjunction with a prescribed diet.** Researchers in Russia and Italy found Plantain reduced intestinal absorption of lipids.

A study published in the *Lancet* described several people who contracted **poison ivy rash.** They were immediately treated with Plantain leaf. The itching subsided and did not return.

PLEURISY ROOT

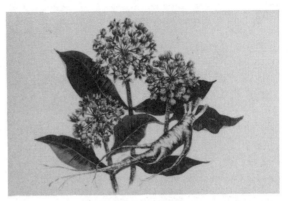

Pleurisy Root

SCIENTIFIC NAME: *Asclepias tuberosa*
PARTS USED: Root

DOSAGE:

Root: For medicinal use, 1 teaspoonful of the powdered root is used per 1½ pints of boiling water; boil in a covered container for about ½ hour at a slow boil. Allow liquid to cool slowly in the *closed* container. Drink cold, 1 swallow or 1 tablespoon at a time, 1 to 2 cups per day.

PLEURISY ROOT: *In both Native American and domestic American practice, this root was used to treat respiratory ailments.*

Traditional Usages

The root of the Butterfly Weed, or Pleurisy Root, derives its name from its effectiveness as an **expectorant**, helping to expel phlegm from the bronchial and nasal passages. It was employed in a variety of respiratory ailments besides **pleurisy**, including **cough, consumption,** and **bronchitis.** Because of its claimed **antispasmodic properties**, the dried and powdered root was administered to cure **infant colic.** Adults likewise drank a herb tea of the root as an aid in eliminating flatulence.

The Natchez drank a tea of the boiled roots as a remedy for **pneumonia.** The same preparation was used by the Catawbas for **dysentery.** The fresh root was chewed by the Omahas for bronchitis and other respiratory complaints.

Prior to the advent of synthetic drugs, Pleurisy Root was widely employed by medical practitioners in the United States. Medical journals frequently carried scientific articles on the effectiveness of Pleurisy Root preparations as a diaphoretic, expectorant, emetic, and cathartic. The specific effect was dependent on the amount of the preparation used. Pleurisy root was in the *U.S. Pharmacopoeia* from 1820 to 1905 and in the *National Formulary* from 1916 to 1936. The active principle responsible for these effects, however, remains unknown.

Recent Scientific Findings

Pleurisy root has yet to have a fair trial in the laboratory and would appear to be a good candidate for renewed research.

POMEGRANATE

SCIENTIFIC NAME: *Punica granatum*
PARTS USED: Bark, rind, and fruit

DOSAGE:

Root bark: 1 teaspoonful of root bark, chopped small, to 1½ pints of boiling water; slow boil in a covered container for about ½ hour. Allow liquid to cool slowly in the *closed* container. Drink cold, 1 mouthful at a time, over the day, to a maximum of 1 cup total.

POMEGRANATE: *This tasty fruit's root bark has long been an effective remedy for intestinal worms.*

Traditional Usages

The fruit of this small shrubby tree is eaten and its juice is used to make refreshing drinks, particularly in the Middle East. In Israel, the fruit has been cultivated for 5,000 years. The powdered root rind was held to be **astringent**, and was utilized to treat **diarrhea**, excessive perspiration, as a **gargle for sore throats**, for intermittent fevers, and for leucorrhea.

The root bark was administered by the ancients to rid the intestines of worms. This medicinal usage was overlooked by Europeans until 1804, when a practitioner in India who had cured an Englishman of a tapeworm was persuaded to share his secret remedy. Nausea and vomiting sometime accompanied the purgative action of this plant; consequently, patients were advised

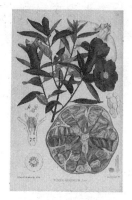

Pomegranate

to fast for 12 hours prior to treatment. Two hours after administration of the remedy, a brisk cathartic was given to expedite discharge of the remains of the worm. The remedy was repeated day after day, sometimes as many as four times, until success was achieved.

Recent Scientific Findings

Of all types of intestinal worm infestations, Pomegranate root bark is most useful in cases of **tapeworm**. The active principle, discovered in 1878, is the liquid alkaloid pelletierine, which was used in human medicine for a number of years, and then became relegated to veterinary use. **Thus, it is well established that root bark preparations of Pomegranate would be effective when used to expel worms from the intestinal tract.**

Anyone who has bitten into the peel of a Pomegranate fruit can testify to the highly astringent nature of this material. In fact, it is known that the fruit peel contains about 30 percent of tannin, which is the active astringent substance.

POPLAR

SCIENTIFIC NAME: *Populous nigra,*
P. balsamifera

PARTS USED: Leaf buds

DOSAGE:

> **Leaf buds:** A handful of buds, macerate in olive oil, and apply sparingly externally.

POPLAR: *At one time, the leaf buds were part of popular European ointment.*

Traditional Usages

Poplar leaf buds are covered with a resinous exudate; their smell is balsamic and pleasant, the taste bitterly aromatic. Poplar buds have been used for the same purposes as the Turpentines and other balsams. Macerated in oil, they were applied externally as a liniment for the treatment of **rheumatism**. A popular salve was made in France of equal parts (100 grams) of Poppy, Belladonna, Henbane, and Black Nightshade, moistened with 400 grams of alcohol, rested for 24 hours, then heated with 4,000 grams of lard for 3 hours, after which 800 grams crushed Poplar buds were added and the mixture was heated for 10 more hours, then strained. This anodyne ointment was used to treat painful local afflictions including sores and burns. Known as "Pommade de Bourgeons de Peuplier," it was widely used throughout Europe. There were several different ways to concoct this ointment, using the same plant materials.

In tincture form the buds have been given for chest complaints and in the treatment of **inflammation of the kidneys.**

Recent Scientific Findings

Poplar buds are rich in chemical substances having actions similar to aspirin, such as salicin and mixtures of phenolic acids. Thus, Poplar buds taken *internally* would be useful in minor rheumatic pains. The phenolic acids would contribute to the effectiveness of extracts being used for **coughs** as well. We can find no rationale for the application of Poplar bud extracts externally to relieve rheumatism symptoms, since the active chemicals are not known to be absorbed through the skin.

PRICKLY ASH

SCIENTIFIC NAME: *Aralia spinosa*
　　　　　　　　Zanthoxylum
　　　　　　　　Clava-Herculis,
　　　　　　　　Zanthoxylum
　　　　　　　　fraxineum
PARTS USED: Bark and berries

DOSAGE:

Berries: Women suffering from chronic pelvic diseases used this plant as a counter-irritant, applying hot packs of 2-4 ounces of fluidextract *zanthoxylum*, mixed with 1 ounce of tincture of cayenne pepper to 2 quarts of water, to the external pelvic area, to relieve their distress.

Bark: A decoction may be prepared using 1 teaspoon of the bark, boiled in a covered container with 1½ pints of boiling water for about ½ hour at a slow boil. Allow liquid to cool slowly in the *closed* container. Drink cold, 1 swallow or 1 tablespoon at a time, 1 to 2 cups per day.

PRICKLY ASH: *Called the "toothache tree," the dried bark was in the U.S. Pharmacopoeia as a rheumatism treatment.*

Traditional Usages

Numerous Native American tribes employed the pulverized root and/or the bark for **toothache.** In domestic American medicine, the bark was simply chewed raw, or inserted into cavities. Indeed the southern variety was once known as the "toothache tree."

Prickly Ash was also a popular remedy for **chronic rheumatism**, and was utilized extensively in the United States for this purpose. This plant is a **stimulant** and was also used to produce perspiration.

The bark and roots were boiled in water and the decoction drunk as a cure for venereal disease. J. Carver's *Travels through the Interior Parts of North America* includes an account of a Winnebago chief who cured a white trader of gonorrhea. During the 19th century Prickly Ash bark was used to treat typhoid pneumonia. The dried bark was official in the *U.S. Pharmacopoeia* from 1820 to 1926 as a treatment for rheumatism. The berries were listed in the *National Formulary* from 1916 to 1947 for their **antispasmodic, stimulant**, and **antirheumatic** purposes.

Prickly Ash bark was also employed in the treatment of **flatulence** and **diarrhea.** The berries are aromatic in addition to the above properties, and were used medicinally only in this connection.

Recent Scientific Findings

Prickly Ash has been the subject of only limited laboratory or clinical testing. To date, it has exhibited **analgesic** and **diaphoretic** properties as well as promoting saliva. It also may prove useful as an **insecticide.**

PSYLLIUM

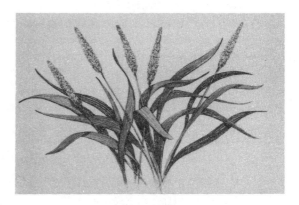

Psyllium

SCIENTIFIC NAME: *Plantago ovata*
PARTS USED: Seed

DOSAGE:

One-half teaspoon of seeds after breakfast.

PSYLLIUM: *The seeds have exhibited some extraordinary effects as a dietary supplement.*

Traditional Usages

Psyllium was esteemed by Indian, Persian, and Arab physicians of the Middle Ages as a lubricating agent for the lower intestinal tract. It also was used as an emollient.

Recent Scientific Findings

Psyllium proves to have a remarkable variety of positive applications as a dietary supplement.

Psyllium is commonly used to manage diarrhea, not only in the short-term, but also for long-term management of irritable bowel syndrome. For instance, in one clinical trial conducted over a several month period, patients undergoing treatment remained in remission. Interestingly, patients on placebo who had relapsed, became asymptomatic upon resumption of the treatment. Also those for whom treatment was curtailed relapsed but then recovered upon resumption.

Recent research has found that Psyllium's ability to manage diarrhea may also be useful for patients in intensive care who are being fed intravenously. Diarrhea is a major complication for tube-fed patients. In one study involving 49 patients at a large medical center, Psyllium significantly reduced diarrhea.

Psyllium's hypocholesterolemic effects are well established. Hypercholesterolemia is a significant risk factor for coronary heart disease. There are numerous clinical trials attesting to Psyllium's cholesterol-lowering effects. One double-blind study of 163 men and women with high serum cholesterol levels supplemented the American Heart Association's recommended diet with Psyllium. The results showed that Psyllium "significantly enhances the American Heart Association diet effects." Another study involving 59 subjects came to the same conclusion regarding Psyllium supplementation to the Phase I diet.

A randomized double-blind, placebo-controlled study involving 58 male patients confirmed that Psyllium cereals are "an effective and well-tolerated part of a prudent diet in the treatment of mild to moderate hypercholesterolemia." Another double-blind study involving 75 patients as well as a two-stage study with 14 individuals also concluded that Psyllium was an effective adjunct to diet. An eight week study of 26 men stated that "the reductions in total cholesterol and LDL cholesterol became progressively larger with time, and this trend appeared to be continuing at the eighth week. Psyllium treatment did not affect body weight, blood pressure, or serum levels of high-density lipoprotein cholesterol, triglycerides, glucose, iron, or zinc."

In a longer term study, over a one year period 176 ambulatory elderly patients used psyllium hydrophilic mucilloid (PHM) while 741 patients did not use PHM. The researchers concluded that "the dose of PHM administered was significantly correlated with the change in serum cholesterol."

While it is not known exactly how Psyllium reduces cholesterol, preliminary findings indicate that Psyllium lowers cholesterol absorption and increases the rate of cholesterol transformation to bile acids.

Psyllium added to the diet has also been found to possibly be helpful for **diabetics**. In a crossover study 18 non-insulin-dependent diabetics were given Psyllium before breakfast and dinner. The results showed that Psyllium reduced glucose levels following the meals.

Preliminary research raises the possibility that Psyllium may also indirectly protect the colon from cancer by providing protection for colonocytes.

Caution: Severe allergic reactions to Psyllium have occurred, especially among individuals sensitized by occupational exposure, such as health care workers.

PUMPKIN

SCIENTIFIC NAME: *Cucurbita pepo*
PARTS USED: Seeds

DOSAGE:

Seeds: From 1 to 2 ounces Pumpkin seeds, as fresh as possible (shelled) beaten to a paste with finely powdered sugar, and diluted with water or milk, when taken; no food to be eaten for 24 hours *prior* to taking this remedy. Three or four hours afterward, 1 or 2 tablespoons of castor oil should be taken.

The seed oil was also given (as an alternative to the above) in doses of 1/2 ounce, repeated once or twice at an interval of 2 hours and followed in 2 hours more by a dose of castor oil.

PUMPKIN: *For centuries pumpkins seeds have been used to remove intestinal worms.*

Traditional Usages

Pumpkin seeds have been used in almost every culture in the world for centuries **as an aid to remove intestinal worms (vermifuge) from the body, or more specifically, to rid the body of tapeworms (taeniafuge).**

In 1820 a Cuban physician reported that 3 ounces of fresh flesh of the Pumpkin would accomplish the death and expulsion of the tapeworm exactly as the recommended dose of 1 1/2 ounces of seeds. However, the Pumpkin flesh dosage has to be repeated to be effective, whereas the treatment with the seeds, following a 12-hour fast, followed in 1 hour by a cup of tea, and by a brisk cathartic an hour after that, and finally by a hearty meal in 2 hours, effectively expelled the tapeworm without repeating the dose. Medicinal knowledge of Pumpkin was first introduced into the United States in 1851 by Richard Soule.

Recent Scientific Findings

The amount of Pumpkin seeds used for vermifuge purposes ranges from 10-200 grams per dose in humans. Studies in China, Russia, and elsewhere have shown that Pumpkin seeds are very effective in removing worms from both animals and humans. **The active anthelmintic agent in Pumpkin seeds has been known for some time; it is an unusual amino acid known as cucurbitin.** Cucurbitin is present in Pumpkin seeds in quantities ranging from 0.18 to 0.66 percent.

Purified cucurbitin was studied in 150 patients with various types of intestinal worm infestations. It was shown to be unusually safe when given by mouth, especially against the beef and pork tapeworm, and pinworms. No contraindications were recommended for the use of cucurbitin as a result of the study. A small number (3 percent) of the patients (5/150) had mild side effects from the drug, including nausea, dizziness, and weakness.

Other studies in the United States have shown that when 30-65 grams daily of Pumpkins seeds are taken by mouth, a slight decrease in the amount of urine excreted occurs. On the other hand, daily elimination of urea and uric acid in the urine was increased. Thus, we can once again point out a rational basis for the use of a centuries-old herbal remedy, based on animal and human studies.

> Pumpkin also exhibited interesting results as a psychological treatment. L-tryptophan had been long-established as a safe, effective treatment for anxiety, depression, and sleep disorders when it was abruptly withdrawn from the market, for capricious reasons. A 1988 study reported on a 44 year-old man successfully treated with an alternate source of this amino acid, pumpkin seeds.

The patient suffered from "recurrent unipolar depressions." He could not tolerate pharmaceutical antidepressants; in 1985 he was put on L-tryptophan as an alternative. He was so sensitive that on 4.5 grams per day he became hypomanic. When the dose was reduced to 1.5 grams per day he was stabilized and discharged from the clinic. For five years the man remained well "apart from a bout of depression with biological features every three months or so. At these points he took about 1.5 grams of L-tryptophan over two days and found that this quickly restored his well being." Unfortunately, the patient was unable to self-treat his latest bout of depression due to this product's withdrawal from the marketplace.

Seeking an alternative this innovative psychiatrist drew on the work of another patient, a physician who had cured his own sleep problem with L-tryptophan from Pumpkin seeds. This patient was given about 200 grams of these seeds, equal to about 1 gram of L-tryptophan and "within 24 hours . . . he felt quite transformed. He was no longer anergic or depressed and happily returned to work the following day."

QUASSIA

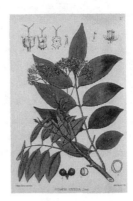

Quassia

SCIENTIFIC NAME: *Picrasma excelsa*
PARTS USED: Wood

DOSAGE:

Wood: The medicinal dose is prepared by using one teaspoon of granulated wood per 1½ pints of boiling water, boiled in a separate container for about ½ hour, at a slow boil. Allow liquid to cool slowly in the *closed* container. Drink cold, 1 mouthful at a time, 1 cup per day. When used as a tincture or fluidextract the dose was 0.32 to 0.65 gram.

QUASSIA: *Named for a healer from Surinam, this bitter tonic has been a popular appetite stimulant in Europe.*

Traditional Usages

Quassia was brought to Stockholm in 1756 by a Swede who had purchased it in Surinam from a native healer named Quassi. While the drug soon became popular, the Quassia of Surinam was eventually superseded by *P. excelsa* from the West Indies. A powerful simple bitter tonic, the medicine was widely used in Europe for gastric upsets, as an appetite stimulant, and as a **laxative** in cases of chronic constipation in convalescents.

In overdoses, Quassia causes vomiting. It has been thought by some to possess narcotic properties, since it acts as a narcotic poison on flies, and perhaps on higher animals as well. "Flypaper" used for trapping and killing flies was once made of an infusion of Quassia sweetened with sugar.

Recent Scientific Findings

Quassia wood contains extremely bitter chemical substances known as "qaussinoids," the major one being called quassin. These bitter principles are very poorly soluble in water, and for this reason the wood has been used to prepare "Quassia cups." A Qaussia cup is filled with hot water and the water is allowed to cool somewhat before being drunk. This results is a liquid that is very bitter and thus acts to stimulate the appetite. Quassia cups can be used in this way for a number of years and will retain an ability to produce a bitter water extract.

We have found no laboratory evidence for the folkloric claim that Quassia preparations will have an expectorant effect.

QUERCETIN
(a bioflavonoid)

PARTS USED: Bioflavonoid found in many plants

DOSAGE:

1.0 to 2.0 grams in capsule or tablet form as a dietary supplement daily.

QUERCETIN: *This common bioflavonoid possesses remarkable anti-inflammatory effects.*

Recent Scientific Findings

Here we briefly look at a bioflavonoid found in many, many plants. In my many years of searching the tropical jungles for new plant remedies I've often watched local healers as they prepared and administered various folk-cures. Seeing cases of badly inflamed skin treated with plant medicine made me wonder if the almost instantaneous **anti-inflammatory** effects were due to the flavonoids found in the various salves and infusions.

Quercetin achieves these "blocking" actions by inhibiting IgE mediated allergic mediator release from mast cells. In simpler terms this type of naturally occurring flavonoid acts as an antihistamine. Quercetin works best when combined with vitamin C. Like quercetin, substantial evidence supports the use of vitamin C in allergic diseases.

In addition, quercetin inhibits lipoxygenase, an enzyme involved in the metabolism of arachidonic acid (AA) in cells. Recall, AA is required for the inflammatory response to occur, via the production of prostaglandins and leukotrienes. Bioflavonoids such as quercetin can block the production of leukotrienes and other pro-inflammatory AA metabolites. They also act as anti-oxidants, scavenging dangerous free-radicals and protecting cells.

Suppressing inflammation and allergies are only some of the effects of Quercetin. This potent phytopharmaceutical, made by nature and found in many plants has **also been found to stimulate the immune system and kill viruses.**

Where can we find this remarkable herbal compound? As we stated, it is widely distributed in the vegetable kingdom. Quercetin (and other flavonoids) is found in fruits, vegetables, seeds, nuts, leaves, flowers, roots and bark.

RASPBERRY, RED

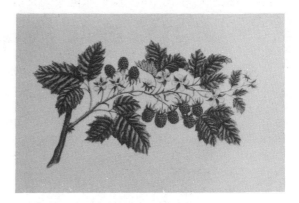

Red Raspberry

SCIENTIFIC NAME: *Rubus spp.*
PARTS USED: Leaf

DOSAGE:

Leaves: One teaspoon of the leaf is used per cup of boiling water. Drink cold, 1 to 2 cups per day. During pregnancy: steep ½ ounce with 1 pint of boiling water 3-5 minutes, drink warm, 1 pint per day.

Root bark: The root bark is used in the proportion of one teaspoonful of chopped root bark per 1½ pints of water; boil down to 1 pint, and administer 1 to 2 ounces cold, 3 or 4 times per day.

RED RASPBERRY: *The leaves of this tasty fruit are the source of a tea often drunk during pregnancy to relieve morning sickness.*

Traditional Usages

Five varieties and a form have been distinguished of this common plant that is found in dry or moist woods, fields, and roadsides, north to Alaska, south to New England, Pennsylvania, Indiana, Iowa, and in the west to Arizona.

The Pawnee, Omaha, and Dakota tribes used a boiled decoction of black raspberry roots for dysentery. The fruit was listed in the *U.S. Pharmacopoeia* from 1882 to 1905 as a flavoring.

Recent Scientific Findings

Red Raspberry leaves contain high concentrations of tannins, which is most likely responsible for the antinauseant, antivomiting, antidiarrheal, and astringent effects of this plant. A vast literature exists supporting the numerous folkloric claims for this interesting plant genus. **Various species of Raspberry have been shown to: induce ovulation, relax the uterus, act as a diuretic, stimulate immunity, kill viruses (including herpes), control glucose-induced high blood sugar, promote insulin production, kill fungi, and stimulate interferon induction.**

Red Raspberry leaf or root tea is an excellent astringent remedy for diarrhea, and will also allay nausea and vomiting. The leaf tea is also drunk during pregnancy to facilitate childbirth, and, as indicated above, will help with "morning sickness."

As the scientific evidence indicates, many species of Raspberry are "super-useful" for a myriad of women's problems. One study showed that

Raspberry leaf prevented the typical hyper-growth effects of chronic gonadotrophin on ovaries and uterus, while another study demonstrated that Raspberry leaf relaxes uterine muscles. In the latter study tea concentrates were tested on several species of animal. If the smooth muscle of the uterus was "in tone," the water extract of Raspberry leaf relaxed it. If the muscle was relaxed, the herb caused contractions.

Other studies have found antiviral activity in cell culture against vaccinia virus and strong antiviral activity (in cell culture) against herpes virus II; also antiviral activity has been found against soxsackie virus, influenza virus, polio virus I, and reovirus I.

REISHI MUSHROOM

SCIENTIFIC NAME: *Ganoderma lucidum, G. japonicum*

PARTS USED: Cap and stem

DOSAGE:

2 to 3 grams, in capsule or tablet form, once per day.

REISHI MUSHROOM: *This "lucky fungus," which has been eaten in Japan for at least 3,000 years, now is being discovered by Americans.*

Traditional Usages

The Japanese names for this member of the basidiomycetes are *mannentake*, meaning "tens of thousand year fungus," *saiwaitake* "happy fungus," or *kisshotake*, "lucky fungus." Originally utilized in China as a food "to lengthen life," the reishi mushrooms have been eaten in Japan for at least 3,000 years.

In traditional Chinese medicine this almost magical fungus has long been prized to "prevent serious damage or recover quickly from disease." In other words, Reishi is able to work both as a *preventive* herb as well as to treat seriously ill people.

Recent Scientific Findings

Long regarded with suspicion by Americans, the mushrooms are now receiving renewed attention owing to the health promoting compounds found in several species. While most of the results reported thus far are based on animal studies, the historical reverence assigned reishi mushrooms by the Japanese tends to support the contention that human studies will produce equally exciting results.

Reishi mushrooms are commercially available in several varieties. *G. lucidum*, the red variety, is the type preferred in Japan. *G. japonicum*, which is darker and softer as well as cultured varieties are also sold. Chinese herb doctors tend not to distinguish these species, using them all, however, only *G. lucidum* has been the subject of intensive research.

A recent study from Korea showed that *Ganoderma* elicited immunopotentiation in mice. **Antitumor activity** in mice of polysaccharide fractions of these mushrooms was reported from Japan, while Chinese scientists described adaptogenic activity, again in mice. According to this Chinese study a hot water extract was found to enhance a **self-protecting mechanism of the central nervous system, improve heart function and correct parasympathetic nerve function. Perhaps most interestingly this study also demonstrated an anti-radiation effect from a polysaccharide fraction.**

The **immune-enhancing effects** ascribed to Reishi mushrooms by the Korean scientists noted above were described as enhancing macrophages and polymorphonuclear leucocytes (two types of fighting cells). Many studies have reported potent antiallergic activity, including antihistamine actions. And, it is now well-established that mushrooms such as **Reishi can significantly reduce serum cholesterol and "thin" the blood in a manner similar to aspirin by reducing agglutination of platelets.**

A 1990 study involved 15 healthy volunteers and 33 patients with atherosclerotic diseases. When a watery soluble extract was added to the platelets in vitro, the healthy volunteers showed platelet inhibition in relation to dosage.

From the above documentation it appears that the claims of healing properties in these (and other) mushrooms are based on fact not myth. Fears of toxicity should be allayed by the finding that reishi has an LD_{50} of greater than 5,000 mg/K, with no toxic effect at this high level of consumption even after 30 days of consumption. No toxic effects in humans are to be expected even if a person were to eat 350 grams a day, between 40-300 times the therapeutic dose.

RHUBARB

SCIENTIFIC NAME: *Rheum officinale*
PARTS USED: Root and rhizome

DOSAGE:

Root: The root is prepared for medicinal use in the proportion of 1 teaspoon of granulated root per 1½ pints of boiling water. Drink cold, 1 cup per day, a mouthful at a time.

RHUBARB: *The roots have the unique properties of combining cathartic and astringent effects.*

Traditional Usages

Rhubarb is an unusual medicine in that it **combines cathartic with astringent properties;** since the purgative effect precedes the astringent, the latter does not interfere with the former. **It is for these well-balanced opposite actions that Rhubarb is so valuable as a cathartic gentle enough even for infants. First it relieves constipation, then checks bowel evacuation through its astringent property.**

As a tonic and stomachic in small doses, Rhubarb invigorates the powers of digestion. In strong doses, Rhubarb has a tendency to cause painful griping of the bowels; in order to avoid this problem it is often mixed with aromatics such as Anise, Ginger, Peppermint, and Spearmint.

When Rhubarb is roasted or boiled long enough, the purgative property is largely destroyed, while the astringency remains. It is thus treated when used as a remedy for diarrhea, when no purging is desired.

Recent Scientific Findings

Rhubarb is generally employed in combination with other laxatives, rendering it more effective. The powder is applied to indolent ulcers.

Rhubarb preparations are used as cathartics, and also to control diarrhea (antidiarrhetic). This paradox deserves an explanation. It is known that when small doses of Rhubarb preparations are taken internally, the predominant action is to produce a laxative effect. This is due to the predominant effect of the anthraquinones and anthraquinone sugar derivatives. However, when large amounts are taken, the action of the astringent tannins in the Rhubarb root predominate. Hence, in large doses, an antidiarrheal effect results.

Rhubarb extracts have also cured upper digestive tract bleeding. One hospital studied three kinds of alcoholic extracted tablets of Rhubarb for a period of 10 years. Employing a double-blind method, patients in each of the three groups showed an efficiency of over 90% in curing the bleeding.

In 1987 a research team investigated extracts of 178 Chinese herbs for antibacterial activity against one of the major microorganisms in human intestinal flora. Only Rhubarb was found to be have significant activity.

Rhubarb preparations applied topically to wounds and sloughing ulcers are often beneficial since the tannins afford a covering to the affected area, and the body then proceeds to heal the wound by normal processes.

A word of caution here is required. In the past a favorite method for treating burns was to cover them with an ointment or cream containing tannin or tannic acid. Although this was very effective, there have been reports of severe reactions in some persons undergoing such treatment. These adverse effects are only noted when large areas of the body have been burned, for example, if 40 percent or more of the body surface area is burned. The reason for the toxic effect is that enough of the tannic acid is absorbed by the body through the burned area, enters the bloodstream, and eventually goes to the liver. Tannins are not compatible with the liver, and severe reactions often result. Thus, if one applies Rhubarb, which contains tannins, to small body areas to alleviate sloughing ulcers, there would be no adverse effects, but application to extensive areas of the body should be avoided.

> *Caution:* The leaf-blades, but not the petioles, of the plant are poisonous, containing oxalic acid and oxalates. Several cases of deaths have been reported in humans who have eaten the cooked leaf-blades.

ROSE

SCIENTIFIC NAME: *Rosa gallica*
PARTS USED: Unexpanded petals and buds

DOSAGE:

Buds and Petals: Approximately ½ ounce of buds and petals to 1 pint of water. Boil water separately and pour over the plant material and steep for 5 to 20 minutes, depending on the desired effect. Drink hot or warm, 1 to 2 cups or more per day, at bedtime and upon arising.

ROSE: *Since ancient times, the petals of these beautiful flowers have been employed for their astringent properties.*

Traditional Usages

The use of Rose petals dates from very ancient times. Early writers considered the petals purgative, astringent, and tonic, and used them in chronic catarrhs, hemoptysis, diarrhea, and leucorrhea. Avicema and other physicians after him recommended the petals in pulmonary phthisis.

The medicinal properties of the petals was generally considered very mild. The buds and petals have a pleasantly astringent and bitter taste, and were formerly prepared as a simple tonic. Their medicinal application ultimately dropped off entirely, and they remained in use only as an elegant vehicle for tonic and astringent medicines, due to their coloration and flavor qualities.

The essential oil, because of its powerful aroma, has been believed since early times to exert an effect on the nervous system. Hippocrates recommended the oil in diseases of the uterus.

Recent Scientific Findings

It is known that Rose buds and petals are a **rich source of vitamin C**, astringent tannins, and related phenolic compounds. They are thus used to advantage as tonics and astringents.

ROSEMARY

SCIENTIFIC NAME: *Rosmarinus officinalis*
PARTS USED: Leaf and flowers

DOSAGE:

0.5 to 1.0 grams per day of the ground leaf on food, or in capsule or tablet form taken orally.

ROSEMARY: *Once a subject of superstition, it is official in the U.S. Pharmacopoeia.*

Traditional Usages

Rosemary's history is rich with superstitions concerning its power. Ancient Greek students wore Rosemary to improve their memory. During the Middle Ages, it was believed that Rosemary warded off evil spirits. Medicinally, the flowers were steeped in water and drunk as a tonic. The legendary Rosemary water was reputed to cure paralysis. The burning of Rosemary branches was thought to prevent the Plague. More recently, herbalists prescribed Rosemary leaves as a stomachic, astringent, and expectorant. Externally, an ointment from oil of Rosemary was used for rheumatism and minor wounds and bruises.

Recent Scientific Findings

Rosemary's volatile oil is used in rubefacients and carminatives. It is official in the *U.S. Pharmacopoeia*. A recent study suggested that a Rosemary extract **may be a chemopreventive agent for breast cancer.** A dietary supplement of the extract "resulted in a significant (47%) decrease in mammary tumor incidence compared to controls."

RUE

SCIENTIFIC NAME: *Ruta graveolens*
PARTS USED: Herb

DOSAGE:

Herb: The traditional medicinal dose of 1 teaspoon of the herb, chopped fine, per cup of boiling water, boiled separately and pour over the plant material and steep for 5 to 20 minutes, depending on the desired effect. Drink cold, 1 teaspoon at a time, 1 cup per day. *Caution should be exercised with the use of this herb.*

RUE: *This herb has a long history of use as an abortifacient.*

Traditional Usages

A powerful local irritant, in proper dosages, Rue has been valued since the time of the early Greeks for its stimulant properties on the **nervous and uterine systems.** Pliny wrote that painters and carvers ate Rue to improve their eyesight. It has been used to treat **hysteria** and **colic**, and to provoke menstruation as well as to correct excessive or protracted menstrual bleeding. It has also been employed as an anthelmintic, and the oil has been used externally as a rubefacient.

For ages Rue was considered beneficial in warding off contagion; even in recent times it has been employed to keep off noxious insects. **Rue is one of the most popular of all herbal abortifacients.** It also is used to induce menstruation in cases of amenorrhea.

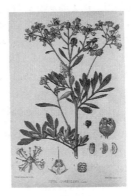

Rue

Recent Scientific Findings

The source of Rue's medicinal properties is a volatile oil that is a powerful local irritant. Handling the fresh leaves can cause redness, swelling, and even blistering of the skin. Care should be exercised when using Rue as an internal medicine, as it can cause, in sufficient quantity, violent gastrointestinal pains and vomiting, as well as convulsive twitching. **Large doses may also produce abortion.**

A number of animal experiments have shown that various types of Rue extracts will cause abortion, and this is probably due to a direct stimulant effect on uterine muscle. The agent responsible for this effect is the furoquinoline alkaloid skimmianine.

However, a number of cases of human poisoning have been reported when Rue extracts were used to induce menses and/or abortion. Apparently, in order to cause these effects, large doses must be taken. It must be that in large doses, some chemical constituent of the plant other than skimmianine has a predominant toxic effect.

There are a number of chemical constituents present in Rue that can cause a person to become extremely sensitive to light. Overexposure to sunlight after taking Rue preparations would result in severe sunburns. Rue also is known to cause severe dermatitis in some individuals.

> Thus, even though there is a rational basis for the abortifacient and menstrual inducing effects of Rue, the incidence and potential severity of side effects following its use should be sufficient to warn us to refrain from using it for any prolonged period of time.

SAFFLOWER

SCIENTIFIC NAME: *Carthamus tinctorius*
PARTS USED: Flowers

DOSAGE:

Flowers: The medicinal dose is 1 teaspoon of flowers, granulated, steeped for 5-20 minutes in 1 cup of boiling water. Drink cold, 1 tablespoon at a time, one cup per day.

SAFFLOWER: *The flowers of this herb are the source of Safflower oil.*

Traditional Usages

In large doses, Safflower is thought to have **laxative** value, and when given as a warm infusion to have a **diaphoretic** effect.

Carthamus flowers are sometimes fraudulently mixed in commerce with much more costly Saffron, which they resemble in color, but they may be distinguished by their tubular form and by the yellowish style and filaments which they enclose. Like Spanish Saffron (*Crocus sativus*), *Carthamus* is used in treating measles, scarlatina, and other inflammatory eruptions of the skin, including those of viral origin, in order to promote and hasten eruption. Saffron, in addition, was extensively employed by the ancients and by medieval physicians as a highly stimulant antispasmodic and to relieve menstrual cramping and pain.

This annual herb is the source of Safflower oil, much used in recent years for cooking. The fruits are edible and when fried are used to make chutney.

Recent Scientific Findings

Numerous animal studies have been conducted recently comparing Safflower oil with other fatty oils. In one study Safflower oil was not as beneficial as Perilla oil in suppressing carcinogenesis, allergic hyperreactivity, thrombotic tendency, apoplexy, and hypertension.

A comparison of groundnut, coconut, mustard, and safflower oils found that rats fed Safflower and mustard oils had higher cholesterol content and a higher degree of unsaturation in the membrane fatty acid composition. The researchers believe the higher cholesterol levels with Safflower oil are due to its linoleic and arachidonic acid content.

In a dietary study with rabbits, plasma cholesterol levels doubled after two weeks and remained elevated when diet supplemented with mixture of corn, palm, and safflower oils. A rat study found that oral administration of Safflower oil significantly increased awake systolic blood pressure. Interestingly, Evening Primrose oil prevented this increase.

SAGE

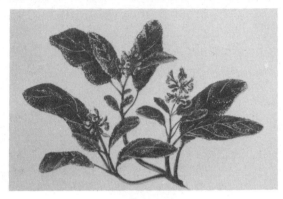

Sage

SCIENTIFIC NAME: *Salvia officinalis*
PARTS USED: Leaves and flowering tops

DOSAGE:

    Leaves: Steep 1 teaspoon leaves in $1/2$ cup water for 30 minutes; take 1 cup per day, 1 tablespoon at a time.

SAGE: *Believed by the ancients to prolong longevity, the Chinese variety of this herb may be an ideal tranquilizer.*

Traditional Usages

An ancient Arabian proverb said, "How shall a man die who has sage in his garden?" **Since ancient times, Sage was believed to prolong longevity.** During the Middle Ages, Sage was one of the main ingredients of longevity tonics. As late as the 17th century, the English botanical writer John Evelyn claimed that the use of sage would render a man immortal.

California Sage was used by Native Americans to prevent drying of the nasal mucous. The ground seeds were stirred in water, and the resulting mucilate was slowly sucked. On the East Coast, the Catawbas pounded wild Sage roots into a salve to be applied to sores. From 1842 to 1916, *Salvia officinalis* was official in the *U.S. Pharmacopoeia*, where it was recommended for its **tonic, astringent,** and **aromatic properties, given in dyspepsia.**

The mint-like Asian variety of this herb is classified as a "blood regulator" in Chinese medicine and is said to "facilitate blood circulation, dissolve clots, and keep the blood vessels soft and supple." *Salvia militiorrhiza,* a member of the Labiatae family, has a long history in Chinese folk medicine as a treatment for insomnia, cerebrovascular diseases, and coronary heart diseases.

Recent Scientific Findings

The "minor" tranquilizers such as Valium® and Librium®, classified as benzodiazepines, have been widely prescribed since 1960 to treat epilepsy, muscle spasms, sleep problems, and anxiety. They are very effective but quite addictive, with physical dependence demonstrated in humans who have used these agents repeatedly.

If only humankind could have that "perfect" anti-anxiety agent! It would calm without sedating, be non-addictive, and not induce strong muscle relaxation. Does this sound like SOMA, the mythic perfect drug sought for ages? **According to a team of Japanese scientists, the common Chinese variety of Sage may contain the perfect tranquilizing compound within its roots.** A single compound found in this plant may become the source of a new tranquilizing agent, acting like Valium without the troublesome side-effects noted above.

The Benzodiazepines act at pharmacologically specific sites in the central nervous system, the central B_2 receptors, to inhibit nerve transmission by enhancing the neurotransmission of GABA (an inhibitor of neurotransmission). The plant-derived compounds described in the above study also interact with the central B_2 receptors. Determined to be diterpene quinones, so-called tanshinones, they chemically differ from all the other known natural and synthetic B_2 receptors yet discovered.

The most potent of these tanshinones is Miltirone. In experiments with mice it was found to diminish anxiety *without* producing sedation or muscle relaxation, and without diminishing performance or producing addiction.

Other studies have found Sage to be of some use in soothing and regulating menopausal problems, possessing antibacterial activity in vitro against several human pathogens, and exhibiting anti-yeast activity in vitro against Candida albicans and antiviral activity in cell culture against herpes simplex virus II, influenza virus A2, vaccinia virus, and polio virus II.

ST. JOHN'S WORT

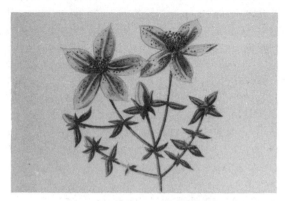

St. John's Wort

SCIENTIFIC NAME: *Hypericum perforatum*
PARTS USED: Tops and flowers

DOSAGE:
> *Not recommended for internal use.*

ST. JOHN'S WORT: *At one time ascribed magical properties, this herb is the source of hypericin, which may work against the HIV virus.*

Traditional Usages

St. John's Wort was valued by the ancients and continued to enjoy a good reputation among the earlier modern physicians. Galen and Discorides recommended St. John's Wort as a diuretic, emmenagogue, and for killing internal worms. The famous herbalist Gerarde, wrote that "St. John's Wort, with his flowers and seed boyled and drunken, provoketh urine, and is right good against stone in the bladder . . . " It is possible that the employment of St. John's Wort as a remedy for wounds was originally suggested, according to the "doctrine of signatures," by the red juice of its capsules, which was taken as a signature of human blood.

The plant's name came about because the peasantry of Europe assigned the plant magical powers. They gathered it on St. John's Day, June 24, for special cures. At one time, it was believed that this plant could be used to drive devils out of a person possessed; however, this may have been based on the observation of its usefulness in treating hypochondriasis and insanity. The plant was a popular charm against witchcraft and evil spirits.

Recent Scientific Findings

Although the USFDA has included this plant in their (out-of-date) March 1977 "unsafe herb list," it has been used beneficially for thousands of years, especially for **wounds** and **bruises**, administered both internally and externally. Evidently, the FDA included St. John's Wort on the list based on reports of toxic reactions in cattle, not humans.

An oil extract is recommended as a good external salve for **burns, sores, bruises,** and **skin problems.** German scientists applied an ointment containing St. John's Wort to burns and reported that first degree burns healed in 48 hours and second and third degree burns healed three times faster than burns treated conventionally. In Russia, two widely prescribed St. John's Wort remedies are Novoimanine and Imanine. Both have been found effective against *Staphylococcus aureus* infection in laboratory tests.

St. John's Wort's chemical constituents include tannins, flavonoids, xanthones, terpenes, phloroglucinol derivatives, and carotenoids. An extract, hypericin, has been found to be an **anti-depressant**. A 1984 clinical trial with this extract involved six depressive women between the ages of 55 and 65. The researchers measured metabolites of noradrenaline and dopamine in urinalysis. After taking the hypericin extract, there was a significant increase in 3-methoxy-4-hydroxyphenylglucol, which is a chemical marker for anti-depressive reactions. These same researchers conducted another study with 15 women. **Results showed an improvement in symptoms of depression, anxiety, insomnia, dysphoric mood, and self-esteem. No side effects were reported.**

Hypericin has recently generated much interest as an AIDS drug. Researchers at both New York University and the Weizmann Institute of Science in Israel found that hypericin possessed antiviral activity. Mice given the extract had the damage from viruses alleviated and the proliferation of the virus was decreased. They stated that "When the compounds interact with the infecting particles shortly after *in vivo* administration, disease is completely prevented." The researchers noted that the extract seemed to have potent activity against HIV-1, declaring "Preliminary *in vivo* studies with pseudohypericin indicate that it can reduce the spread of HIV."

Anecdotal reports have claimed hypericin is beneficial for persons with the HIV virus. Some individuals have decided on their own to take hypericin extract and dramatic improvements have been reported in certain cases. There are also preliminary indications that hypericin extract works synergistically with AZT against HIV. Further clinical research in these areas is currently in progress.

However, at this time, there have still been no clinical studies of hypericin's effect on HIV in humans. Indeed, there is no standardized hypericin extract available. Also what may be an effective dose is unknown.

Caution: It has been firmly established that hypericin is a phytotoxic constituent. After taking the plant or its extracts, and following exposure to sunlight, light-skinned individuals may suffer a dermatitis, severe burning, and possibly blistering of the skin. The severity of these effects will depend on the amount of plant consumed and the length of exposure to sunlight. Therefore, individuals with fair skin should avoid sunlight while taking St. John's Wort. Some authorities recommend that all individuals avoid sunlight when using *hypericin*, especially when taking large quantities. Considering the extensive use of *hypericin* extracts in Europe, consumers should not be in danger as long as they confine their use to moderate doses and restrict their exposure to sunlight.

SARSAPARILLA

SCIENTIFIC NAME: *Smilax aristolochiaefolia, S. medica, S. officinalis*

PARTS USED: Root

DOSAGE:

Root: Boil 1 teaspoon of the root in a covered container of 1½ pints of water for about ½ hour, at a slow boil. Allow liquid to cool slowly in the *closed* container. Drink cold, 1 swallow or 1 tablespoon at a time, 1 to 2 cups per day.

SARSAPARILLA: *At one time a popular remedy for a variety of ailments, the root is now considered a mild diuretic.*

Traditional Usages

Sarsaparilla was used extensively by various Native Americans, who transmitted their knowledge to whites. The Penobscots made a **cough remedy** from pulverized Sarsaparilla roots in combination with Sweet Flag roots. In the Pacific Northwest the Kwakiutl prepared a cough medicine with the pulverized root and an unspecified oil. The cough remedy of the Pillager Ojibwas was a decoction of pulverized root boiled in water. While Native Americans generally utilized Sarsaparilla by itself, popular commercial drinks featured Sarsaparilla root mixed with the roots of several other plants.

Sarsaparilla was introduced into European medicine in the mid-sixteenth century as a treatment for syphilis and

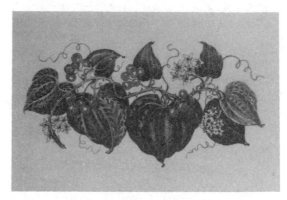

Sarsaparilla

subsequently discarded for that purpose. Thereafter it was utilized for many chronic diseases, such as **rheumatism** and **scrofula.** The smoke of Sarsaparilla was even inhaled by asthmatic patients.

Mexican Sarsaparilla (*S. aristolochiaefolia*), one of the commercial sources of the "drug," is utilized extensively in that country. Some tribes use a root decoction to lower fevers, and for kidney troubles, while it is also generally used externally for skin diseases and rheumatism.

Recent Scientific Findings

Commonly regarded as tonic, diaphoretic, and diuretic, Sarsaparilla in actuality is probably no more than a mild gastric irritant due to its saponin content.

Sarsasapogenin and smilagenin are steroidal aglycones with potential use as precusors for the synthetic production of cortisone and other steroidal drugs. The plant possesses **diuretic** action, stimulating the excretion of uric acid. Sarsaparilla **root extracts have been observed to have anti-tubercle bacillus activity in culture studies.**

SASSAFRAS

SCIENTIFIC NAME: *Sassafras albidium*
PARTS USED: Root bark

DOSAGE:

Root bark: For those who may wish to defy the official ban, it is interesting to note that in former times this plant was very frequently used as a spring tonic. One cup of boiling water was added to a teaspoonful of the granulated root bark. It was taken cold, a mouthful at a time, to a maximum of 1 cup daily. useful externally for poison ivy and poison oak.

SASSAFRAS: *The refreshing aromatic teas from this plant have long been popular.*

Traditional Usages

Sassafras has rarely been used alone in medicine; its main use seems to have been to make less agreeable tasting, more efficient medicines more palatable. The root bark, combined with Sarsaparilla and Guaiacum, was given for chronic rheumatism, skin diseases, and syphilitic affections. In domestic medicine Sassafras tea has been a popular "tonic" for high blood pressure and to promote perspiration. The mucilaginous and rather gummy pith was used as a soothing application for inflamed eyes and was given for dysentery, catarrhs, and nephritis.

Most of the tribes of the eastern United States utilized Sassafras for various ailments. The Houmas and Rappahannocks drank an infusion of Sassafras roots to lower

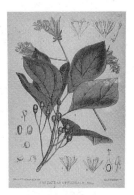

Sassafras

fever and promote the eruption of the measles rash. During Colonial times, Sassafras was an important export, especially to England, where it was used for colic, venereal disease, pain, and other ailments.

Rural general practitioners commonly administered Sassafras tea to treat high blood pressure and to promote perspiration in colds. A tea from the flowers was used by the Pennsylvania Germans to reduce fevers. The root bark was official in the *U.S. Pharmacopoeia* from 1820 to 1926 when its volatile oil was used as a pain reliever.

> Despite its reputation for gentle action, Sassafras in overdose has been reported to produce narcotic poisoning and accidental abortion, although it was apparently never used as an abortifacient.

Recent Scientific Findings

The aromatic oil is still utilized as an antiseptic and as a flavoring agent. The essential oil from the root bark of Sassafras has been experimentally determined to have antiseptic properties, and if applied externally would undoubtedly have such an effect, as reported in folkloric use.

Water extracts of Sassafras root bark continue to be used widely, especially in North America, as refreshing aromatic teas. Such teas contain small amounts (about 7-10 milligrams per cup) of a chemical compound known as safrole. In the early 1960s it was found that safrole, when fed to rodents in their diet, resulted in liver damage, and more specifically, liver cancer, in a high percentage of animals. This caused the U.S. Food and Drug Administration to prohibit the sale of safrole-containing materials, such as Sassafras root bark, for use in foods and flavors. However, despite an official ban, Sassafras root and root bark remain as an item of commerce in the United States, and are still widely used.

Of importance is that safrole itself does not produce cancer in animals. It must be converted by the animal to a substance containing one additional hydroxy group, i.e., 1-hydroxysafrole. The latter substance is termed a proximate carcinogen. 1-hydroxysafrole is produced by several animal species, including rats, mice, and digs, when safrole is administered orally.

Interestingly enough, in 1977 the results of a study conducted in Switzerland was published in which safrole was taken orally by one human adult, and the proximate carcinogen 1-hydorxysafrole could be found in the urine of this individual. It is well known that chemical compounds may be converted differently by different species. If additional confirming experiments are carried out in humans, and it is found that safrole is not changed to a carcinogen, the official ban on the sale of Sassafras root bark may be removed.

SAW PALMETTO

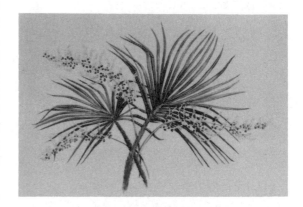

Saw Palmetto

SCIENTIFIC NAME: *Serenoa repens*
PARTS USED: Fruit

DOSAGE:
1.0 to 2.0 grams of dried plant material per day, in capsule or tablet form.

SAW PALMETTO: *Recent research has confirmed the berries folkloric use for prostate problems.*

Traditional Usages

The tea of the berries of Saw Palmetto has long been employed for genitourinary conditions. **In the early years of the 20th century, it was commonly used to treat prostate problems and as a mild diuretic.** Indeed, Saw Palmetto was called the "plant catheter" because of its tonic effect on the neck of the bladder and the prostate.

Saw Palmetto also was used as an aphrodisiac as well as to **increase sperm production,** and **by women to enlarge breasts.** It was also used as a nutritive tonic and for respiratory diseases. Southern slaves fed livestock with Saw Palmetto and the practice was copied by whites.

Saw Palmetto was official in the *U.S. Pharmacopoeia* from 1905 to 1926 and *The National Formulary* from 1926 to 1950. **It was most commonly prescribed for frequency of urination and excessive night urination due to inflammation of the bladder and prostate enlargement.**

Recent Scientific Findings

Until recently, Saw Palmetto was generally considered by the scientific community to have no therapeutic value. Recent studies have contradicted this earlier skepticism. Several extracts from the berries have been the subject of research, exhibiting estrogenic activity and inhibiting the enzyme testosterone-5-alpha-reductase in mice experiments. The dried berries of Saw Palmetto contain high amounts of sitosterols.

Also the folkloric claims of benefits to prostate problems have been substantiated. Benign prostatic hyperplasia (BPH) is considered to be caused by testosterone accumulating in the prostate. The testosterone is then converted to dihydrotestosterone (DHT), which causes the cells to multiply too quickly and leads to enlargement of the prostate. The Saw Palmetto extract prevents testosterone from converting to dihydrotestosterone. It also inhibits DHT from binding to cellular receptor sites and so increase DHT's breakdown and excretion.

Several double blind trials have been conducted. One study involved 110 patients with each receiving either a placebo or a hexane extract of Saw Palmetto for a period of one month. The researchers found a statistically significant improvement for those patients receiving the extract. Despite the improvement, the reduction in residual urine was not enough to remove the symptoms.

Another long-term study was also conducted. For a period ranging from seven to 30 months 32 patients received the Saw Palmetto extract while 15 received a placebo. The researchers found that 37 of the 40 patients available for follow-up had improved. Unfortunately, the authors were unclear how many of the patients were in the group receiving the extract and how many the placebo.

A randomized, double-blind, placebo-controlled study of 30 patients suffering from prostate adenoma also found statistically significant differences between the treated group and placebo. However, once again the improvement was only minimal. So while Saw Palmetto may provide some relief from prostate symptoms, it does not seem to be meaningful enough to be an effective treatment. For this reason, in 1990 the FDA refused to grant the drug OTC status.

There is preliminary evidence that Saw Palmetto aids those suffering from thyroid deficiency.

SCHIZANDRA

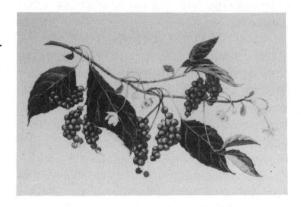

Schizandra

SCIENTIFIC NAME: *Schizandra chinensis*
PARTS USED: Berry

DOSAGE:
1 to 2 grams per day in tablet
or capsule form.

SCHIZANDRA: *This is the source for several Oriental medicines and a registered medicine in Russia.*

Traditional Usages

Schizandra is the source of several Oriental medicines, including "gomishi" in Japan, where it is utilized for tonic and antitussive purposes. Classed as an adaptogen (like Ginseng), Schizandra has a long history of folkloric use in China and Tibet and more recent folk applications in Russia.

Throughout the ages various groups of people have enjoyed the benefits of Schizandra. For example, in Northern China there lives a hunting tribe known as the Nanajas. Their hunting lifestyle means that they often set out on long and exhausting hunting trips under harsh conditions. But they always take along dried Schizandra fruit. A handful of the small red berries gives them the strength to hunt all day without eating. To this day hunters in the wilds of Eastern Siberia use the berries, stalks and roots of this plants in the form of tea to provide them with extra energy when hunting.

This amazing fruit helped Russian pilots to withstand lack of oxygen in their flights during the forties. In more recent years Schizandra has contributed to the successes of the Swedish skiing team. In Russia, Schizandra is a registered medicine for vision difficulties, i.e. short-sight and astigmatism, etc.

The principle active compounds found in Schizandra are lignans known as *schizandrin, gamma-schisandrin,* and *deoxy-schisandrin,*

Recent Scientific Findings

This interesting plant has many biological activities including: **antibacterial** (equivocal results), **sympathomimetic** (stimulant), **resistance stimulation, liver-protective, anti-toxic, antiallergenic, antidepressant**, and **glycogenesis stimulant**.

In addition, and perhaps most interesting from the point of view of it being a folkloric "tonic," this herb protected against the narcotic and sedative effects of alcohol (ETOH) and pentobarbital (PB) and exposure to the highly toxic ether, in mice. As a result of these data, the authors concluded that **Schizandra may be a useful** clinical agent for reversal of CNS depression.

They based this **antidepressant** activity on the reasoning that depression may be due, in part, to adrenergic exhaustion following severe psychogenic stress. It is known that MAO (monoamine oxidase) inhibitors, as well as other selected compounds that increase noradrenergic neurotransmission within the CNS (such as imipramine), have proven benefit in depression.

> This herb is also being promoted for its stimulating effect on the nervous system without being excitatory like amphetamine or caffeine. There are some proponents who claim "the higher the degree of exhaustion, the greater is the stimulating effect."

A very interesting study on performance in race horses tends to confirm the folkloric claims. Polo horses given the berry extract of this species showed a lower increase in heart rate (during exercise), a quicker recovery of respiratory function, a reduction of plasma lactate, and improved performance.

A 1990 study reported that a lignan component of Schizandra fruit *suppresses* the arachidonic (AA) cascade in macrophages. The AA cascade pushes the production of leukotrienes, which may play a role in inflammatory diseases. By inhibiting the arachidonic acid cascade, Schizandra both protects the liver and stimulates the immune system—two key roles of an ideal adaptogen.

An interesting non-Western 1991 study tested the "tonifying and invigorating yang" powers of Schizandra and other herbs in mice. The researchers measured the animals body weight, thymus weight, leukocyte count, and other parameters of "yang." They observed a direct correlation between the amount of herb ingested (as hot water extracts) and improved immunocompetence. They also noticed a distinct **anti-fatigue quality**, which was measured by reduced excitability of the parasympathetic nervous system. No toxicity was reported.

It appears that this creeping herb from the Far East has valid claims to the title of a "new" anti-fatigue agent which possibly helps to accelerate restorative processes within the human body. Traditional Chinese Medicine continues to offer new candidates to the annals of World Medicine. As we in the West are slowly learning, "traditional" or "folk" medicine really is the medicine of the people.

Caution: While Schizandra is a very safe herb with much historical usage one supplier of a standardized extract recommends that this herb be avoided by: epileptics, those with high intracranial pressure or severe hypertension, and those with "high acidity."

SCULLCAP

SCIENTIFIC NAME: *Scutellaria laterifolia*
PARTS USED: Whole plant

DOSAGE:

Leaves: One teaspoon of granulated leaves per cup of boiling water. Repeat as often as you like.

SCULLCAP: *At one time named "Mad Dog Scullcap" when it was used to treat rabies, recent studies indicate promising action against pulmonary infections.*

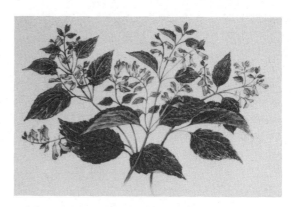

Scullcap

Traditional Usages

Employed rather commonly as a tonic and **general relaxant** in times of excitement, Scullcap tea was a **very mild and safe nervine.** In the Thomsonian system of medicine it was used in the treatment of delirium tremens, St. Vitus' dance, convulsions, lockjaw, tremors, and was given to **teething babies.**

Beginning with a series of experiments in 1772 by Dr. Van Derveer, the sedative and antispasmodic properties of this perennial herb were applied widely in the treatment of rabies. This use earned the plants its nickname "Mad Dog Scullcap." The dried herb was entered into the *U.S. Pharmacopoeia* in 1863 and remained until 1916 when it was shifted to the *National Formulary.*

Recent Scientific Findings

Scullcap contains the flavonoid glycosides scutellarin and scutellarein.

Scullcap preparations have been shown to have a **relaxant effect on uterine tissue** in test-tube studies.

A survey of 60 patients with pulmonary infection (mainly pneumonia) compared the effect of a Scullcap compound with a placebo. The patients were randomly divided into two groups of thirty with no different in clinical data prior to beginning the treatment. The total effective rate was over 70%. The researchers concluded that their results indicate that further investigation is warranted.

Animals studies have demonstrated *Scutellaria* species to have diuretic, bile-stimulating, anti-fever, and depressant activity, and to lower blood pressure. In Chinese studies, a root extract demonstrated central nervous system depressant activity in humans.

SEAWEEDS

SCIENTIFIC NAME: *Geldium, Gracilaria,* and *Pterocladia* spp. (Agar-Agar); *Lyngbya lagerheimii* and *Phormidium tenue* (Blue-Green Algae), *Laminaria* spp. (Brown Algae, Kelp), *Chlorella* spp. (Chlorella), *Chondrus crispus* (Irish Moss)

PARTS USED: Whole plant

DOSAGE:

Agar: It should be eaten daily as a cereal in the amount of 7 to 15 grams.

Other Species: Follow the label directions of commercial preparations.

Dextran sulfate should be taken under medical supervision.

SEAWEEDS: *Used in Oriental medicine for centuries, these sea vegetables are yielding some fascinating discoveries; a great deal of recent interest has been generated by the possibility that the extract dextran sulfate may inhibit the HIV virus.*

Traditional Usages

Seaweeds, especially Brown Kelp, have been used in Oriental medicine for centuries. They were applied externally for **skin diseases, burns,** and **insect bites.** Internally, they are most widely known for their use as a **cancer treatment.** But a host of ailments were also treated. These include bronchial problems, disorders of the digestive and urinary systems, and rheumatic diseases.

Agar-Agar is the dried mucilaginous substance extracted from marine algae. It has been widely used to treat **chronic constipation.** It has also been employed for its emollient and demulcent properties.

Irish Moss was used by the New England colonists as a **bulk laxative.**

Recent Scientific Findings

An entire book has been written that is devoted to "marine algae in pharmaceutical science." Marine flora are shown to possess numerous medicinal properties, including **antibiotic, antiviral, antimicrobial** in general, and **antifungal.**

Japanese food is in vogue in Western nations, primarily because of the low fat, low calorie, high-fiber aspects. Wakame (a brown kelp, Undaria), Kombu (*Laminaria*), and *Nori* (*Porphyra*) which is used to wrap around rice for *sushi*, all contain active anti-tumor compounds.

These sea vegetables protect us against cancers of the digestive tract due to at least four known factors:

1. The alginic acid content swells in the intestine thus diluting potential carcinogens.

2. Some contain beta-sitosterol, a potent anti-cancer compound.

3. They may contain antibiotic compounds which inhibit the growth of several different gram-positive and gram-negative bacteria known to potentiate carcinogens in the colon.

4. They may possess anti-oxidant activity.

Agar-Agar

This sea plant has a very high concentration of polysaccharide mucilage, which swells and is very slimy when moistened. This mucilage is responsible for the laxative effect of agar, exerting a type of lubricant effect.

When used as a laxative, Agar should be taken with large amounts of water, and never dry. It usually will not produce a laxative effect with a single dose, but must be used regularly. Its function is very similar to that of vegetable cellulose foods and of bran. As a good bulk laxative, it may also be added to cereals, soups, cakes, or any other food without altering its effect. If the constipation is stubborn, Cascara (see *Cascara Sagrada*) bark is added to precipitate action.

Blue-Green Algae

Most of the recent attention to the Seaweeds has centered around dextran sulfate's possible action against the **AIDS** virus. Dextran sulfate is created when dextran is boiled with chlorosulfonic acid. It is a sulfate ester not a sulfonic acid. Dextran sulfate has been used for more than 30 years in Japan, primarily as an intravenous drug that **reduces clotting and lowers blood cholesterol. Dextran sulfate also inactivates the herpes simplex virus.**

In a 1987 letter to *The Lancet*, two Japanese researchers reported that dextran sulfate blocked the binding of HIV-1 to T-lymphocytes as well as blocking the transfer of HIV from cell to cell by cell fusion. The authors followed this with another paper that maintained that dextran sulfate could work synergistically with AZT *in vitro*.

Recently, Dr. K. R. Gustafson and other scientists at the National Cancer Institute (U.S.) reported that cellular extracts from cultured Blue-Green Algae protected human T cells from infection with the AIDS virus. In test-tube experiments pure compounds extracted from these algae also proved to be "strikingly active against HIV-1."

These algae were originally collected in Hawaii and the Palau Islands (Micronesia) and then cultured. The original technique for culturing such marine organisms and producing an extract (which later proved to be cytotoxic) was pioneered by my first professor of pharmacology, Dr. T.R. Norton. It was in 1968 in Dr. Norton's basement laboratory at Leahi Hospital of the University of Hawaii School of Medicine where I was first introduced to the search for medicines from plants.

The AIDS virus killing compounds just discovered in the Blue-Green Algae are classified as sulfolipids. These lipids are found within the structures of chloroplast membranes and occur widely in other algae, higher plants and microorganisms which conduct photosynthesis.

Initial clinical trials with dextran sulfate treatment for HIV indicate a fairly frequent improvement of general well-being. Consistent changes in T-cell counts were not noted. A John Hopkins University study confirmed the initial results from a study at San Francisco General Hospital that dextran sulfate is poorly absorbed when given orally.

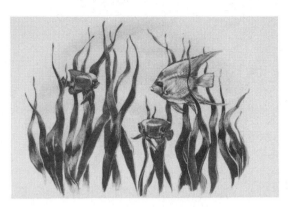

Brown Algae, Kelp

Brown Algae

I first learned of the **anti-cancer** and **antithrombotic effects** of the brown algae from a Japanese colleague. True, I had long believed that mankind would once again "return to the sea," by adding the aquatic plants to his armamentarium of terrestrial medicinals. But my attention was not galvanized until I learned about fucoidan.

Recent research has shown that the main active component with **antitumor activity in edible seaweeds** is likely a type of sulphated polysaccharide, fucoidan. The same compound has been shown to be responsible for **anticoagulant** and **fibrinolytic activities** in animal studies.

Another researcher, utilizing epidemiological and biological data, speculates that **the brown kelp seaweed *Laminaria* is "an important factor contributing to the relatively low breast cancer rates reported in Japan."**

Brown algae also contains dextran sulfate. See the above discussion under Blue-Green Algae for further information.

Chlorella

These microscopic species of algae possess distinct biological activities and are certain to take their place among the better-known marine organisms. All that has been said about the other species of seaweed is also applicable to the various unicellular marine algae, especially species of *Chlorella*.

Numerous animal studies have demonstrated **antitumor activity, antiviral activity, and interferon inducing effects**. The antitumor activity was observed specifically against mammary tumors, against leukemia, ascitic sarcoma, and liver cancer. A glycolipid fraction was tested which showed immune-enhancing effects in mice, most likely it was chlorellin.

An extract of Chlorella was found to have antiviral activity against cytomegalovirus (in mice) and against equine encephalitis virus (horse).

Immune stimulation by extract of Chlorella was observed due to induction of interferon production in mice infected with estomegalovirus (murine) and enhanced natural killer cell production was observed in mice infested with estomegalovirus as well as in mice with lymphoma-YAC-I.

Antihypertensive and antihyperlipedimic activity were observed with the protein fraction derived from Chlorella.

Irish Moss

Irish Moss is commonly used as a stabilizer in various foods, especially dairy products.

Experimental results have shown

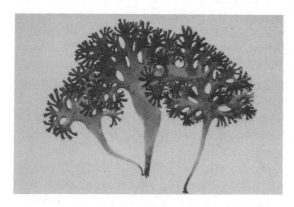

Irish Moss

that Irish Moss **may reduce high blood pressure.**

A product has been patented containing an extract of Irish Moss. The manufacturers claim the extract treats **ulcers.**

Other promising areas that have been observed in preliminary testing and warrant further investigation include Irish Moss' properties as a **demulcent, an anti-inflammatory,** an **immune-stimulant, antibacterial activity** against Streptococcus mutans, and lymphocyte blastogenesis stimulant activity.

SENEGA SNAKEROOT

SCIENTIFIC NAME: *Polyala senega*
PARTS USED: Root

DOSAGE:

Root: The medicinal dose is 1 teaspoon of granulated root, boiled in a covered container with 1 1/2 pints of water for about 1/2 hour, at a slow boil. Allow liquid to cool slowly in the *closed* container. Drink cold, 1 tablespoon at a time, 1 cup per day. For purging, 1 cup is drunk hot in the morning.

SENEGA SNAKEROOT: *As its name says, this was a popular remedy for rattlesnake bites in the 18th century.*

Traditional Usages

It is said that Senega was originally introduced into practice as a remedy for rattlesnake bite. Like most snakebite remedies, the roots were chewed and then applied directly to the bite. In 1735, a Scotch physician, John Tennent, noted that the Senecas successfully employed this plant for rattlesnake bites. He persuaded the Senecas to show him the root. Since the symptoms of snakebite were similar in certain aspects to pleurisy and latter stages of peripneumonia, Tennent tried the root on those diseases. After successful experiments, he wrote an epistle that was printed in Edinburgh in

1738, leading to the drug's acceptance in Europe and the beginning of cultivation in Britain in 1739. However, it came to be recognized of questionable value in treating venomous bites.

The primary application of Senega has been as an expectorant, to help the expulsion of mucus from the respiratory tract, in cases of bronchitis, asthma, and where otherwise indicated in similar pulmonary conditions. The 23rd edition of the *Dispensatory of the United States* describes the plants use in bronchitis and asthma, attributing the therapeutic value to the saponins contained in the dried root. It was official in the *U.S. Pharmacopoeia* from 1820 to 1936.

In larger doses the plant has been used as an irritant poison to produce vomiting and purging of the intestinal tract, but this usage was very infrequent, there being more desirable plants available for this purpose.

Recent Scientific Findings

Extracts of Senega Snakeroot have been shown experimentally to have expectorant properties when administered orally to a variety of animals, including cats, guinea pigs, and rabbits. it is thus reasonable to believe that tea prepared from the roots of this plant would have similar beneficial effect in humans.

SENNA

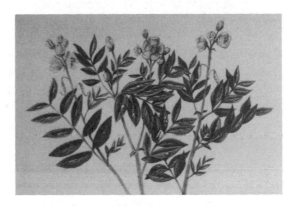

Senna

SCIENTIFIC NAME: *Cassia senna,*
Cassia acutifolia
(Alexandrian Senna),
C. angstifolia
(Indian Senna)

PARTS USED: Dried leaflets

DOSAGE:

Leaves: One teaspoon of the leaves per cup of boiling water, *steeped* (not boiled) for ½ hour. Taken ½ cup at bedtime, 1 tablespoon 3 times a day.

SENNA: *For over a thousand years this has proven to be an effective gentle laxative.*

Traditional Usages

Senna is an Arabic name, and the first recorded medical uses appear in Arabic writings from the 9th century. Its Chinese name, *Fan-Hsieh-Yeh,* means "foreign country laxative leaf;" most likely it was introduced to the Orient by Arabic traders. Senna is highly valued as a cathartic, working particularly on the lower bowel. It is consequently utilized on cases of chronic constipation. Senna was official in the *U.S. Pharmacopoeia* from 1820 to 1882.

American Senna was utilized by Native Americans in a variety of ways, none of them as a laxative. The Cherokees drank a decoction to **reduce fevers** and applied the root to sores. Other tribes employed Senna as a **sore throat remedy**.

Recent Scientific Findings

The leaflets and pods of *Cassia acutifolia* and *C. angustifolia* are popular laxative preparations that have the advantage over most other laxatives of being less "harsh," or producing less "intestinal griping." The reason for the laxative effect is that the leaves and pods contain varying amounts of complex anthraquinones known as sennosides (sennoside A and B are the two major active constituents). Many laxative preparations combine sennosides with a stool softener, but the combination has not proved more effective than the sennosides alone to the best of our knowledge.

Senna is recommended for persons suffering from looser stool constipation who only need to increase frequency of bowel movement. Senna is often combined with aromatics such as Anise, Fennel, Ginger, Nutmeg, and Peppermint to further reduce the tendency to produce intestinal griping. Its nauseous taste can be removed by preparing the plant as an alcoholic extract.

Caution: Not for use by persons suffering from "tension-related" or "nervous" constipation; may cause dehydration if over-used.

SHEPHERD'S PURSE

SCIENTIFIC NAME: *Capsella bursa-pastoris*
PARTS USED: Whole herb

DOSAGE:

Herb: 1 teaspoonful of herb per 1 cup of boiling water. Steep 3-5 minutes. Drink cold, 1 tablespoon at a time, 1 to 2 cups per day.

SHEPHERD'S PURSE: *This common plant may have anti-ulcer properties.*

Traditional Usages

This insignificant-looking little plant, which grows so plentifully almost everywhere, has long been a popular medicinal.

It was used in English domestic medicine for **diarrhea**.

Shepherd's Purse was administered for the alarming symptom of blood in the urine (hematuria). This condition can be caused by a lesion of the urinary tract, contamination during menstruation or during the 6 weeks following childbirth, prostate disease, tumors, poisoning, and toxemia.

Recent Scientific Findings

Shepherd's Purse extracts have been shown to **prevent duodenal ulcer** formations induced by stress in rats, and to show marked **anti-inflammatory** activity under a variety of test conditions in animals. Extracts of this plant have also shown significant **antitumor** activity against several experimental tumor systems in laboratory animals.

One study has shown that extracts of this plant inhibit the growth of bacteria in test tube experiments. There is also reasonable evidence, in animals and humans, that this plant has **hemostatic properties**. To date, high quantities of vitamin C have not been reported present in Shepherd's Purse, and thus, although it has been used as a remedy for scurvy, this antiscorbutic claim may not be warranted.

SHIITAKE MUSHROOM

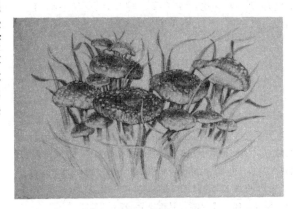

Shiitake Mushroom

SCIENTIFIC NAME: *Lentinus edodes*
PARTS USED: Cap and stem

DOSAGE:

Whole Plant: Approximately 1 ounce of the chopped mushroom to 1 pint of water. Boil water separately and pour over the mushroom and steep for 5 to 20 minutes, depending on the desired effect. Drink hot or warm, 1 to 2 cups per day.

SHIITAKE MUSHROOM: *This fungus has been found to possess antitumor and antiviral properties.*

Traditional Usages

Shiitake mushrooms traditionally were utilized in the diet as a strengthener.

Recent Scientific Findings

When I first studied medical mycology, over 20 years ago, Wilson and Plunkett's classic text provoked such fear and revulsion through the color photos of rare fungous diseases of man that I vowed to never eat another mushroom! All fungi became a source of dread for me.

Within the past few years I have since changed my view of these "lower" plants. The mushrooms are not only acceptable to me but have become highly coveted, owing to their documented **immuno-stimulant, cholesterol-lowering**, and **antitumor activities**.

Extracts of Shiitake have been shown to inhibit a number of different cancerous tumors in animal experiments. A principle antitumor compound isolated from this species *lentinan* does not appear to kill tumor cells directly but inhibits tumor growth by stimulating immune-function.

Lentinan appears to function by activating macrophages which then engulf cancerous cells. This activation is again via an indirect route—T-helper cells are stimulated which increase the effectiveness of macrophages.

The AIDS epidemic has fostered interest in any helpful compounds and lentinan is now a high priority item. A highly publicized letter to the prestigious medical journal *The Lancet* (October 20, 1984) was signed by Robert Gallo, one of the co-discoverer of the HIV Virus, and two French researchers from the Pasteur Institute. In it the authors concluded that lentinan "may prove to be effective in AIDS or pre-AIDS or for HIV carriers." After intravenous administration of lentinan with two Japanese patients, HTLV-I and HTLV-III antibodies disappeared.

The use of lentinan to treat AIDS is still in its early stages. In Japan, a few hemophiliacs infected with HIV have been administered lentinan. After several months treatment, there was a modest boost in T4 cells while macrophages and NK cells showed increased activity.

Unfortunately, despite repeated requests to subject this drug to human trials, based on its long history of usage for cancer treatment in Japan, nothing much has been done by governmental authorities in the U.S.

This is odd considering the long list of studies showing lentinan's antiviral properties; interferon inducing, natural killer cell enhancing, phagocytosis rate enhancing, as well as numerous antitumor studies. The *in vitro* inhibition of HIV by an extract of this mushroom is not, of itself, highly significant owing to the many substances known to kill this virus. However, taken together with all of the above evidence, it is safe to assume that Shiitake is all that it is claimed to be.

Caution: Skin and respiratory allergic reactions have been observed in workers involved in the commercial production of Shiitake.

SKUNK CABBAGE

SCIENTIFIC NAME: *Symplocxarpus foetidus (Spathyema foetida)*

PARTS USED: Root, rhizome, and seeds

DOSAGE:

Root: For medicinal use 1 teaspoon of granulated root is slowly boiled with 1 pint of water, for approximately ½ hour in a covered container. Take 1 tablespoon at a time, 1 cup per day.

SKUNK CABBAGE: *In the 19th century, the rootstock was official in the U.S. Pharmacopoeia.*

Traditional Usages

The Skunk Cabbage is a very curious plant, the only one of the genus to which is belongs. Credited with **antispasmodic, emetic, diuretic,** and **narcotic** properties, Skunk Cabbage has been used to treat asthma, chronic dry coughing spells and other upper respiratory problems, chronic rheumatism, nervous affections, muscular spasms and twitchings, hysteria, and dropsy (water retention). Externally, it has been utilized as an ointment or salve for skin irritations.

The Menominees boiled skunk cabbage root hairs and applied them to stop external bleeding. The leaf bases were applied in a wet dressing for bruises by the Meskwakis. The Winnebago and Dakota utilized Skunk Cabbage to stimulate the removal of phlegm in asthma. As employed in respiratory and nervous disorders, rheumatism, and dropsy, the rootstock was official in the *U.S. Pharmacopoeia* from 1820 to 1882.

The roots are an excellent emergency food, especially good baked or fried.

SLIPPERY ELM

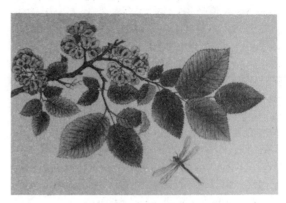

Slippery Elm

SCIENTIFIC NAME: *Ulmus fulva*
PARTS USED: Bark

DOSAGE:

Bark: One teaspoon of the bark, boiled in a covered container with 1 1/2 pints of water for about 1/2 hour, at a slow boil. Allow liquid to cool slowly in the *closed* container. Drink cold, 1 swallow or 1 tablespoon at a time, 1 to 2 cups per day.

SLIPPERY ELM: *The bark continues to be a useful treatment for sore throats.*

Traditional Usages

The demulcent properties of Slippery Elm bark led to its application in a number of ailments. The Ojibwas of North America made a tea from the inner bark to treat **sore throat**. The tea is also reportedly helpful for **coughs**. One pint of warm tea, administered as an **enema**, was given to babies to soothe the bowels after they had been cured of constipation or colic by repeated enemas. The bark was also eaten after convalescence, both for its soothing effects on the stomach and intestines, and for its nutritional value. Drunk combined with milk, it was easily digested, assimilated and eliminated.

Used as an ointment, Slippery Elm sap was employed in Thomsonian medicine during labor as a lubricant for the midwife's hand when she ascertained the presentation of the infant internally. The Thomsonian system also used a poultice of Slippery Elm, Lobelia, and a little soft soap as a means of bringing abscesses and boils to a head. These were then lanced and drained. Mausert considered this one of the most mild and harmless laxatives for children, causing no pain.

Slippery Elm sticks were used in some North American Indian tribes to provoke abortion by inserting them into the cervix.

Recent Scientific Findings

All of the effects indicated for Slippery Elm bark are explained on the basis of an abundance of mucilage-containing cells surrounding each fiber of the bark. When the bark, in strips or powdered form, comes into contact with water, the mucilage cells swell enormously and thus produce a lubricating, demulcent, emollient, and/or laxative effect when administered locally or by mouth. Powdered Slippery Elm bark is especially useful to soothe sore throats, and it has a pleasant, aromatic odor and taste as well.

Narrow strips of Slippery Elm bark, when soaked in water for a few minutes, become very slippery and pliable. For this reason, it has been reported that some pregnant women have attempted to induce abortion by inserting a long strip of moistened bark into the cervix. This is an extremely dangerous practice, since many deaths have results due to uncontrollable hemorrhaging. Serious infections can also be expected due to the unsanitary conditions under which this type of practice is carried out.

In some states in the United States, the law requires that Slippery Elm bark be broken into pieces no longer than 1.5 inches in length before being sold. The intent of such laws is obviously to discourage the use of Slippery Elm bark for the induction of abortion.

SOAPWORT

SCIENTIFIC NAME: *Saponaria officinalis*
PARTS USED: Root and leaves

DOSAGE:

Rhizome and Root: 1 teaspoon of rhizome or root, boiled in a covered container with 1 pint of water for about 1/2 hour, at a slow boil. Allow liquid to cool slowly in the *closed* container. Drink cold, 1 swallow or 1 tablespoon at a time, 1 to 2 cups per day.

Leaves: Approximately 1/2 ounces of leaves to 1 pint of water. Boil water separat;y and pour over the plant material and steep for 5 to 20 minutes, depending on the desired effect. Drink hot or warm, 1 to 2 cups per day.

SOAPWORT: *Named due to its lathering action, its saponins may possess anti-cancer properties.*

Traditional Usages

The name of the Soapwort is derived from the fact that when agitated in water, the rhizomes and roots form a lather, like a solution of soap.

Many Native Americans pounded the root and mixed it with water as a **hair shampoo. The Kiowa considered it an effective treatment for dandruff and skin irritations.** The Pomos prepared a lotion of the soapy juice and rubbed it on the **poison oak rash.** Soapwort was prescribed by medieval Arab physicians for **leprosy** and other skin complaints. The leaves, soaked for a short time, yield an extract which has been used to promote sweating, as a remedy against **rheumatism**, and to purify the blood.

Recent Scientific Findings

The active principle responsible for Soapwort's lathering effect is saponin, which carries the detergent as well as the medicinal properties of this plant. In 1917 in China there were reportedly eleven species of trees that contained saponin which were utilized in the formation of detergents for the purpose of laundry washing.

A 1991 study examined the effect on human breast cancer cells of Saporin 6, a protein purified from Soapwort seeds. **The results showed that the breast cancer cells were highly sensitive to Saporin 6.**

Another 1991 study conducted by a different research team investigated Saporin 6 for its effect on leukemia cells.

SOLOMON'S SEAL

SCIENTIFIC NAME: *Polygonatum officinale*
PARTS USED: Root

DOSAGE:

Root: For external as well as internal use, a decoction is prepared, using 1 teaspoonful of the root, boiled in a covered container with $1\frac{1}{2}$ pints water for about $\frac{1}{2}$ hour, at a slow boil. Allow liquid to cool slowly in the *closed* container. Drink cold, 1 swallow or 1 tablespoon at a time, 1 to 2 cups per day, when taken internally.

SOLOMON'S SEAL: *The roots contain allantoin, an anti-inflammatory agent.*

Traditional Usages

The root was formerly used for its emetic properties, and externally for bruises, especially near the eyes, as well as for treatment of tumors, wounds, poxes, warts, pimples, etc. Taken internally, it was thought to be effective in assisting the knitting of broken bones.

In 16th century Italy Solomon's Seal was esteemed as a cosmetic wash which would maintain healthy skin and prevent freckles, sunburn, pimples, and the mottling of old age.

Recent Scientific Findings

The roots of Solomon's Seal contain allantoin, a substance well known for its **healing and anti-inflammatory effects. Extracts of the root of this plant lower blood sugar levels in rabbits, lower blood pressure, and have a cardiotonic action, indicating possible usefulness in heart conditions.**

SPEARMINT

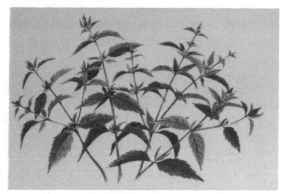

Spearmint

SCIENTIFIC NAME: *Mentha spicata*
PARTS USED: Leaves and flowering tops

DOSAGE:

Leaves and Flowering tops: Approximately ½ ounce of leaves and flowering tops to 1 pint of water. Boil water separately and pour over the plant material and steep for 5 to 20 minutes, depending on the desired effect. Drink hot or warm, 1 to 2 cups or more per day.

SPEARMINT: *Like the other mints, the tea is one of our most pleasant carminatives.*

Traditional Usages

Much the same as Peppermint, without the cooling sensation in the mouth which accompanies the ingestion of the plant, Spearmint is an **aromatic stimulant.** It is used for **mild indigestion,** to cure **nausea**, to relieve spasmodic stomach and bowel pains, help the expulsion of stomach and intestinal gas, and to otherwise remedy the deleterious effects of too much food or an improper diet. Spearmint it also combined with other less palatable medicines to make them more agreeable or to allay their tendencies of producing nausea or griping effect.

Recent Scientific Findings

The leaves and flowering tops of Spearmint owe their pleasant and aromatic properties, as well as characteristic taste, to a volatile oil. The major active principle in the oil is a simple terpene derivative, carvone.

Refer to Peppermint, for further information. This plant is the same in action, only weaker due to the fact it does not contain menthol. Its use is largely a matter of taste preference.

SPINDLE TREE (WAHOO)

SCIENTIFIC NAME: *Euonymus atropurpureus*

PARTS USED: Bark, root, fruit, and seeds

DOSAGE:
> *Extremely toxic:* No dosage is recommended for home use.

SPINDLE TREE: *Though this is an extremely toxic plant, it was at one time a popular remedy for a variety of ailments.*

Traditional Usages

Despite its toxicity, all parts of this tree have been employed at one time or another in traditional medicine. Native Americans used the Wahoo for a variety of purposes, including **uterine problems**, as an **eye wash** and a **physic**. The bark became a popular **diuretic** soon after its introduction to early settlers. The dried root bark was believed to be stimulant, laxative, and diaphoretic (producing sweating). As a result of this latter characteristic it was employed in the treatment of dropsy (water retention). The oil expressed from the seeds was utilized for its emetic and purgative properties. The fruits were held to be diuretic. However, in light of their toxicity in even small quantities, the dosage must have been minute. The inner bark was utilized in treating eye diseases.

In 1912 a report was published that this species effects a digitalis-like action on the heart, which caused Wahoo to become a popular heart medicine in domestic practice.

Recent Scientific Findings

This is one plant which deserves its place on the USFDA 1977 unsafe herb list. The fruits are terribly toxic; ingestion of as few as 3 or 4 can prove fatal to a child and can cause an adult extreme pain and discomfort, as they function as a drastic purgative.

Wahoo fruit and seeds contain cardiac glycosides, which would be expected to produce a diuretic effect in persons with cardiac insufficiency. Large amounts would also be predicted to cause emesis. These cardiac glycosides, however, are not present in other parts of the plant.

SQUAW VINE (PARTRIDGE BERRY)

SCIENTIFIC NAME: *Mitchella repens*
PARTS USED: Vine

DOSAGE:
Vine: One teaspoon of the ground vine is used per cup of boiling water; steep for 5-10 minutes, and drink cold, 1 to 2 cups per day, 1 tablespoon at a time.

SQUAW VINE: *Used by Native Americans to facilitate childbirth, this vine was in the National Formulary from 1926 to 1947.*

Traditional Usages

Also called partridge berry, Squaw Vine was administered by Native American women as a tea to facilitate childbirth. As was common for plants employed for "female troubles," Native Americans were reluctant to provide much information about their methods of preparation and specific applications of Squaw Vine. The Cherokee informed one investigator they used a tea made from the leaves. The Penobscots of Maine used the same preparation. In the few weeks prior to the expected date of delivery, frequent doses of the tea were taken. All aspects of labor, delivery of the child and the afterbirth, stimulation of the uterus, and so forth, were thought to be assisted by drinking tea brewed from this plant.

(Pipsissewa and Squaw Vine are thought to have similar properties.)

Squaw Vine became quite popular as a home treatment to speed labor. It was admitted into the *National Formulary* in 1926, where it remained until 1947. The leaves were used for their tonic, astringent, and diuretic properties.

Recent Scientific Findings

Experimentally, Squaw Vine fluid-extract has been tested for uterine stimulant activity against guinea pig pregnant and nonpregnant uterus, and was without effect. Thus, most likely the claims for this plant to be useful in facilitating parturition are unfounded. **The plant contains tannins, which probably account for its beneficial effects as a local astringent. We have found no experimental basis for the use of Squaw Vine as a diuretic.**

SQUILL

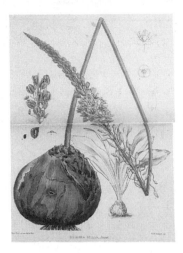

Squill

SCIENTIFIC NAME: *Urginea maritima*
(*U. scilla*)
PARTS USED: Bulbs, divested of outer coats and centers

DOSAGE:
Potentially lethal: No recommended home use dose.

SQUILL: *An ancient Egyptian papyrus described the cardiotonic effects that have been substantiated in this popular European heart medicine.*

Traditional Usages

The Ebers Papyrus (14th century B.C.) is the first indication that the bulb of Squill has **cardiotonic** effects. Squill was used by Greek physicians to treat **dropsy**, which is a manifestation of congestive heart failure.

In small doses, Squill reportedly acted as an expectorant and diuretic, in large doses as an emetic and purgative, and in overdose as a poison. There are two varieties of Squill, White Squill and Red Squill.

Recent Scientific Findings

Squill is quite a dangerous plant, and makes an excellent rat poison. Here is one herb that belongs on the USFDA unsafe herb list, but it is not to be found there! Obviously not for home use, Squill may prove valuable in the hands of the skilled herbalist-physician for its digitalis-like effect on the heart. It can be useful in treating heart disease, but overdose will cause death due to heart paralysis.

White Squill contains active cardiac glycosides similar in structure and action to those present in Foxglove (in Foxglove article see remarks on *Digitalis purpurea*). The major active substances are scillaren A and scilaren B. Currently, Squill preparations are used in medical practice in Europe, but not in the United States. Squill has essentially the same effects as *Digitalis* on the heart, and the only advantage over *Digitalis* is that Squill can be used in those parents who cannot tolerate the latter drug.

Red Squill has been used as a raticide; 250,000 kilograms were imported annually into the United States prior to World War II. It is curiously toxic to rats, other animals either refusing to eat it, or they apparently always vomit and are thus otherwise unaffected by it (unless the herb is disguised in a mixture!). Since rats do not vomit, they retain the plant material and it eventually kills them. Red Squill is 500-1,000 times more toxic to rats than White Squill. The active poison in Red Squill is called scilliroside.

SQUIRTING CUCUMBER

SCIENTIFIC NAME: *Ecballium elaterium*
PARTS USED: Juice sediment from fruit

DOSAGE:
This plant is not recommended for home use, due to its toxicity in accidental overdose.

SQUIRTING CUCUMBER: *The juice has been called the most powerful known cathartic.*

Traditional Usages

The Wild or Squirting Cucumber owes its name to its fruit. Shaped like a small oval cucumber, the fruit separates from its peduncle when ripe and expels its juice and seeds with considerable force through an opening at its base. The sediment from the juice of the fruit, known as elaterium, traces its name back as far as Hippocrates, who used the term to signify any active purge. The plan was known to the ancients for its **purgative** effects, and was also used by them to stimulate menstruation. In Turkey, the juice is a well-known folk remedy for **sinusitis**.

Recent Scientific Findings

Elaterium has been called the most powerful hydragogue cathartic known, effective in extremely small doses. The fruit juice of the Squirting Cucumber is well known to cause a powerful hydragogue cathartic effect in humans. This effect is caused by the major principles in the juice, a mixture of compounds referred to as cucurbitacins.

There is evidence from animal experiments that the juice of the Squirting Cucumber has an effect on the heart that would suggest a useful application in humans to treat dropsy (congestive heart failure). However, human experiments are lacking to support this contention. Further, the toxicity of the cucurbitacins must be taken into account when considering the use of Squirting Cucumber for any condition requiring long-term use, such as in dropsy.

We have found no experimental evidence that this plant would be useful in treating mania and melancholy, as reported by some herbalists. In large doses it would probably have an emetic effect due to the cucurbitacins, but experimental evidence to support this is lacking.

Cucurbitacin B, an extract isolated from the juice, showed significant anti-inflammatory activity in a 1988 animal study.

Ecballine, a compound derived from the fruits, is used in treating baldness as well as a cure against scalp diseases.

STAR ANISE

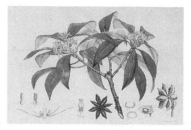

Star Anise

SCIENTIFIC NAME: *Illicum verum*
PARTS USED: Fruit

DOSAGE:

Fruit: An infusion of the dried fruit is made using 1 teaspoon to 1 cup of boiling water.

STAR ANISE: *Used in Chinese medicine for centuries, this aromatic fruit is a satisfying carminative.*

Traditional Usages

The fruit of the Chinese Star Anise is remarkable among the herbal remedies for its unusual appearance and its characteristic aroma. If we were to stumble upon this plant without being aware of its medicinal virtues we would undoubtedly try it out. It has been employed in Chinese medicine for centuries, particularly to cure **rheumatism** and **lumbago**. The seeds and oil have **stimulant, carminative, diuretic,** and **digestive properties;** Star Anise is also used to soothe inflamed mucous membranes of the nasal passages.

In China the seeds are applied locally to treat **toothache,** while the essential oil is given for **colic** in children. **Experimentally, alcoholic extracts of the fruit were effective against gram-positive and gram-negative bacteria and against twelve species of fungi.**

Recent Scientific Findings

Star Anise owes much of its therapeutic effect to the essential oil present in the fruits. **About 90 percent or more of the essential oil is comprised of anethole, which produces a carminative and mild internal stimulant effect, if taken internally.** Thus there is ample justification for the use of Star Anise infusions or decoctions as a carminative or mild stimulant.

The fruit is now popularly employed in several commercial brands of herbal tea.

STROPHAN-THUS

SCIENTIFIC NAME: *Strophanthus kombe, S. hispidus*

PARTS USED: Seeds

DOSAGE:

> *Not recommended.* Too variable in effects for home use.

STROPHANTHUS: *The seeds are a potent cardiac medicine similar to digitalis.*

Traditional Usages

Strophanthus was originally used by natives in the region of Lakes Tanganyika and Nyasa for arrow poison.

Recent Scientific Findings

Strophanthus is formally recognized as a **cardiac stimulant.** Its action is very similar to that of digitalis, but it exerts its effect more rapidly, diminishes its action in less time, and does not reduce the pulse rate to the same levels as does digitalis.

All parts of these two species, particularly the seeds, are known to contain cardiac glycosides quite similar in chemical structure and also in their effects on the body to the *Digitalis* glycosides. Strophanthus preparations thus exert a strengthening action on the heart by causing it to slow down and function with stronger force. This confirms the usage long reported in folklore.

Strophanthus is less dependable than digitalis due to its irregular absorption through the intestinal tract. A reported side effect of Strophanthus is **diarrhea**, produced by increased peristalsis of the intestines. The plant was also felt to be **diuretic** and has therefore been widely used in cases of chronic heart weakness coupled with dropsy (water retention).

Because it functions more rapidly than digitalis, Strophanthus is of great benefit during an emergency heart failure. In such cases it has been administered intravenously by injection.

SUMAC

SCIENTIFIC NAME: *Rhus glabra*
PARTS USED: Bark and fruit

DOSAGE:

Berries: Boil 1 teaspoon of the berries in a covered container with 1½ pints water for about ½ hour, at a slow boil. Allow liquid to cool slowly in the *closed* container. Drink cold, 1 swallow or 1 tablespoon at a time, 1 to 2 cups per day.

SUMAC: *The berries contain high concentrations of tannins and are an excellent gargle for sore throats.*

Traditional Usages

Of this genus there are several species that possess poisonous properties, and should be carefully distinguished from that here described. This species of *Rhus*, called variously Smooth Sumac, Pennsylvania Sumac, and Upland Sumac, is an indigenous shrub from 4 to 12 feet high. The leaves are smooth petioles and consist of many pairs of opposite leaflets, with an odd one at the extremity, all of which are lanceolate, acuminate, acutely serrate, glabrous, green on their upper surface and whitish beneath. In autumn their color changes to a beautiful red. The flowers are greenish-red, and disposed in large, erect, terminal, compound thyrses, which are succeeded by clusters of small crimson berries covered with a silky down.

Sumac berries were given as a **gargle** in decoction form and believed to be helpful during attacks of **anginal pain**. The decoction was also gargled for throat irritations, or by persons suffering from any inability to breathe easily, such as asthmatics. The high tannin content of the bitter berries made them valuable in the alleviation of **diarrheas**. The root was chewed by some North American tribes for mouth sores.

Recent Scientific Findings

Sumac berries contain high concentrations of tannins, which as indicated previously have an **astringent** effect on mucous membranes. Thus, when water extracts of Sumac berries are used as a gargle, or applied to other mucous membranes, the medicinal effect that is experienced has a rational explanation.

SWEET FERN

SCIENTIFIC NAME: *Polypodium vulgare*
PARTS USED: Root

DOSAGE:

Root: 1 teaspoon of the root, boiled in a covered container with 1½ pints water for about ½ hour, at a slow boil. Allow liquid to cool slowly in the *closed* container. Drink cold, 1 swallow or 1 tablespoon at a time, 1 to 2 cups per day.

SWEET FERN: Its flavor lives up to its name.

Traditional Usages

Not surprisingly, the taste of this fern is sweet; the rhizome is reminiscent of the Licorice root in shape. Its medicinal virtues are rather mild, although it was lavishly praised by the ancients for melancholic conditions and visceral obstructions. While the resin is considered **anthelmintic**, Sweet Fern is also a useful **purgative**. Its **demulcent** properties prevent it from being a strong medicine. **A very strong decoction is necessary for the expulsion of intestinal parasitic worms.** Sweet Fern is reportedly useful in alleviating coughs and other chest complaints, and is a useful tonic in dyspepsia and loss of appetite.

Recent Scientific Findings

Aqueous extracts of Sweet Fern root have produced CNS depressant activity.

SWEET FLAG

SCIENTIFIC NAME: *Acorus calamus*
PARTS USED: Oil and root

DOSAGE:

> **Oil:** The essential oil is not recommended, pending further scientific investigations.
> **Root:** *Avoid.*

SWEET FLAG: *Though this has been used in various countries for centuries, a single study of one variety of this plant led to an FDA ban that has discouraged further research.*

Traditional Usages

The Sweet Flag, or Calamus, was known for its medicinal virtues to ancient Greek and Arabian physicians. Calamus has been valued for centuries by the native practitioners of India and elsewhere as a feeble aromatic aiding digestion and regular elimination. **The root is used in powdered form in India and Ceylon as a remedy for expelling parasitic worms from the intestines.** The candied fresh root is chewed in Turkey and India as a treatment against epidemic diseases. In European countries the root was masticated to clear the voice. In North America, the Plains Indians chewed it for toothache. The Meskawakis applied the boiled root to burns. **An insecticide is produced from the essential oil.**

Recent Scientific Findings

The efficacious nature of Sweet Flag decoction or infusion as carminative and aromatic is well established, based on animal and human experiments. If highly concentrated amounts of the active principles in this plant are taken, effects other than those indicated could be unpleasant.

Even though the use of Sweet Flag has a rational basis of action, it has been disapproved for human use in any form because of studied reported in 1968 by the U.S. Food and Drug Administration. In a two-year rodent feeding study, using *Acorus calamus* essential oil, cancerous lesions were found in a significant number of the test animals. However, only the Jammu (Indian) variety of *Acorus calamus* oil was tested, and it is known that varieties of Calamus from other parts of the world than India are significantly different in their chemical composition.

> In view of this, the FDA has banned the use of all varieties of *A. calamus* intended for human use, until such time as it has been determined that varieties other then the one from Jammu do not cause this carcinogenic effect. Since 1968, no reports have been published regarding this problem.

TAMARIND

SCIENTIFIC NAME: *Tamarindus indica*
PARTS USED: Fruit

DOSAGE:

Fruit: The fruit is eaten as needed.

TAMARIND: *This refreshing fruit is one of nature's most gentle cathartics.*

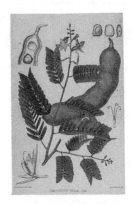

Tamarind

Traditional Usages

The Tamarind tree is the only species of this genus. Tamarind's medicinal properties were first discovered by Arab physicians. The Arabs imported Tamarind stock from India to Europe, where it became extensively cultivated.

Mildly cathartic, Tamarinds have long been considered a beneficial addition to the convalescent diet. It is often mixed with Senna and chocolate and administered to infants when a **gentle cathartic** is necessary. Tamarind is therefore a useful drink in feverish conditions, as well as being a popular cooking beverage in hot countries.

Recent Scientific Findings

The pulp of the fruit contains citric, tartaric, and malic acids, which give it cooling properties. **The fruit of Tamarind owes its laxative, mild cathartic and refrigerant effects almost totally to a high sugar concentration.** The types of sugars are not absorbed to a high degree, when in the intestinal tract. Because of this, they cause water to migrate from the surrounding tissues into the lumen of the intestines. This causes the intestines to expand, which **results in a nonirritant type of bowel movement.**

TANSY

SCIENTIFIC NAME: *Tanacetum vulgare*
PARTS USED: Herb

DOSAGE:

Not recommended for internal use.

Herb: For external use as a flea and lice killer, prepare by adding 1 pint of boiling water to 1 teaspoonful of the herb. Apply locally when cold, by soaking cloth or towels in the infusion.

TANSY: *At one time, this was commonly used in England to induce menstruation.*

Traditional Usages

Tansy's name comes from the Greek work for immortality. At one time Tansy was rubbed on corpses as well as wrapped in the shrouds of the dead to repel the onslaught of worms after burial. **The principal use of Tansy has been to expel worms from the intestines. Externally, the plant is a useful home remedy to kill fleas and lice.**

This herb has also been used as a sudorific (to promote perspiration) and to generate a comfortable internal feeling. In Europe a bitter tea tonic was recommended "in the hysteria, especially when this disease is supposed to proceed from menstrual obstructions." Tansy was officially employed to induce menstruation in England. When Tansy was introduced from Europe, Native Americans used it to induce abortion as well as menstruation. Conversely, it was also an old folk remedy for the prevention of miscarriage.

Recent Scientific Findings

The active constituent of Tansy, tanacetin, is toxic to animals, and, in overdoses, to humans. Among the striking symptoms of poisoning in humans are convulsions, spasms, frothing at the mouth, dilated pupils, and rapid and feeble pulse. **Its usage as a home remedy is absolutely to be avoided.**

The plant contains an essential oil, borneol, thujone, camphor, and resins. Experimentally, various plant parts exhibit much biological activity, as follows: antiseptic (flowers, volatile oil); antibacterial (flowers, roots, and root stocks); antifungal (volatile oil); liver functions (whole plant); and bile stimulation (leaves, flowers and stems).

TEA TREE

SCIENTIFIC NAME: *Melaleuca alternifolia*
PARTS USED: Leaf oil obtained from steam distillation

DOSAGE:

Used externally in various commercial preparations such as salves, ointments, hair care products, natural cosmetics, etc. Used internally only via throat lozenges and toothpastes. We recommend the consumer buy commercially prepared preparations instead of concocting their own recipes from raw material.

TEA TREE OIL: *Has currently become a very well respected major ingredient of many preparations used to treat a variety of external skin complaints ranging from* **Dandruff and Herpes** *to* **Acne and Fungal Infections.**

Traditional Usages

The Tea Tree is native to Australia, where is was well respected for its many applications to a variety of ailments, most notably ailments affecting the skin. It was thought to be antiseptic as well as antifungal and to possess rejuvenating properties.

Recent Scientific Findings

The active constituents of Melaleuca are Cineole and Terpinol. The balance of these two constituents determines the efficacy of the plant oil. It is desirable to have a Cineole level below 15% and a Terpinol level above 30% to achieve the best results. (The Australian Government Standard Requirement mandates these specifications, as well.)

Current research is underway to determine the efficacy of Tea Tree Oil for the following problems. While the reported results are not yet in, we feel this herb is receiving **significant** attention and will prove its efficacy via lengthy scientific studies, results of which should be published in the near future.

Aching Muscles, Diaper Rash, Sore Throat, Gingivitis, Burns, Heat Rash, Acne, Ear Infections (Antiseptic), Cuts and Abrasions, Mouth Ulcers, Athlete's Foot, Yeast Infections (Anti-Fungal), Dandruff, Sunburns, and Sinus and Bronchial Congestion; all are among the list of potential validated scientific applications of Melaleuca.

THYME

SCIENTIFIC NAME: *Thymus vulgaris*
PARTS USED: Herb

DOSAGE:

Herb: Approximately ½ ounce of herb to 1 pint of water. Boil water separately and pour over the plant material and steep for 50 to 20 minutes, depending on the desired effect. Drink hot or warm, 1 to 2 cups per day, at bedtime and upon awakening.

THYME: *This common spice contains thymol, which has disinfectant and anti-inflammatory properties.*

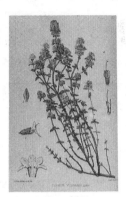

Thyme

Traditional Usages

This popular spice has also been used as a medicinal since ancient times. The Greeks Pliny, Dioscorides, and Theophrastus all make reference to this tasty herb.

It has been utilized for coughs, bronchitis, asthma, and whooping cough; for flatulence, colic in infants, to produce sweating to break a fever, for anemia, and for all kinds of stomach upsets.

The oil, applied locally to carious teeth, has been used as a means of relieving **toothache**. The herb has also been employed as an **antiseptic** against tooth decay.

Externally the leaves have been applied in fomentation (cloth or towels dipped in infusion or decoction and applied locally) for **aches** and **pains**.

Recent Scientific Findings

The active principle, a simple terpene, thymol or thymic acid, has been shown to have **disinfectant properties** equal to those of carbolic acid. Thymol has been shown to have **antiseptic value**, expectorant and bronchodilator effects in animal as well as human experiments. Thymol additionally releases entrapped gas in the stomach and relaxes the smooth muscle of that organ. **This explains the use of Thyme to alleviate the symptoms of colic and flatulence.**

Externally, thymol and thymol-containing plants act as rubefacients. That is, thymol causes an increased blood flow to the area of application, which then **results in relief of inflammation and pain.**

TOADFLAX

SCIENTIFIC NAME: *Linaria vulgaris*
PARTS USED: Herb, leaves

DOSAGE:

Leaves and Herb: Approximately 1/2 ounce of leaves or whole herb to 1 pint of water. Boil water separately and pour over the plant material and steep for 50 to 20 minutes, depending on the desired effect. Drink hot or warm, 1 to 2 cups per day, at bedtime and upon awakening.

TOADFLAX: This was once used for a vareity of ailments.

Traditional Usages

A very common herb, Toadflax was valued for its external and internal usages. To treat hemorrhoids a poultice or fomentation of the fresh plant was applied locally. This method was used on various skin diseases. In addition, the flowers were sometimes mixed with vegetable oils to make a liniment.

Taken internally, an infusion of the leaves was used to eliminate kidney stones, the effects being diuretic and cathartic. This remedy was often given to treat dropsy and jaundice, being a favored herb for disorders of the pneumo-gastric region.

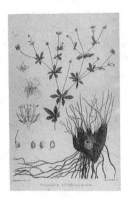

Tormentil

TORMENTIL

SCIENTIFIC NAME: *Potentilla tormentilla, P. erectus*
PARTS USED: Root

DOSAGE:

Root: 1 teaspoon, boiled in a covered container of 1 1/2 pints of water for about 1/2 hour, at a slow boil. Liquid allowed to cool slowly in the *closed* container. Drink cold, 1 swallow or 1 tablespoon at a time, 1 to 2 cups per day. Note: Brew stronger for external, weaker for internal usage.

TORMENTIL: *The roots high concentrations of tannins make them a powerful astringent.*

Traditional Usages

Tormentil is a **powerful astringent,** and has been **used primarily to treat diarrhea and hemorrhage.** Additionally, it was considered by the ancients to promote sweating and was thought helpful in curing plague. It was administered to treat syphilis, fevers, smallpox, measles, and a vast list of other disorders. As a treatment for **warts**, a piece of linen was soaked in a strong decoction of Tormentil, placed on the wart, and repeated frequently until success was achieved. **The decoction was also gargled to cure mouth ulcers and spongy gums.**

The herbalists Gerard and Culpepper both employed Tormentil for **toothache**, comparing it favorably with Cloves. In Europe, a tincture is frequently utilized for intestinal disorders and in brandy for stomach disorders.

As is the case with most strong astringents, the root was also utilized for tanning leather, in this case in the Orkney Islands of Scotland. The masticated root was used to dye leather red by the Laplanders.

Recent Scientific Findings

The dried root contains chinovin, tormentilic acid, and chinova acid. However, **the anti-diarrhetic and anti-dysenteric effect of this perennial herb is due to the astringent and mildly antiseptic action of the tannins present in the rhizomes of virtually all** *Potentilla* **species.**

TURMERIC

SCIENTIFIC NAME: *Curcuma longa*
PARTS USED: Rhizome

DOSAGE:
1 to 2 grams per day in food or take capsules/tablets.

TURMERIC: *This common spice of Indian cuisine may be a potent anti-mutagenic agent.*

Traditional Usages

The wisdom of ethnic diets continues to amaze me. Time tested, *authentic* ethnic foods and food combinations evolved slowly and would not have survived as part of a culture were it not for the health-benefits experienced through trial and error. In the case of East Indian cuisine it has long been the unique use and preparation of freshly ground seasonings that set these dishes apart; the *vasana,* or aroma, of food is key.

Turmeric, ginger, pepper and chili are the major spices found in Indian food. But the list of all the spices used is quite large: cardamon, cloves, cinnamon, mace, nutmeg, saffron, various peppers, dill, cumin, fennel, bay leaf, mustard, coriander and, of course, garlic.

The Turmeric rhizome, or underground rootlike stem, is also widely utilized in traditional medical systems, mainly for treating various inflammatory conditions such as **arthritis**. In Ayurvedic medicine, Turmeric was prized for its aromatic, stimulant, and carminative properties.

Recent Scientific Findings

Currently, Turmeric is used in India to treat anorexia, liver disorders, cough, diabetic wounds, rheumatism, and sinusitis. In one study Turmeric extract was tested for its anticarcinogenic and antimutagenic properties. **Laboratory (non-human) experiments it was found that this ancient spice reduced both the number of tumors in mice and the mutagenicity of benzo(a)pyrene (BP) and two other potent mutagens, NPD and DMBA.**

Preventing cancer now receives the attention it has long deserved. Numerous biochemical and epidemiological studies have demonstrated diet's role in modulating the development of cancer. Laboratory experiments have established that the active principle of Turmeric (curcumin) is a **potent anti-mutagenic agent.**

For those interested in *how* curcumin may act to prevent cancer we turn again to the by-now all pervasive theory of free-radical inactivation. The test carcinogens BP and DMBA are metabolically activated to proximate mutagenic/carcinogenic epoxides, which then bind to macromolecules. One study's authors concluded that since curcumin is a potent anti-oxidant, it may scavenge the epoxides and prevent binding to macromolecules. In other words, this spice's cell-protective properties are similar to nutrient anti-oxidants, vitamins C and E, which inhibit free radical reactions.

This type of herb is known as a non-steroidal anti-inflammatory (NSAID). Curcumin inhibits cycloxygenase and lipoxygenase enzymes. Curcumin has three main mechanisms of action: 1) anti-oxidant activity; 2) lipoxygenase inhibitor; and 3) cyclooxygenase inhibition. By inhibiting the associated biochemical pathways, inflammation is curtailed. Modern science thus confirms what traditional healers have known for centuries. **Namely, that the fresh juice from the rhizome will reduce swelling in recent bruises, wounds and insect bites; and that the dried powdered root kills parasites, relieves head colds and arthritic aches.** (Interestingly, this spice has sometimes been used to adulterate ginger.)

A 1991 pharmacological review confirmed many of Turmeric's folkloric effects, including wound healing, gastric mucosa protection, antispasmodic activity, reduction of intestinal gas formation, protection of liver cells, increasing bile production, diminishing platelet aggregation (i.e. blood clumping), lowering serum cholesterol (at very high doses), antibacterial properties, antifungal properties, and potential antitumor activity. While most of the above effects were demonstrated with intravenous extracts in animals, they do parallel folkloric claims in humans and are not to be dismissed as "experimental" or "trivial."

Turmeric's benefits for arthritis treatment have been demonstrated in human clinical trials. A herbal formula of Turmeric, Ashwagandha, and Boswellin was evaluated in a randomized, double-blind, placebo-controlled study. After a one-month evaluation period 12 patients with osteoarthritis were given the herbal formula or placebo for three months. The patients were evaluated every two weeks. After a 15 day wash-out period, the treatment was reversed with the placebo patients receiving the drug and vice versa. Again results were evaluated over a three month period. **The patients treated with the herbal formula showed a significant drop in severity of pain and disability score.**

TURPENTINE TREE

SCIENTIFIC NAME: *Pistacia terebinthus,*
Pinus, Abies, and
Larix species

PARTS USED: Sap

DOSAGE:

Sap: As an enema, ½ to 1 ounce of oil to 1 pint of warm soapsuds.

TURPENTINE TREE: *At one time, "spirits of turpentine" were used as everything from an expectorant to a an ointment for rheumatism.*

Traditional Usages

The term *turpentine* is now generally applied to certain vegetable juices, liquid or concrete, which consist of resin combined with a peculiar essential oil called oil of turpentine. They are generally procured from different species of Pine, though other trees afford products known by the same general title, such as *Pistacia terebinthus,* which yields the Chian turpentine.

Pistacia terebinthus is the Terebinth, a small tree native of Greece. It flourished in the islands of Cyprus and Chio, the latter giving its name to the turpentine obtained from the tree. The annual product of Chian turpentine is very small. Therefore, the turpentine commanded a high price and very little of it reached North America. It is frequently adulterated with other less costly coniferous turpentines.

White Turpentine is the common American variety and is procured chiefly from *Pinus palustris*, partly also from *Pinus taeda*, and some other species inhabiting the Southern states. In former times, large quantities were collected in New England. However, the turpentine trees of that area have been largely exhausted and more recently other parts of the United States have been the source of supply.

"Spirits of turpentine" is the volatile oil distilled with water from the concrete oleoresin. This oil (or "spirits") is locally irritant and feebly antiseptic. It was commonly employed as a stimulating expectorant. As it irritated the mucous membranes, it helped to expel phlegm and was a useful treatment in bronchitis. It stimulates kidney function and was sometimes used in mild doses as a diuretic; in large doses, it is dangerous to the kidneys. It was used as a carminative, and was considered one of the most valuable remedies for flatulent colic. Terebinth was also utilized to treat chronic diarrhea and dysentery, typhoid fever, internal hemorrhage, purpureal fever and bleeding, helminthiasis, leucorrhea, and amenorrhea.

Turpentine baths, arranged in such a way that the vapors were not inhaled by the patient, were given in cases of chronic rheumatism. Applied externally as a liniment or ointment, it has been used in rheumatic ailments such as lumbago, arthritis, and neuralgias. It was also applied locally to treat and promote the healing of burns and to heal parasitic skin diseases.

Recent Scientific Findings

Unfortunately, research has not been conducted to confirm or deny Turpentine's folkloric claims.

VALERIAN

SCIENTIFIC NAME: *Valerian officinalis*
PARTS USED: Root

DOSAGE:

   Root: Use *fresh* material! One teaspoonful to 1 cup of boiling water.

VALERIAN: *Used since antiquity, this root may be our safest and most effective tranquilizer.*

Traditional Usages

Valerian root has been used since ancient times in the treatment of **epilepsy**, particularly when the seizures are brought on by emotions such as fear and anger. Warriors of the Thompson tribe made several different preparations of American Valerian to treat wounds. The fresh pulverized roots were applied directly to injured areas, while the dried root was utilized as an antiseptic powder.

In more recent times Valerian has been employed as a **stimulant** and **antispasmodic**. Combined with Cinchona it has been given to treat intermittent fevers.

Valerian has been used as a tranquilizing agent since antiquity. It is all too tempting to observe the present frequency of tranquilizer use as indicative of doomed, exhausted populations crushed by machine civilization. Surely the pace and noise of present life create tension in biological man, but what do you make of this curious entry, recorded in 1831 by Samuel Thomson, a practicing botanic family physician.

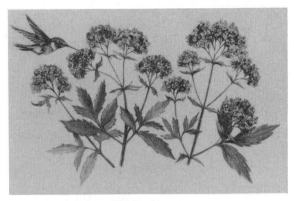

Valerian

This powder [Valerian] is the best nervine known; I have made great use of it, and have always found it to produce the most beneficial effects, in all cases of nervous affection, and in hysterical symptoms; in fact, *it would be difficult to get along with my practice in many cases without this important article.*

Apparently, even then, nervousness was a complaint all too frequently brought before the attention of healers. Thomson recommended half a teaspoon in hot water, sweetened, to promote sleep and leave the patient at ease.

Recent Scientific Findings

In an age of anxiety, when tranquilizing agents reign supreme, it may be wise to reconsider the natural sedatives. Of the many plants employed to calm nervous patients, quiet hysteria, or allay the fears of hypochondriacs, none seems to come forward with such recommendations as this root.

Valerian is clearly a non-narcotic, perfectly safe herbal sedative, highly recommended in anxiety states. While the unground dried root is presently available in most herb stores, and very popular (the powdered root is much more potent than the chipped bark), most users are experiencing only a trace, or a remnant of the effects of the fresh root, which is far more potent.

The roots of Valerian contain a complex mixture of substances known a valepotriates, which are known to have sedative and tranquillizing properties. Other important chemical constituents, known as esters, are unstable and are lost during the drying process. For this reason the drug's effects vary considerably, so much so that physicians largely abandoned it by the end of the 19th century.

A far more potent action is had by using the juice of the fresh root, in dosages of 1 to 3 tablespoonfuls. Of course, in Europe, Valerian tincture is freely available and a very popular natural "tranquilizer."

As expected, a remedy so prevalent in ancient and recent usage has proven itself under the sometimes too caustic rituals of the modern pharmacologist. Petkov and associates in Bulgaria recently demonstrated that an extract of the root has central nervous system sedative effects and the ability to steady an arrhythmic heart in lab animals.

Perhaps more interesting is Cavazzuti's work in Italy, which demonstrated that a mixture of Valerian, Passionflower, Chamomile, Hawthorn (fluidextract), sucrose, and orange essence was effective in treating children, "one- to twelve-year olds with psychomotor agitation and non-adaptation disorders." By the all too infrequently applied double-blind method (rarely applied in evaluating herbs), this herbal mixture displayed genuine effects in treating **hyperactivity** and **insomnia.** Unlike other hyperactivity medications, **Valerian showed no side effects.**

Another research team performed a double-blind study of Valerian's effect on **poor sleep.** Of the patients given the Valerian preparation, 44% reported perfect sleep and 99% reported improved sleep. Again, no side effects were observed.

Caution: Valerian may produce sensations of "strangeness" in some individuals. These persons should not use Valerian.

VIRGINIA SNAKEROOT

SCIENTIFIC NAME: *Aristolochia serpentaria*
PARTS USED: Rhizome and root

DOSAGE:

Root: The medicinal use was generally 1 teaspoon of the granulated root per pint of boiling water, steep for 1/2 hour. One tablespoon, 3 to 6 times per day, was the dosage. However, the *potential toxicity noted below recommends against use of the plant for self-medication.*

VIRGINIA SNAKEROOT: *At one time, this was the most popular remedy for snakebites.*

Traditional Usages

Virginia Snakeroot was the most renowned of the Native American treatments for the bites of poisonous snakes. Native Americans chewed the root and applied it to the snakebite. Its reputation spread rapidly among European settlers. It was admitted to the London *Pharmacopoeia* as early as 1650. Although it was originally introduced into regular medicine for this purpose, its efficacy against snakebite has never been conclusively demonstrated, and the most valuable application of Serpentaria seems to have been as a tonic for persons suffering from **intermittent fevers**, such as malaria. For this purpose it was often utilized as an adjunct to Cinchona (Quinine). Another usage was in the treatment of **dyspepsia** and **indigestion** arising from other disease conditions.

Recent Scientific Findings

Within the United States, three species contribute indiscriminately to furnish the Snakeroot of the shops: *A. serpentaria, A. tomentosa,* and *A. hastata.*

In larger doses the plant can cause nausea, vomiting, griping bowel pain, and dysenteric tenesmus. However, in the proper dosage it may be beneficial. It is known to be an appetite stimulant.

Virtually all the many species of *Aristolochia* that have been chemically investigated contain two materials in common. The first is an essential oil that holds a number of antiseptic compounds. The second constituent is a toxic material known as aristolochic acid. Aristolochic acid has been carefully studied in human subjects and is known to be extremely toxic to the kidneys and liver. Undoubtedly, the aristolochic acid content of these plants accounts for most of the uses alleged for them. **However, it cannot be recommended that *Aristolochia* species be used for any purpose, primarily on the basis of potential severe toxic reactions that could result.**

WALL GERMANDER

SCIENTIFIC NAME: *Teucrium chamaedrys*
PARTS USED: Tops and leaves

DOSAGE:

Tops and Leaves: Approximately ½ ounce of tops or leaves to 1 pint of water. Boil water separately and pour over the plant material and steep for 50 to 20 minutes, depending on the desired effect. Drink hot or warm, 1 to 2 cups per day.

WALL GERMANDER: *This was once a major ingredient of a popular patent medicine, Portland Powder.*

Traditional Usages

The Wall Germander was recommended by ancient herbalists for its **vulnerary** properties (ability to heal wounds), and continues to be a folk remedy for **ulcers** and **sores**. It is also recommended for general use as a tonic for digestion. Other ailments that have reportedly been treated with this plant are **anemia, asthma, bronchitis**, and other **chronic respiratory diseases**.

It is astringent, antiseptic, diuretic, and stimulant, and has been used in the treatment of **jaundice, dropsy, gout**, and ailments of the **spleen**. The Egyptians utilized the plant for treating intermittent fevers; interestingly, it was given as a preventive, the dose being taken one hour in advance of the paroxysm which was known to reoccur at four hour intervals.

At one time this herb was part of a popular patent medicine for the treatment of **gout** and **arthritis**, known as Portland Powder, which contained equal parts *Aristolochia rotunda* root, *Gentiana lutea* root, tops and leaves of Germander and *Erythroea centaurium*, and leaves of *Ajuga chamoepitys*, the Ground Pine.

Recent Scientific Findings

Studies on a closely related species, *Teucrium polium*, showed **anti-inflammatory action**.

WALNUT, BLACK

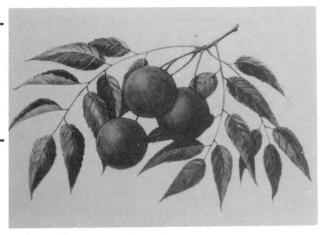

Black Walnut

SCIENTIFIC NAME: *Juglans nigra*

PARTS USED: Hulls and inner bark

DOSAGE:

Bark: 1 teaspoon of the inner bark, boiled in a covered container of 1½ pints of water for about ½hour at a slow boil. Allow liquid to cool slowly in the *closed* container. Drink cold, 1 swallow or 1 tablespoon at a time, 1 to 2 cups per day.

BLACK WALNUT: *This tree's inner bark has long been valued as a mild laxative, while researchers have also found it lowers blood pressure.*

Traditional Usages

Known in different sections of the U.S. by the various names of Butternut, Oilnut, and White Walnut, the inner bark and the root are the medicinal portions. Walnut root was formerly recommended in *U.S. Pharmacopoeia*. It should be collected in May or June.

On the living tree, the inner bark when first uncovered is a of a pure white, which becomes immediately on exposure a beautiful lemon color, and ultimately changes to deep brown. It has a fibrous texture, a feeble odor, and a peculiar bitter, somewhat acrid taste. Its medical virtues are entirely extracted by boiling water. Gathered in the autumn, the bark contains resins, juglandin, jugloine, juglandic acid, and essential oil.

The bark has been valued as one of the mildest and most certain laxatives given us by nature; it operates without causing nausea, irritation, or pain, and does not impair the digestive function. During the Revolutionary War it was commonly used as a habitual **laxative** and was also considered quite valuable in the treatment of liver disorders.

The Menominees ate the syrup of white walnut, or butternut, as a remedy for digestive disorders. A tea from the inner bark was drunk by the Potawatomis for upset stomach, while the Meskwakis used a tea as a mild laxative.

The common European Walnut, *J. regia*, is also used medicinally. The hull of the fruit has been utilized as a **vermifuge** and as a treatment for syphilis and ulcers, and the oil of the fruit is reportedly **anti-parasitic** and **has cured tapeworm**, as well as being employed as a laxative. The Chinese employed this plant to treat **asthma, lumbago, beriberi, impotence,** and **constipation.**

Information on the effectiveness of Walnut preparations for hepatic congestion has not been found in the scientific literature. However, folkloric use for liver complaints is reported.

Recent Scientific Findings

The inner root owes all of its pharmacologic effect either to the presence of tannins or the simple quinone compound juglone. These have **astringent**, **antiseptic**, and **vermifuge** properties, especially juglone.

The chemical constituents are iron, iodine, calcium, silica, the Quinone Juglone, tannins, and ellagic acid. Using large doses, researchers at the University of Missouri in the 1960s found that ellagic acid paradoxically both lowered blood pressure and prevented other agents from lowering blood pressure. This same group of researchers also found that several constituents of Black Walnut had **anti-cancer properties**.

Based on data from mice experiments, the alkaloid fraction of Black Walnut may prevent tumor formation (specifically in mammary glands).

WATER LILY

SCIENTIFIC NAME: *Nymphaea alba* and other *Nymphaea* spp.

PARTS USED: Rhizome

DOSAGE:

To depress the sexual function, seek out a white Water Lily and meditate on its purity.

WATER LILY: *These beautiful flowers were once used to treat a variety of skin problems.*

Traditional Usages

Although all colors of Water Lilies were employed in folk medicine, the white Water Lily in particular was valued, due to its purity, rising out of the often murky marsh, stream, or pond.

It was used as an anaphrodisiac (depress the sexual function). This concept most likely originated with the romantic notion of the purity of the flower rising from the muck more than any true folkloric belief in such abilities. This power was likely attributed only to the white *Nymphaea*.

Externally, white and yellow Water Lilies were used to treat various skin disorders, such as **boils**, **inflammation**, **tumors**, and **ulcers**. It was also employed for **diabetes**. The rootstocks contain much starch, useful as a food in emergencies.

A 1989 article maintains the Water Lily was used by the ancient Egyptians as an integral part of shamanistic healing. The author argues that Water Lily and Mandrake were used to induce shamanistic trance and used both medicinally and ritualistically.

Recent Scientific Findings

No research exists to support the folkloric claims for Water Lily.

WHEAT GRASS (COUCH GRASS)

SCIENTIFIC NAME: *Agropyron, var. spp.*
PARTS USED: Root and rhizome

DOSAGE:

Root: 1 teaspoon, boiled in a covered container of 1½ pints of water for about ½ hour, at a slow boil. Liquid allowed to cool slowly in the *closed* container. Drink cold, 1 swallow or 1 tablespoon at a time, as much as desired.

WHEATGRASS: *For centuries herbalists have employed this plant to treat urinary-tract disorders.*

Traditional Usages

Dogs and cats, when they are ill, will seek out and eat this plant in preference to any other field grasses. The roots possess both **diuretic** and **demulcent** properties, and have been used by herbalists for centuries to treat inflammation of the bladder, frequent or painful urination, blood in the urine, and other urinary-tract diseases.

An old home remedy for coughing, the roasted rootstocks have also long been utilized as a coffee substitute and as a source of bread in times of famine.

Recent Scientific Findings

The roots of Couch Grass contain mucilage, which accounts for the plant's soothing and demulcent action on mucous membranes. Animals studies in Rumania showed that Couch Grass rhizome preparations had a **diuretic** effect in rats. In Tanzania researchers found **strong central nervous system depressant activity in mice.** Extracts have also been shown to have **antibiotic effects against bacteria and molds.**

Water extracts of the roots of *A. repens* have been studied in laboratory animals and when administered orally give rise to **pronounced diuretic effects.**   In addition, the extracts are known to have **antibiotic** effects against a variety of bacteria and molds.

Couch Grass is very valuable in disorders of kidneys and bladder and in urinary troubles that originate with colds or catarrhal inflammation of these organs. It induces the proper flow of the urine and tends to relieve painful, scanty but frequent urination. Its blood-purifying properties are also quite pronounced.

WILLOW, WHITE

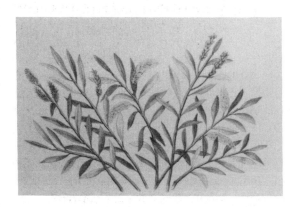

White Willow

SCIENTIFIC NAME: *Salix alba*
PARTS USED: Bark

DOSAGE:

Bark: Boil 1 teaspoon of bark in a covered container of 1 1/2 pints of water for about 1/2 hour, at a slow boil. Liquid allowed to cool slowly in the closed container. Drink cold, 1 swallow or 1 tablespoon at a time, as needed to promote sweating in chills and fever.

WHITE WILLOW: *For centuries, Willow bark has been revered as one of the safest and most effective means for pain relief and lowering fevers.*

Traditional Usages

Most of the willows have been utilized

for their **pain-relieving** and **fever-lowering** properties since antiquity. Ancient Egyptian, Assyrian, and Greek texts refer to Willow bark; the Greek physicians Hippocrates and Dioscorides (circa A.D. 60) used it to combat pain and fevers.

Willows were employed throughout their range of growth in the United States. The Pomos boiled the inner root bark of the California Willow and drank the resulting tea to promote sweating in cases of chills and fever. In the South, the Natchez used Red Willow bark in their fever remedies, while the Alabama and Creeks plunged into Willow root steam baths to alleviate fever. The use of willow is also reported among tribes from the Pima of Arizona to the Penobscots of Maine. In the mid-1700s the bark enjoyed immense popularity in colonial America as a fever treatment.

For thousands of years people were known to chew the leaves or inner bark of Willows or other shrubs in the spirea sub-family of plants. All of the above contain salicylic acid; in 1838, using Willow bark, Rafaele Piria prepared the first pure form of salicylic acid. As obtained from various species of Willow, Salicin was official in the *U.S. Pharmacopoeia* from 1882 to 1926. Salicylic acid was used to produce acetyl-salicylic acid, which was dubbed aspirin (a-spirin) to denote that it did not utilize plants from the spirea sub-family.

Recent Scientific Findings

Willow bark contains salicin which probably decomposes into salicylic acid in the human system. The structural formulas for Acetylsalicyclic acid (aspirin) and salicylic acid are quite similar. Aspirin-like compounds, the nonsteroidal, anti-inflammatories (NSAID's) have been found to inhibit the manufacture of certain prostaglandins (PG's) from their precursor, the fatty acid arachidonic acid (AA). Prostaglandins play a key role in the regulation of immune function.

Aspirin is a prostaglandin (PGE2) inhibitor. When we take aspirin, or like compounds, we may stimulate our immune system by blocking PGE2 production. Although salicylic acid is only a *weak* cycloxygenase inhibitor its potency within the body is about equal to aspirin. It is speculated that salicin (from Willow) does not cause gastric or intestinal upset or bleeding because unlike acetylsalicylic acid (aspirin) this natural product does not block prostaglandins in the stomach or intestine. Instead Salicin bypasses the stomach or intestine and does not have prostaglandin blocking effects until it reaches the liver where the acetyl-group is metabolically picked up.

It should be noted, though, that the immune system is not a one way path. Both enhancement *and* suppression of immunological functions have been reported for PG's! For the sake of this small discussion, it is sufficient to note that PG's and the metabolites of AA are involved in immune reactions.

Aspirin is now receiving wide usage to prevent heart attacks in men over 50. This may be due to the fact that cycloxygenase inhibitors prevent platelet aggregation or blood clots. The spread of tumor cells is also thought to be associated with platelet clumping. Several tumor cell types can aggregate platelets and form a metastasis. So, along with preventing heart attacks, the aspirin-like compounds, including salicin may also help prevent the spread of cancer.

WINTER-GREEN

SCIENTIFIC NAME: *Gaultheria procumbens*
PARTS USED: Leaves and flowering tops

DOSAGE:

> **Leaves and Flowering tops:**
> One teaspoon of the plant to 1
> cup of boiling water, steep for 5 to
> 20 minutes and drink cold, 1 cup
> per day, 1 mouthful at a time.

WINTERGREEN: *This aromatic herb is still listed in the U.S. Pharmacopoeia for its astringent, diuretic, and stimulant properties.*

Traditional Usages

The name wintergreen has been ascribed to many different plants, including *Pyrola*, *Chimaphila*, and *Moneses*. However, *Gaultheria* is the most popular in domestic American medicine. Thoreau describes imbibing the leaves as a tea prepared by his Native American guide. The Montagnais of Labrador and southeastern Canada drank Wintergreen tea to treat **paralysis**.

An old favorite, Wintergreen tea is **diuretic** in small doses; large doses are emetic. It is an aromatic stimulant with astringent properties, and consequently is of assistance in cases of **chronic diarrhea. It has been used to promote menstruation and increase milk production in nursing mothers.** Oil of Wintergreen has been used as an **external application**, in the form of cloths soaked in the aromatic liquid and tied to the painful part, in the treatment of **body aches and pains**. Wintergreen leaves were official in the *U.S. Pharmacopoeia* from 1820 to 1894. Oil of Wintergreen is still listed for its **astringent, diuretic**, and **stimulant** properties.

Recent Scientific Findings

Some of the medicinal actions can be explained on the basis of the methyl salicylate contained in the oil, which is closely related to acetylsalicylic acid, or aspirin.

WITCH HAZEL

SCIENTIFIC NAME: *Hamamelis virginiana*
PARTS USED: Bark, twigs, and leaves

DOSAGE:

Leaves and Bark: 1 teaspoon of leaves or bark, granulated, to 1 cup boiling water. Applied cold or gargled as a mouthwash.

WITCH HAZEL: *Once ascribed occult powers, this plant is an ingredient in many cosmetic face creams and lotions.*

Traditional Usages

This plant was named by those who ascribed occult powers to it. The forked branches were used as divining rods to find water and gold.

North American tribes used this shrub as a sedative application to external inflammations, and so we inherited yet another valuable gift of nature from the indigenous American. A decoction of boiled twigs was employed as a cure for aching backs. The Potawatomi treated muscular aches with a steam created by placing the twigs in water with hot rocks. In 1744 it was observed that the Mohawks treated bruised eyes with a wash of steeped Witch Hazel bark. In 1850 the American Medical Association listed Witch Hazel as a treatment for eye inflammations, internal hemorrhages, and piles. Witch Hazel leaves were listed in the *U.S. Pharmacopoeia* from 1862 through 1916, and in the *National Formulary* from 1916 to 1955.

Internally, it was at one time recommended as a fluidextract in the treatment of **varicose veins** and internal bleedings. **Itching hemorrhoids** were treated with a soothing ointment made of lard and a decoction of Apple tree bark, Witch Hazel bark, and White Oak bark.

Recent Scientific Findings

Witch Hazel is utilized today largely as described above, and as a **liniment for body aches and pains.** Witch Hazel extracts contain astringent tannins that explain the beneficial effects of water extract in reducing inflammation when applied externally. **Commercially available "witch hazel extract," however, does not contain tannins.** When the extract is prepared the plant is mixed with water and distilled. The distillate is a clear, colorless liquid having an aromatic odor. It contains a mixture of aromatic substances that have not been well studied. Yet, that this extract is **soothing and refreshing** when applied externally can be verified by anyone who has used it.

Many cosmetic face creams and lotions contain Witch Hazel.

WOLFSBANE

SCIENTIFIC NAME: *Aconitum napellus*
PARTS USED: Root

DOSAGE:
   Dangerous: Avoid internal use.

WOLFSBANE: *Also known as Aconite, this plant was adopted by conventional medicine from homeopathic practitioners.*

Traditional Usages

Wolfsbane, or Aconite, possesses sedative, anodyne, diuretic, and inflammation reducing properties. **But in overdose it and all its relatives are swift and fatal poisons.** Nevertheless, in 1762 a Viennese physician, Baron Störck, published experiments proving the value of this plant in the materia medica, claiming success in treating **gout, rheumatism, intermittent fevers,** and **scrofulous swellings.**

By the time the twentieth edition of the *U.S. Dispensatory* was issued (1918), **Aconite was recognized as a valuable circulatory sedative in heart problems, since it reduced excessive heart action and decreased arterial tension.** Concomitant with the reduction of blood pressure Aconite was also noted for its ability to induce sweating.

Aconite is a highly valued homeopathic remedy; in fact, it was originally crossed over into regular medicine from homeopathic practice as a substitute for the widespread and sometimes fatal practice of bloodletting that prevailed through the 19th century. **Homeopathic practitioners** also used Aconite in the treatment of pains, to promote a sense of calm, and, parallel to the observations of the *U.S. Dispensatory,* to produce and increase perspiration.

Used externally as a liniment, the plant has proved useful in the treatment of **neuralgia** and **rheumatic pains.**

Recent Scientific Findings

The active principle, aconitine, was discovered in 1833. Although it is exceedingly toxic in even very small quantities, there have been reports of people being able to eat the boiled leaves without harm. We cannot substantiate, however, that boiling destroys the fatally dangerous principle, and it should be noted that a decoction of this herb was employed to execute the condemned in early times.

It is well known that the leaves and roots of Wolfsbane contain very potent alkaloids that have been studied in animals and are known to produce sedative and painkilling effects. However, the amount of these alkaloids that will produce these effects is nearly the same as the amount that will produce serious poisonous effects. Thus, one must be cautioned that Wolfsbane is a potentially dangerous plant when considered for any use in humans. An overdose will cause adverse effects on the heart (fibrillations).

WOOD BETONY

SCIENTIFIC NAME: *Stachys officinalis*
PARTS USED: Leaves and root

DOSAGE:

Leaves: Approximately 1 ounce to 1 pint of water. Boil water separately and pour over the leaves and steep for 5 to 20 minutes, depending on the desired effect. Drink hot or warm, 1 to 2 cups or more per day.

Root: 1 teaspoonful powdered or ground root boiled in 1½ pints of water in uncovered container for ½ hour; boiled down to 1 pint. Drink cold, 1 cup per day, 1 to 2 tablespoons at a time.

WOOD BETONY: *Once a very popular remedy, this is now a flavoring for herbal teas.*

Traditional Usages

Highly esteemed by the ancients, Betony was extolled as a remedy for a wide variety of ailments. The root is both **emetic** and **purgative. It was also used to expel intestinal worms.**

The leaves are quite mild, possessing aperient (mildly laxative), cordial, aromatic, and astringent properties. **A tea brewed from the plant has been used in the treatment of stomach disorders, gout, headaches, and disorders of the spleen.** An infusion was a popular remedy for bladder and kidney problems.

Recent Scientific Findings

Betony's major use today is not as a medicinal but as a flavoring agent in herbal tea blending. It is thought to be a **valuable nervine** by some people in the herbal tea industry.

Animal experiments have shown **antihypertensive** activity and an **antihistamine effect** (SRSA antagonist).

WORMWOOD
or
QING HAO

SCIENTIFIC NAME: *Artemisia* species
PARTS USED: Leaves & flowering tops

DOSAGE:

Leaves and Flowering tops: Approximately ½ ounce of the leaves or flowering tops to 1 pint of water. Boil water separately and pour over the plant material and steep for 5 to 20 minutes, depending on the desired effect. Take ½ cup per day, 1 teaspoon at a time.

WORMWOOD: *Long utilized to invigorate the internal organs, modern research reveals additional uses for this member of the rose family.*

Traditional Usages

Wormwood was formerly utilized in several ways, the most important being as an **anthelmintic** (to expel tapeworms and other intestinal worms)—hence the common name for the plant. It was considered a **powerful local anesthetic,** and has been **applied externally to relieve rheumatic pains,** as well as for sprains, bruises and local irritations. Taken internally, it was additionally utilized as a tonic and cathartic. Various Amerind tribes employed Wormwood for bronchial ailments. Before the introduction of quinine (Cinchona bark), it was highly regarded as a remedy in intermittent fevers.

In Chinese medicine, Sweet Wormwood (*A. annua*) has been written about since 168 BC and is prescribed for "summer colds," malaria, "heat excess;" in other words as an antipyretic, to reduce fevers. It is *not* used to kill parasites.

Near relatives, *A. indica* and *A. chinensis,* were utilized in China to produce moxas. These agents are small combustible masses used to cause sloughing following cauterization. They are caustics, used in skin diseases, to destroy infected tissue and to counteract the bites of animals and insects.

Wormwood has gained an unfavorable reputation among many as an herbal remedy because of the toxicity of the essential oil prepared by distilling the above-ground portions of the plant. The liqueur absinthe, made from oils of Wormwood, Angelica, Anise, and Marjoram, contains a high concentration of thujone, which is a convulsant poison and narcotic when taken in large amounts. Absinthe is banned in virtually every country in the world. Unlike ordinary alcoholism, Absinthism also produces "restlessness at night, with disturbing dreams, nausea and vomiting in the morning with great trembling of the hands and tongue, vertigo, and a tendency to epileptiform convulsions."

Recent Scientific Findings

Species of *Artemisia* are now receiving much attention for their purported anti-parasitic properties. Experimental evidence supporting such claims is weak or non-existent.

We have been unable to find experimental evidence to corroborate the anthelmintic or anti-parasitic effect of Wormwood but water extracts given to animals by mouth have been shown to produce a cathartic action. A tea of Wormwood would be bitter, and most bitter substances act as tonics by increasing gastric secretion. Mausert prescribed this herb for liver complaints, since it promoted the flow of bile. Being an active medicinal, it must be carefully dosed.

However, a great deal of research has recently been undertaken concerning Wormwood's anti-malarial properties. Malarial parasites have developed resistance to synthetic antimalarial agents, leading to a resurgence in the use of quinine. There's also been renewed attention in finding new antimalarial drugs. A sesquiterpene lactone isolated from Wormwood, artemisinin, has been the subject of a great deal of new preliminary research. The World Health Organization has developed Artemether, a potent derivative of artemisinin, as the drug of choice.

Wormwood has been used to make a herbal tea containing only a very small amount of absinthe, and hence thujone, in the final beverage. Thujone has a very low water-solubility; thus it would be difficult to experience the adverse effects of absinthe when the plant is used in the form of a normally brewed herbal tea.

YAM, WILD

SCIENTIFIC NAME: *Dioscorea villosa*
PARTS USED: Rhizome

DOSAGE:
   Rhizome: 2-4 milliliters, given either in the form of a decoction or a fluidextract.

WILD YAM: *Once used by Southern slaves for rheumatism, modern research is confirming its anti-inflammatory properties.*

Traditional Usages

As the common names clearly indicate (Colic Root, Rheumatism Root), the Yam has been considered a remedy for bilious colic, and Southerners once used it as a treatment for **rheumatism**. The root is diuretic and expectorant, but only in large doses. It is also antispasmodic, which would explain its efficacy in treating bilious colic.

Recent Scientific Findings

All species of Wild Yam examined to date contain varying amounts of a steroid-like material known as diosgenin. Diosgenin has been shown experimentally to inhibit inflammation in laboratory animals, and thus the **Wild Yam could have beneficial effects in rheumatism, as claimed in folklore.**

A natural oral contraceptive agent due to a steroidal content of 40% diosgenin and 50-60% of other related sapogenins, Yam is utilized as a basis of commercial birth-control product sex hormone production (conversion of Diosgenin to progesterone).

YARROW

SCIENTIFIC NAME: *Achillea millefolium*
PARTS USED: Flowering tops and leaves

DOSAGE:

Leaves and Flowering tops: Approximately ½ ounce of the leaves or flowering tops to 1 pint of water. Boil water separately and pour over the plant material and steep for 5 to 20 minutes, depending on the desired effect. Drink hot or warm, 1 to 2 cups or more per day, at bedtime and upon awakening. Externally, as needed.

YARROW: *Both the ancient Greeks and Native Americans used this plant to heal wounds.*

Traditional Usages

The genus name, *Achillea,* is derived from the Greek hero of the *Iliad*, Achilles, who according to mythology healed the wounds of his comrades-in-arms with a relative of this plant. Yarrow was known to the Greeks as a styptic, vulnerary, and astringent, and hence was utilized in hemorrhagic complaints.

Native American warriors also used Yarrow to treat cuts, bruises, and other minor injuries. The Ute name for Yarrow is translated as **"wound medicine."** The Zuni used it to treat **burns.** The dried leaves and tops were listed for promoting menstruation and as a stimulant in the *U.S. Pharmacopoeia* from 1863 to 1882.

Yarrow has been used both locally and internally in the treatment of

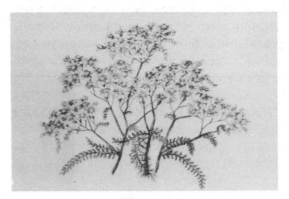

Yarrow

hemorrhoids, and has also been given for bladder conditions such as involuntary urination in children. In weak doses, it has been employed as a mild aromatic, sudorific, tonic, and astringent, the leaves being employed for the latter purpose. Its most noteworthy usage was in menstrual irregularities.

In the Scandinavian countries Yarrow was at one time substituted for Hops in beer and was probably felt to have sedative properties.

Recent Scientific Findings

The use of decoctions or infusions of Yarrow flowers as a tonic has been studied experimentally in humans. It has been confirmed that oral extracts of this plant stimulate gastric juices. This would lead to a tonic effect with improved digestion of foods. The effect is due to the presence of bitter principles (azulenes, sesquiterpenes) in the flowers.

Animals studies have shown that extracts of Yarrow can reduce inflammation, and have a calming effect. Thus, the use of the juice of this

plant for the treatment of ulcers and hemorrhoids has a rational basis. Extracts of Yarrow are also known to have antibiotic effects when evaluated in test tubes. Thus, at least for external applications, one would expect that a person suffering from boils or other microbial infections of a minor nature would receive beneficial results by the external application of Yarrow preparations.

YELLOW DOCK

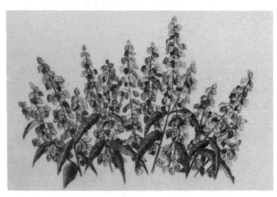

Yellow Dock

SCIENTIFIC NAME: *Rumex crispus*
PARTS USED: Root and rhizome

DOSAGE:

Root: Dock root is given in powder or decoction. Two ounces of the fresh root, bruised, or 1 ounce of the dried, may be boiled in a pint of water, of which 2 fluid ounces may be given as a dose, repeated as the patient can bear it.

Avoid the leaves because of their toxicity. Externally, apply powder as needed.

YELLOW DOCK: *A root decoction was a popular remedy for a variety of ailments in the 19th century.*

Traditional Usages

The roots reputedly have an unusual ability to take up whatever iron is present in the soil, and consequently, Yellow Dock root has been a valued remedy for **anemia**. The root is also **laxative, tonic**, and **astringent**, and has been recommended in skin conditions. When the gums are spongy the powdered root is a recommended **dentrifice**.

Though imported from Europe, Yellow Dock was a popular plant in Native American medicine. The Teton Dakota tribes tied crushed Yellow Dock leaves to boils to bring about a discharge of pus. The Ojibwas applied the pulverized root to cuts. By the late 1800s a root decoction was found "useful in dyspepsia, gouty tendencies, hepatic congestion, scrofula, syphilis, leprosy, elephantiasis, and various forms of scabby eruptions . . . (and) is also considered an excellent dentrifice, especially where the gums are spongy." This lengthy list of uses is not included here as proof of the gullibility of 19th century physicians. Rather it illustrates how when a remedy proved itself in the treatment of one complaint, it was then tried on a variety of other illnesses and probably successfully in some cases. This might be called the empirical method of healing.

The roots were in the *U.S. Pharmacopoeia* from 1863 to 1905. However, the *Dispensary of the United States* later stated that Dock root "has no real value."

Recent Scientific Findings

The leaves are valued as a cure for scurvy. However, they contain oxalic acid, and there are reported cases of death due to oxalic acid poisoning from the ingestion of the leaves. Caution is therefore advised concerning the use of too many leaves, since there are far safer sources of vitamin C to be found.

The roots are rich in a complex mixture of anthraquinones and anthraquinone glycosides, similar to the types of chemical found in Cascara bark and Frangula berries. It is these anthraquinone derivatives that produce the laxative effect characteristic of the roots of Yellow Dock.

Yellow Dock roots are also rich in tannins, which are responsible for the astringent effect of preparations from this plant when applied externally. **Thus, external applications for various skin conditions have a valid scientific base.**

Caution: Oxalate ingestion (large amounts) may cause kidney damage (cases of death have been reported).

YERBA SANTA

SCIENTIFIC NAME: *Eriodictyon californicum*
PARTS USED: Leaves

DOSAGE:

Leaves: 1 teaspoon of the leaves in a cup of boiling water, steep for 1/2 hour. Drink warm, one-half cup before retiring, or a mouthful 3 times per day.

YERBA SANTA: *The "Holy Herb" may contain chemopreventive compounds.*

Traditional Usages

Yerba Santa was the most highly valued medicinal plant among the Native Americans of Mendocino County, California. The leaves were taken as a tea for colds, or smoked and chewed to treat **asthma**. A **natural mouthwash** was prepared by rolling the leaves into balls and then allowing them to dry in the sun. After chewing, one drank water. As one user put it, "It makes one taste kind of sweety inside."

Yerba Santa was quickly adopted by the Spanish missionaries and then later settlers. V.K. Chestnut in his valuable paper on herb usage describes how it was employed as a cure for **grippe**, as a blood purifier, and as a cure for **rheumatism, consumption**, and **catarrh**.

In 1875, Dr. J.H. Bundy introduced Yerba Santa to the medical profession. Parke-Davis & Co. researched the drug and it was official in the *U.S. Pharmacopoeia* first from 1894 to 1905, then again from 1916 to 1947. Since then, Yerba Santa has been recognized in the *National Formulary*.

The leaves of this shrub have been used as a bitter tonic, and to disguise the bitterness of quinine. They were particularly valued for their expectorant properties, making this **a very popular remedy for asthma, chronic bronchitis, and colds**. Yerba Santa was also felt to be helpful in cases of **chronic genito-urinary inflammations**. For treating respiratory ailments, the leaves were sometimes smoked, but they could also be administered as an infusion as described above.

Recent Scientific Findings

The "Holy Herb" contains a resin, pentatriacontane, and cerotonic acid.

As dietary factors have become more recognized as one the primary elements in cancer, research on chemopreventive compounds has increased. Chemopreventive compounds include agents that prevent the formation of carcinogen, agents that interfere with the promotion and progression of carcinogen, as well as what are termed blocking agents, which reduce the activation of carcinogens to react with cells and initiate the induction of cancer. **One recent study (1992) found that a Yerba Santa extract "exhibited reproducible inhibition" of a potent cancer-causing chemical.**

YOHIMBE

SCIENTIFIC NAME: *Corynanthe yohimbe (Pausinystalia yohimba)*

PARTS USED: Bark

DOSAGE:

Caution: Although Yohimbine is on the USFDA unsafe herb list of March 1977, many people will no doubt continue to use it. Safer aphrodisiacs are available.

YOHIMBE: *Though there is no scientific evidence to support it, the bark remains a popular aphrodisiac.*

Traditional Usages

Yohimbe bark is one of the most frequently sought out **aphrodisiacs** that the world has ever known, and is still used for this purpose today, particularly in Cameroon.

Recent Scientific Findings

We have carried out an exhaustive search of the scientific literature for publications describing the effects of Yohimbe bark extracts on animals or humans in order to confirm or deny its reputed **aphrodisiac** properties. To our surprise, we were unable to find a single scientific paper that describes any type of effect for this plant in animals or in humans.

However, many papers have been published by scientists attempting to relate the results of experiments in animals with yohimbine (the bark's active derivative) to the alleged aphrodisiac effect of decoctions or infusions of the bark, in man.

To summarize these findings, very clearly Yohimbine causes a dilation of the blood vessels in animals and in man, including those in the genitalia. Thus, in man, an increased flow of blood is routed to the penis, which theoretically should result in an erection, following the administration of yohimbine and also Yohimbe bark. Unfortunately, Yohimbine in doses required to attain this effect also acts as a powerful agent in reducing normal blood pressure due to the dilatory effect on the blood vessels. As would be expected, a person with extremely low blood pressure would no longer have the physical strength to enter into the vigorous sexual experience that would be anticipated as a reason for taking Yohimbe bark, and thus the effect would be nullified.

> Yohimbine, and also Yohimbe bark, are powerful drugs. The effective dose is very close to the toxic dose, and thus one should not experiment with either of them out of curiosity. A person with normal low blood pressure should completely avoid the use of these two substances.

Some investigators have studied yohimbine in animals in order to ascertain whether or not this material affects ejaculation time and/or frequency, and it was found to do neither.

We have never found reference to the use of Yohimbe bark as an aphrodisiac in females, which tends to point out the long-standing male-chauvinistic attitudes in scientific work. Presumably, Yohimbe bark would also have an aphrodisiac effect in females, since it would cause an increased blood flow to the genitalia.

A recent study, however, discovered that Yohimbine is a **moderately effective weight loss agent**. Yohimbine increased thermogenesis and thus helped obese patients lose body mass. Obese patients who were on a low calorie diet (1,000 cal/day) were given a daily dose of 20 mg (5 mg, 4 times a day) of Yohimbine. The patients were told to take this drug at least 90 minutes before a meal. Yohimbine was found to exert a greater weight-reducing effect than placebo.

The study indicated that Yohimbine *blocks* alpha-2 adrenoreceptors in peripheral tissues. Remember that thermogenesis for weight-reducing purposes can also be achieved by stimulating beta adrenergic receptors. This has been tried in Denmark using ephedrine (a beta adrenergic *stimulant*) in a weight loss pill. While it increased thermogenesis, the side effects of sleeplessness, tachycardia, and muscular fibrillations precluded the widespread use of ephedrine.

YUCCA

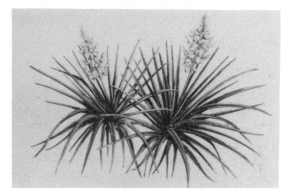

Yucca

SCIENTIFIC NAME: *Yucca brevifolia*
PARTS USED: Leaves

DOSAGE:

Leaves: Approximately 1 ounce of leaves to 1 pint of water. Boil water separately and pour over the plant material and steep for 5 to 20 minutes, depending on the desired effect. Drink hot or warm, 1 to 2 cups per day, at bedtime and upon awakening.

YUCCA: *Native Americans valued this both as food and as a cleanser.*

Traditional Usages

The dried fruits of this plant were valued as an important food for Navajo warriors, especially during long journeys. The roots were crushed and used for soap.

The Hopi especially prized this **natural cleanser**, relating "To **cure baldness**, wash the hair with yucca root and rub with duck grease because ducks have such heavy feathers."

Recent Scientific Findings

There has been inconclusive research which indicates potential usefulness in the treatment of **arthritis**.

CHAPTER 5

REFERENCES

GENERAL REFERENCES

Bender, G.A. *Great Moments in Pharmacy*. Detroit, Northwood Institute Press, 1966.

Carper, J. *The Food Pharmacy: Dramatic New Evidence That Food Is Your Best Medicine*. New York, Bantam Books, 1988.

Chung Shan Medical College. *Kanpo no rinsho oy* (The Clinical Applications of Chinese Herbal Formulas), Tokyo, I-chih-yao shuppansha / Dental and Pharmaceutical Press, 1976.

Flück, Hans. *Medicinal Plants*. W. Foulsham & Co., Ltd, Berkshire, England, 1988.

Holmes, P. *The Energetics of Western Herbs: Integrating Western and Oriental Herbal Traditions*. Boulder, CO, Artemis, 1989.

Hsu, H., et al.,(Eds.) *Oriental Materia Medica: A Concise Guide*, Oriental Healing Arts Institute, Long Beach, CA, 1986.

Hsu, H. *Taiwan ti chu chang chung yao yuao tsai tu chie* (An illustrated guide to the medicinal plants of Taiwan). Taipei, Hsin-chen-yuan, wei-sheng-shu chung-i-yao-wei-yuan hui / Chinese National Health Administration, Committee on Chinese Herbal Medicine, 1972.

Kiangsu New Medical College. *Chung yao ta tsu tien* (Dictionary of Chinese Herbal Drugs), Shanghai, Science and Technology Press, 1978; Hong Kong, Commercial Press Ltd., 1978.

Kidd, P.M. & Huber, W. *Living with the AIDS Virus: A Strategy for Long-Term Survival*. HK Biomedical Inc., 1990.

Lawrence, George H.M. *Taxonomy of Vascular Plants*. Macmillian Company, New York, NY, 1969.

Lust, John. *The Herb Book*. Bantam Books, New York, NY, 1974.

Marderosian, A.D. & Liberti, L.E. *Natural Product Medicine: A Scientific Guide to Foods, Drugs, Cosmetic*. Philadelphia, PA, George F. Stickley Co., 1988.

Mills, Simon Y. *The Dictionary of Modern Herbalism*. Thorsons Publishing Group, New York, NY, 1985.

Millspaugh, Charles F. *American Medicinal Plants*. Dover Publications, Inc., 180 Varick St. New York, NY 10014, 1974 (originally published in two volumes in 1892).

Mowry, D.B. *The Scientific Validation of Herbal Medicine*. Leni, UT, Cormorant Books, 1986.

NAS. *Herbal Pharmacology in the People's Republic of China: A Trip Report of the American Herbal Pharmacology Delegatio*, National Academy of Science, Washington, D.C., 1975.

Ratafia, M. & Purinton, T. The untapped market in plant derived drugs. *Medical Marketing and Media*, 58-68, June 1988.

Spalding, B.J. Modern drugs from folk remedies. *Chemical Week*, 52-53, February 27, 1985.

Takagi, K., et al. *Wakan yakubutsugaku* (The Pharmacology of Medicinal Herbs in East Asia), Tokyo, Nanzando, 1982.

Tyler, V.E., Brady, L.R. & Robbers, J.E. *Pharmacognosy*, 9th Ed. Lea & Febiger, Philadelphia, PA, 1988.

Uphof, J.C.T.H. *Dictionary of Economic Plants*. Verlag J. Cramer, 1968.

Vogel, V.J. *American Indian Medicine*. Norman, University of Oklahoma, 1970, p. 312.

Weiner, M.A. *Secrets of Fijian Medicine*. Government Press, Suva c/o Quantum Books USA, Mill Valley, CA, 1983.

Weiner, M.A. *Earth Medicine-Earth Foods: Plant Remedies, Drugs and Natural Foods of the North American Indian*. New York, Macmillan, 1972; 1980, Ballantine Books, 1990.

Weiner, Michael A. *The Herbal Bible*. Mill Valley, CA, Quantum Books, 1992.

Weiner, M.A. *Maximum Immunity*. Boston, Houghton-Mifflin, 1986.

Weiner, Michael and Janet. *Weiner's Herbal*. Quantum Books, Mill Valley, CA, 1990.

Weiss, R.F. *Herbal Medicine*. Beaconsfield, England, Beaconsfield Publishers Ltd, 1988.

Wood, G.B. & Bache, F. *United States Dispensary*, 20th ed. Lippincott Co., Philadelphia, 1918.

RECENT SCIENTIFIC REFERENCES FOR SPECIFIC PLANTS

AGRIMONY
Swanston-Flatt, S.K., Day, C., Bailey, C.J., & Flatt, P.R. Traditional plant treatments for diabetes. Studies in normal and streptozotopin diabetic mice. *Diabetaolgoia, 33*(8): 162-164, 1990.

ALFALFA
Swanston-Flatt, S.K., Day, C., Bailey, C.J., & Flatt, P.R. Traditional plant treatments for diabetes. Studies in normal and streptozotopin diabetic mice. *Diabetaolgoia, 33*(8): 162-164, 1990.

ANGELICA
Inamori, Y, et al. Antibacterial activity of two chalcones, xanthoangeloi and 4-hydroxyderricin, isolated from the root of Angelica keiskei. *Chemical and Pharmacological Bulletin, 39*(6): 1604-1605, 1991.

Keji, C. Certain progress in the treatment of coronary heart disease with traditional medicinal plants in China, *American Journal of Chinese Medicine, 9*(3):193-196, 1981.

Mei, Q.B., Tao, J.Y., & Cui, B. Advances in the pharmacological studies of radix Angelica sinensis (Oliv) Diels (Chinese Danggui). *Chinese Medical Journal, 104*(9): 776-7871, 1991.

Murakami, S., et al. Inhibition of gastric H+, K(+)-ATPase by chalcone derivatives, xanthoangelol and 4-hydroxyderricin, from Angelica keiskei Koidzumi, *Journal of Pharmacy and Pharmacology, 42*(10), 723-726, 1990.

Okuyama, T., et al. Anti-tumor promotion by principles obtained from Angelica keiskei. *Planta Medica, 57*(3): 242-246, 1991.

Usuki, S. Blended effects of herbal components of tokishakuyakusan on somatomedin C/insulin-like growth factor 1 level in rat corpus luteum. *American Journal of Chinese Medicine, 19*(1): 61-64, 1991.

Usuki, S. Effects of herbal components of tokishakuyakusan on progesterone secretion by corpus luteum in vitro. *American Journal of Chinese Medicine, 19*(1): 57-60, 1991.

Wang, L.R., Li, H.Y., & Xie, C.K. Reverse-phase HPLC determination of coumarin in the traditional Chinese drug bai-zhi (Angelica dahurica forma bai-zhi). *Pharmaceutica Sinica, 25*(2): 131-136, 1990.

Wang, Y.P. Progress of pharmacological research on angelica polysaccharide. *Chinese Journal of Modern Developments in Traditional Medicine, 11*(1): 61-63, 1991.

Yan, Z., Niu, Z. Pan, N., Xu, G, & Yang, X. Analysis of essential oils in roots and fruits of Angelica in Northeast China. *Journal of Chinese Materiamedica, 15*(7): 419-421, 447, 1990.

Yu, S., et al. Research on the processing of Angelica based on the analysis of water soluble constituents. *Journal of Chinese Materiamedica, 16*(3): 148-149, 190, 1991.

Zhuang, X.X. Protective effect of Angelica injection on arrhythmia during myocardial sichemia reperfusion in rat. *Chinese Journal of Modern Developments in Traditional Medicine, 11*(6): 360-361, 326, 1991.

ALOE VERA
Brown, J.S. & Marcy, S.A. The use of botanicals for health purposes by members of a prepaid health plan. *Research in Nursing and Health, 14*(5): 339-350, 1991.

Davis, R.H., et al. Wound healing: Oral & topical activity of Aloe vera. *Journal of the American Podiatric Medical Assoc., 79*(11): 559-562, Nov. 1989.

Davis, R.H., Parker, W.L., & Murdoch, D.P. Aloe vera as a biologically active vehicle for hydrocortisone acetate. *Journal of the American Podiatric Medical Association. 81*(1): 1-9, 1991.

Davis, R.H., Parker, W.L., Sampson, R.T., & Murdoch, D.P. The isolation of an active inhibitory system from an extract of aloe vera. *Journal of the American Podiatric Medical Association. 81*(5): 258-261, 1991.

Fulton, J.E. Jr. The stimulation of postdermabrasion wound healing with stabilizing aloe vera gel-polyethylene oxide dressing. *Journal of Dermatologic Surgery and Oncology, 167*(5): 460-467, 1990.

Hunter, D. & Frumkin, A. Adverse reactions to vitamin E and aloe vera preparation after dermabrasion and chemical peel. *Cutis. 47*(3), 193-196, 1991.

McCauley, R.L., Heggers, J.P, & Robson, M.C. *Postgraduate Medicine, 88*(8): 67-68, 73-77, 1990.

Schmidt, J.M. & Greenspoon, J.S. Aloe vera dermal wound gel is associated with a delay in wound healing. *Obstetrics and Gynecology, 78*(1): 115-117, 1991.

Thompson, J.E. Topical use of aloe vera derived allantoin gel in otolaryngology [letter]. *Ear, Nose, and Throat Journal, 70*(1): 56, 1991.

Thompson, J.E. Topical use of aloe vera derived allantoin gel in otolaryngology [letter]. *Ear, Nose, and Throat Journal, 70*(2): 119, 1991.

ANEMONE
Martin, M.L., San Roman, L., & Dominquez, A. In vitro activity of protaenominin, an antifungal agent. *Planta Medica, 56*(1): 66-69, 1990.

Martin, M.L., et al. Pharmacologic effects of lactones isolated from Pulsatilla alpine subsp apifolia. *Journal of Ethnopharmacology, 24*(2-3_: 185-191, 1988.

Zhang, X.Q., Liu, A.R., & Xu, L.X. Determination of ranunculin in Pulsatilla chinensis and synthetic ranunculin by reversed phase HPLC. *Yao Hsueh Hsueh Pao, 25*(12): 932-935, 1990.

ANISE
el-Shobaki, F.A., Saleh, Z.A., & Saleh, N. The effect of some beverage extracts on intestinal iron absorption. *Journal of Nutritional Sciences, 29*(4): 264-269, 1990.

Moharram, A.M., Abdel-Mallek, A.Y., & Abdel-Hafez, A.I. Mycoflora of anise and fennel seeds in Egypt. *Journal of Basic Microbiology, 29*(7): 427-435, 1989.

Spencer, D.G. Jr., Yaden, S., & Lal, H. Behavioral and physiological detection of classically-conditioned blood pressure reduction. *Psychopharmacology Berlin, 95*(1): 25-28, 1988.

van Toorenenbergen, A.W., Huijakes-Heins, M.I., Leijnse, B., & Dieges, P.H. Immunoblot analysis of IgE-binding antigens in spices. *International Archives of Allergy and Applied Immunology, 86*(1): 117-120, 1988.

ARROWROOT

Rolston, D.D., Matthew, P., & Mathan, V.I. Food-based solutions are a viable alternative to glucose-electrolyte solutions for oral hydration in acute diarrhoea—studies in a rat model of secretory diarrhoea. *Transactions of the Royal Society of Tropical Medicine and Hygiene, 84*(1): 1560159, 1990.

ARTICHOKE

Benveniste, I., Lesot, A., Hasenfratz, M.P., Kochs, G., & Durst, F. Multiple forms of NADPH-cytochrome P450 reductase in higher plants. *Biochemical and Biophysical Research Communications, 177*(1): 105-112, 1991.

Bosque, M.A., Schumacher, M., Domingo, J.L, & Llobet, J.M. Concentrations of lead and cadmium in edible vegetables from Tarragona Province, Spain. *Science of the Total Environment, 95*: 61-67, 1990.

Gabriac, B., Werc-Reichart, D., Teutsch, H., & Durst, F. Purification and immunocharacterization of a plant cytochrome P450: the cinnamic acid 4-hydroxylase. *Archives of Biochemistry and Biophysics, 288*(1): 302-309, 1991.

Gross, K.C. & Acosta, P.B. Fruits and vegetables are a source of galactose: implications in planning the diets of patients with galactosaemia. *Journal of Inherited Metabolic Diseases, 14*(2): 253-258, 1991.

Mereiah, K.A., Bunner, D.L., Ragland, D.R., & Creasia, D.A. Protection against microcystin-LR-induced hetaptotoxicity by Silymarin: biochemistry, histopathology, and lethality. *Pharmaceutical Research, 8*(2): 273-277, 1991.

Tavazza, M., Lucioli, A., Ancora, G., & Benvenuto, E. DNA cloning of artichoke mottled crinkle virus RNA and localization and sequencing of the goat protein gene. *Plant Mol Biol. 13*(6): 685-692, 1989.

ASARABACCA

Bian, R.L., et al. Antianaphylactic components of Asarum forbsii Maxin. *Pharmaceutica Sinica, 25*(11): 824-829, 1990.

Gracza, L. Constituents of Asaraum europeum L. Communication No. 18, Dynamics of the synthesis of flavonoids. *Acta Pharamceutica Hungarica, 61*(2): 86-90, 1991.

Tarada, S., et al. Antiallergic substance from Asarum sagittarioides and synthesis of some analogues. *Chemical and Pharmaceutical Bulletin, 36*(6): 2437-2442, 1987.

Wang, D.Q. & Huang, S.H. Medicinal plants of Asarum in Anhui Province. *Journal of Chinese Materiamedica, 14*(4): 198-200, 253, 1989.

ASHWAGANDHA

Al-Hindawi, M.K., Al-Deen, I.H., Nabi, M.H., & Ismail, M.A. Anti-inflammatory activity of some Iraqi plants using intact rats. *Journal of Ethnopharmacology, 26*(2): 163-168, 1989.

Asthana, R. & Raina, M.K. Pharmacology of *Withania somnifera* (linn) dunal—a review. *Indian Drugs, 26*(5): 199-205, 1989.

Atal, C.K. & Schwarting, A.E. Investigation of amino acids in the berries of *Withania somnifera* Dunal, *Curr. Science, 29*: 22, 1960.

Begum, V.H. & Sadique, J. Long term effect of herbal drug *Withania somnifera* on adjuvant induced arthritis in rats. *Indian Journal of Experimental Biology, 26*(11): 877-882, 1988.

Begum, V.H. & Sadique, J. Effect of *Withania somnifera* on glycosaminoglycan synthesis in carrageenin-induced air pouch granuloma. *Biochemical Medicine and Metabolic Biology, 38*(3): 272-277, 1987.

Bhattacharya, S.K., Goel, R.K., Kaur, R., & Ghosal, S. Antistress activity of sitonindosides VII and VIII, new acylsterylglucosides from *Withania somnifera. Phytotherapy Research, 1*(1): 32-37, 1987.

Brekhman, I.I. Panax ginseng. *Med. Sci Serv.*, 4, 1967, pp. 17-26.

Brekhman, I.I. & Dardymov, I.V. New substances of plant origin which increase non-specific resistance. *Ann. Rev. Pharamacol.*, 9: 419-430, 1969.

Chandra, V., Singh, A., & Kapoor, L.D. Studies on alkaloid-bearing plants. I. *Withania somnifera* dunal. *Indian Drugs Pharm. Ind.*, September-October, 1, 1970.

Elsakka, M., Grigorescu, E., Stanescu, U., & Dorneanu, V. New data referring to chemistry in *Withania somnifera* species. *Revista Medico-Chirurgicala a Societatii de Medici Si Naturalisti Din Iasi, 94*(2): 385-387, 1990.

Elsakka, M., Pavelescu, M., & Grigorescu, E. *Withania somnifera*, a plant with a great therapeutical future. *Revista Medico-Chirurgicala a Societatii de Medici Si Naturalisti Din Iasi, 93*(2): 349-350, 1989.

Ghosal, S., et al. Immunomodulatory and CNS effects of sitoindosides IX and X, two new glycowithanolides from *Withania somnifera. Phytotherapy Research, 3*(5): 201-206, 1989.

Kapoor, L.D. *CRC Handbook of Ayurvedic Medicinal Plants*. CRC Press, Boca Raton, FL, 1990.

Kulkarni, R.R., et al. Treatment of osteoarthritis with a herbomineral formulation: a double-blind, placebo-controlled, cross-over study. *Journal of Ethnopharmacology, 33*(1-2): 91-95, 1991.

Kupchan, S.M., et al. *Journal American Chemistry Society, 87*: 5805, 1965.

Kuppurajan, K., et al. Effect of Ashwagandha (*Withania somnifera* dunal) on the process of ageing in human volunteers.

Singh, N., et al. *Withania somnifera* (Ashwagandha), a rejuvenating herbal drug which enhances survival during stress (an adaptogen). *International Journal Crude Drug Research, 20*(1): 29-35, 1982.

Singh, N. et al. Prevention of urethan-induced lung adenomas by *Withania somnifera* (L.) dunal in albino mice. *International Journal Crude Drug Research, 24*(2): 90-100, 1986.

ASTRAGALUS

Chang, C.Y., Hou, Y.D., & Xu, F.M. Effect of *Astragalus membranaceus* on enhancement of mouse natural killer cell activity. *Chung-kuo I Hsueh K'o Hsueh Yuan Hsueh Pao, 4*(4): 231-234, 1983.

Chu, D-T, Wong W. L. & Mavligit, G. M. Immunotherapy with Chinese medicinal herbs I. Immune restoration of local xenogeneic graft-versus-host reaction in cancer patients by fractionated *Astragalus membranaceous* in vitro. *Journal of Clinical and Laboratory Immunology, 25*:119, 1988.

Chu, D-T, et al. Immunotherapy with Chinese medicinal herbs. II. Reversal of cyclophosphamide-induced immune suppression by administration of fractionated *Astragalus membranaceous* in vivo. *Journal of Clinical and Laboratory Immunology, 25*:125-129, 1988.

Chu, D.T., Wong, W.L. & Mavligit, G.M. Immunotherapy with Chinese medicinal herbs I. immune restoration of local xenogeneic graft-versus-host react cancer patients by fractionated *Astragalus membranaceous* in vitro. *Journal Clin Lab Immunol*, 25(3):119-123, 1988.

Hou, Y., Ma, G.L., Wu, S.H., Li, Y.Y., & Li, H.T. Effect of radix astragali seu hedysari on the interferon system. *Chin Med J*, 94(1): 35-40, 1981.

Li, Y.Y., Liu, X.Y., Shi, L.Y., Li, Y.X., & Hou, Y.D. Induction characteristic of lymphoblastoid interferon. *Chung-kuo I Hsueh K'o Hsueh Yuan Hsueh Pao*, 2: 250-252, 1980.

Peng, J., Wu, S., Zhang, L, Hou, Y., & Colby, B. Inhibitory effects of interferon and its combination with antiviral drugs on adenovirus multiplication. *Chung-kuo I Hsueh K'o Hsueh Yuan Hsueh Pao*, 6(2): 116-119, 1984.

BARBERRY

Amann, M., Nagakura, N., & Zank, M.H. Purification and properties of (S)-tetrahydroprotoberberine oxidase from suspension-cultured cells of *Berberis wilsoniae*. *European Journal of Biochemistry*, 175(1): 17-25, 1988.

Dong, H. Effects of storage time on the berberine content in *Berberis amurensis* Rupr. *Chinese Materia Medica*, 12(9): 19-20, 62, 1987.

Gupta, R.S. & Dixit, V.P. Testicular cell population dynamics following palmitine hydroxide treatment in male dogs. *Journal of Ethnopharmacology*, 25(2): 151-157, 1989.

Morales, M.A., et al. Effects of 7-0-demthylisothalicberine, a bisbenzylisoquinoline alkaloid of *Berberis chilensis* on electrical activity of frog cardiac pacemaker cells. *General Pharmacology*, 20(5): 621-625, 1989.

BEARBERRY

Borkowski, B. Diuretic action of several flavone drugs. *Planta Medica*, 8: 95-104, 1960.

Graham, R.C.B. & Noble, R.L. Comparison of in vitro activity of various species of lithospermum and other plants to inactive gonadotrophin. *Endocrinology*, 56: 239-, 1955.

Jahodar, L., Jilek, P., Patkova, M., & Dvorakova, V. Antimicrobial action of arbutin and the extract from the leaves of *arctostaphylos uva-ursi* in vitro. *Cesk Farm*, 34(5): 174-178, 1985.

Kubo, M., Ito, M., Nakata, H., & Matsuda, H. Pharmacological studies on leaf of Arctostaphylos uva-ursi (L.) Spreng. I. Combined effect of 50% methanol extract from Arctostaphylos uva-ursi. *Journal of the Pharmacological Society of Japan*, 110(1): 59-67, 1990.

Leslie, G.B. A pharmacometric evaluation of nine bio-strath herbal remedies. *Medita*, 8(10): 3-19, 1978.

Matsuda, H., Nakata, H., Tanaka, T., & Kubo, M. Pharmacological studies on leaf of Arctostaphylos uva-ursi (L.) Spreng. II. Combined effect of arbutin and prednisolone or dexamethazone on immuno-inflammation. *Journal of the Pharmacological Society of Japan*, 110(1): 68-76, 1990.

Matsuda, H., Tanaka, T., & Kubo, M. Pharmacological studies on leaf of Arctostaphylos uva-ursi (L.) Spreng. III. Combined effect of arbutin and indomethacin on immuno-inflammation. *Journal of the Pharmacological Society of Japan*, 111(4-5): 253-254, 1991.

May, G. & Willuhn, G. Antiviral activity of aqueous extracts from medicinal plants in tissue cultures. *Arzneim-Forsch*, 28(1): 1-7, 1978.

Namba, T., Tsunezuka, M., Bae, K.H., & Hattori, M. Studies on dental caries prevention by traditional Chinese medicines Part I. Screening of crude drugs for antibacterial action against streptococcus mutans. *Shoyakugaku Zasshi*, 35(4): 295-302, 1981.

Namba, T., *et al.* Studies on dental caries prevention by traditional Chinese medicines (Part IV) Screening of crude drugs for anti-plaque action and effects of artemisia capillaris spikes on adherence of streptococcus mutans to smooth surfaces and synthesis of glucan. *Shoyakugaku Zasshi*, 38(3): 253-263, 1984.

Racz, G., Fazakas, B. & Rac-Kotilla, E. Trichomonacidal and anthelmintic activity in Roumanian folkloric plants. (Abstract). *Planta Medica*, 39: 257A-, 1980.

Schaufelberger, D. & Hostettmann, K. On the molluscicidal activity of tannin containing plants. *Planta Med.*, 48(2): 105-107, 1983.

Swanson-Flatt, S.K., Day, C., Bailey, C.J., & Flatt, P.R. Evaluation of traditional plant treatments for diabetes: studies in streptozotocin diabetic mice. *Acta Diabetologica Latina*, 26(1): 51-55, 1989.

Ueki, H., Kaibara, M., Sakagawa, M., & Hayashi, S. Antitumor activity of plant constituents. I. *Yakugaku Zasshi*, 81: 1641-1644, 1961.

BEE POLLEN

Iarosh, A.A., Macheret, E.L., Iarosh, A.A., & Zapadniuk, B.V. Changes in the immunological reactivity of patients with disseminated sclerosis treated by prednisolone and the preparation Proper-Myll. *Vrachebnoe Delo*, Feb(2): 83086, 1990.

Koshte, V.L., Kagen, S.L., & Aalberse, R.C. Cross-reactivity of IgE antibodies to caddia fly with arthropoda and mollusca. *Journal of Allergy and Clinical Immunology*, 84(2): 174-183, 1989.

Koslik, S. Possible utilization of the favorable effects of bee pollen in patients with chronic renal insufficiency. *Vnitrni Lakarstvi*, 33(8): 633-640, 1987.

Lin, F.L., Vaughan, T.R., Vandewalker, M.L., & Weber, R.W. Hypereosinophilia, neurologic, and gastrointestinal symptoms after bee-pollen ingestion. *Journal of Allergy and Clinical Immunology*, 83(4): 793-796, 1989.

Liu, X. & Li, L. Morphological observation of effect of bee pollen on intercellular lipofuscin in NIH mice. *Journal of Chinese Materiamedica*, 15(9): 561-563, 578, 1990.

Ludianskii, E.A. The use of apiotherapy and radon baths in treating syringomyelia. *Zhurnal Nevropatologii i Paikhiartrii Imani*, 91(3): 102-103, 1991.

Pham-Dalegua, M.H., Etievant, P., & Masson, C. Molecular parameters involved in bee-plant relationships: a biological and chemical approach. *Biochimie*, 69(607): 661-670, 1987.

Profet, M. The function of allergy: immunological defense against toxins. *Quarterly Review of Biology*, 66(1): 23-62, 1991.

Qian, B., Zang, X., & Liu, X. Effects of bee pollen on lipid peroxides and immune response in aging and malnourished mice. *Journal of Chinese Materiamedica*, 15(5): 301-303, 319, 1990.

Sabbah, A., Le Dauphin, C., & Haulin, M.G. Comparative study of ELISA and RIA technics for the detection of specific IpG4. *Allergie et Immunologie*, 20(6): 232-235, 1988.

Wai, J., Cao, S., Liang, N., & Du, Y. Chemical components of bee's pollen from buckwheat (agopyrum esculentum Moench). *Journal of Chinese Materiamedica*, 15(5): 293-295, 318, 1990.

Wojcicki, J., et al. Effect of pollen extract on the development of experimental atherosclerosis in rabbits. *Atherosclerosis, 62*: 39-45, 1986.

BELLADONNA

Fukui, A., Nakashima, Y., & Kimura, K. Anesthetic management of a patient with Sjogren's syndrome associated with an allergic reaction to various antiphlogistics and sedatives. *Japanese Journal of Anesthesiology, 40*(4): 627-631, 1991.

Kushnir, S., et al. Nucleo-cytoplasmic incompatibility in hybrid plants possessing an Atropa genome and a Nicotinaa plastome. *Molecular and General Genetica, 225*(2): 225-230, 1991.

Liu, W.Z. Construction and application of atropine flow-through sensor in flow injection analysis. *Pharmaceutica Sinica, 25*(6): 451-456, 1990.

Terashchenko, A.V., et al. The conservative treatment of children with vesico-urateral reflux. *Uroligiia i Nefrologiia,* Mar-Apr(2): 24-28, 1991.

BETEL NUT

Frawer, L.J. The effect of betel nut on human performance. *Papua New Guinea Medical Journal, 33*(2): 143-145, 1990.

Khrime, R.D., Mehra, Y.N., Mann, S.B., Mehta, S.K., & Chakrabort, R.N. Effect of instant preparation of betel nut (pan masala) on the oral mucosa of albino rats. *Indian Journal of Medical Research, 94*: 119-124, 1991.

Nair, U.J, et al. Effect of lime composition on the formation of reactive oxygen species from areca nut extract in vitro. *Carcinogenesis, 11*(2): 2145-2148, 1990.

Parkin, D.M., et al. Liver cancer in Thailand. I. A case-control study of hepatocellular carcinoma. *International Journal of Cancer, 48*(3): 323-328, 1991.

Rajendran, R., Anil, S., & Vijayakumar, T. A rare human model for oncogenesis. *Singapore Dental Journal, 13*(1): 49-52, 1988.

Srivatanakul, P., et al. Liver cancer in Thailand. II. A case-control study of hepatocellular carcinoma. *International Journal of Cancer, 48*(3): 329-332, 1991.

Stich, H.F., Mathrew, B., Sanakranarayanan, R., & Nair, M.K. Remission of oral precancerous lesions of tobacco/areca nut chewers following administration of beta-carotene or vitamin A, and maintenance of the protective effect. *Cancer Detection and Prevention, 15*(2): 93-98, 1991.

Sundovita, K., et al. Areca-nut toxicity in cultured human buccal epithelial cells. *Iarc Scientific Publications,* (105): 281-285, 1991.

BILBERRY

Bonati, A. How and why should we standardize phytopharmaceutical drugs for clinical validation? *Journal of Ethnopharmacology, 32*(1-3): 195-197, 1991.

Cristoni, A. & Magistretti, M.J. Antiulcer and healing activity of *Vaccinium myretillus* nathocyanosides. *Farmaco, Edizione Pratica, 42*(2): 29-43, 1987.

Fokina, G.I., Frolova, T.V., Roikhel, V.M., & Pogodina, V.V. Experimental phytotherapy of tick-borne encephalilitial. *Voprosy Virusologil, 36*(1): 18-21, 1991.

Magistretti, M.J., Conti, M., & Cristoni, A. Antiulcer activity of an anthocyanidin from *Vaccinium myrtillus. Arzneimeittel-Forschung, 38*(5): 686-690, 1988.

Morazzoni, P., Livig, S., Scilingo, A., & Malandrino, S. *Vaccinium myrtillus* anthocyanosides pharmacokinetica in rats. *Arzneimeittel-Forschung, 41*(2): 128-131, 1991.

Saija, A., et al. Effect of *Vaccinium myrtillus* anthocyanins on triiodothyronine transport into brain in the rat. *Pharmacological Research, 22*(Suppl 3): 59-60, 1990.

BLACK WALNUT

Galay, F.D., et al. Black walnut (*Juglans nigra*) toxicosis: a model for equine laminitis. *Journal of Comparative Pathology, 104*(3): 313-326, 1991.

Galay, F.D., et al. Gamma scintigraphic analysis of the distribution of perfusion of blood in the equine foot during black walnut (*Juglans nigra*)-induced laminitis. *American Journal of Veterinary Research, 51*(4): 688-695, 1990.

Galay, F.D., Beasley, V.R., Schaeffer, D., & Davis, L.E. Effect of an aqueous extract of black walnut (*Juglans nigra*) on isolated equine digital vessels. *American Journal of Veterinary Research, 51*(1): 83-88, 1990.

Minnick, P.D., Brown, C.M., Braselton, W.E., Meerdink. G.L., & Slanker, M.R. The induction of equine laminitis with an aqueous extract of the heartwood of black walnut (*Juglans nigra*). *Veterinary and Human Toxicology, 29*(3): 230-233, 1987.

Uhlinger, C. Black walnut toxicosis in ten horses. *Journal of the American Veterinary Medical Association, 195*(3): 343-344, 1989.

BLOODROOT

Eisenberg, A.D., Young, D.A., Fan-Hsu, J., & Spitz, L.M. Interactions of sanguinarine and zinc on oral streptococci and Actinomyces species. *Caries Research, 25*(3): 185-190, 1991.

Harper, D.S., Mueller, L.J., Fine, J.B., Gordon, J., & Laster, L.L. Clinical efficacy of a dentrifice and oral rinse containing sanguinaria extract and zinc chloride during 6 months of use. *Journal of Periodontology, 61*(6): 352-358, 1990.

Harper, D.S., Mueller, L.J., Fine, J.B., Gordon, J., & Laster, L.L. Effect of 6 months use of a dentrifice and oral rinse containing sanguinaria extract and zinc chloride upon the microflora of the dental plaque and oral soft tissues. *Journal of Periodontology, 61*(6): 359-363, 1990.

Kuftinec, M.M., Mueller-Joseph, L.J, & Kpozyk, R.A. Sanguinaria toothpaste and oral rinse regimen clinical efficacy in short- and long-term trials. *Journal Clinical Dentistry, 1*(3): 59-66, 1989.

Walker, C. Effects of sanguinarine and Sanguinaria extract and microbiota associated with the oral cavity. *Journal Canadian Dental Association, 56*(7 Suppl): 13-30, 1990.

Walker, C. New perspectives on Sanguinaria clinicals: individual toothpaste and oral rinse testing. *Journal Canadian Dental Association, 56*(7 Suppl): 19-30, 1990.

BONESET

Beier, R.C. & Norman, J.O. The toxic factor in white snakeroot: identity, analysis and prevention. *Veterinary and Human Toxicology, 32*(Suppl): 81-89, 1990.

Beier, R.C., Norman, J.O., Irvin, T.R., & Witzel, D.A. Microsomal activation of constituents of white snakeroot (Eupatorium rugosum Houtt) to form toxic products. *American Journal of Veterinary Research, 19*(1): 583=585, 1987.

Chan, M.Y., Zhao, X.L., & Ogle, C.W. A comparative study on the hepatic toxicity and metabolism of *Crotaleria assemica* and *Eupatorium* species. *American Journal of Chinese Medicine, 17*(3-4): 165-170, 1989.

Elema, E.T., Schripaema, J., & Malingra, T.M. Flavones and flavonol glycosides from *Eupatorium cannabrinum* L. *Pharmaceutisch Weekbled, 11*(5): 161-164, 1989.

Hendrika, H., Huizing, H.J., & Bruins, A.P. Ammonium positive-ion and hydroxide negative-ion chemical ionization gas chromatography-mass spectrometry for the identification of pyrrolizidine alkaloids in *Eupatorium rotundifolium* L. var. ovatum. *Journal of Chromatography,* 128(2): 352-356, 1989.

Hirschmann, G.S. & Ferro, E. Indigo from Eupatorium leave. *Journal of Ethnopharmacology,* 26(1): 93-94, 1989.

Lexa, A., et al. Choleretic and hapatoprotective properties of *Eupatorium cannabinum* in the rat. *Planta Medica,* 55(2): 127-132, 1989.

Woerdenbag, H.J., et al. Induction of DNA damage in Ehrlich ascites tumor cells by exposure to eupatoriopicrin. *Biochemical Pharmacology,* 39(11): 2279-2293, 1989.

Woerdenbag, H.J., Lemstra, W., Malingre, T.M., & Konings, A.W. Enhanced pyostatic activity of the sesquiterpene lactone eupotoriopicrin by glutathione depletion. *British Journal of Cancer,* 59(1): 69-75, 1989.

Zhao, X.L., Chan, M.Y., Kumana, C.R., & Ogle, C.W. A comparative study on the pyrrolizidine alkaloid content and the pattern of hepatic pyrrolic metabolite accumulation in mice given extracts of Eupatorium plant species, *Crotaleria assemica* and an Indian herbal mixture. *American Journal of Chinese Medicine,* 15(1-2), 59-67, 1987.

Zhao, X.L., Chan, M.Y., & Ogle, C.W. The identification of pyrrolizidine alkaloid-containing plants—a study on 20 herbs of the Compositae family. *American Journal of Chinese Medicine,* 17(1-2): 71-79, 1989.

BORAGE

Bunce, O.R., Abou, C.L., & Cla, S.H. Ciacosanoid synthesis and ornithine decarboxylase activity in mammary tumors of rats fed varying levels and types of N-3 and/or N-G fatty acids. *Prostaglandins Leukotrienes and Essential Fatty Acids,* 11(2): 105-113, 1990.

Chapkin, R.S. & Carmichael, S.L. Effects of dietary n-3 and N-G polyunsaturated fatty acids on macrophage phospholipid classes and subclasses. *Lipids,* 25(12): 27-34, 1990.

Chapkin, R.S., Somers, S.D., & Erickson, K.L. Dietary manipulation of macrophage phospholipid classes: selective increase of dihomogammalinolenic acid. *Lipids,* 23(8): 766-770, 1988.

Chapkin, R.S., Somers, S.D., Schumacher, L., & Erickson, K.L. Fatty acid composition of macrophage phospholipids in mice fed fish or borage oil. *Lipids,* 23(1): 390-393, 1988.

Engler, M.M., Karanian, J.W., & Salem, N. Jr. Ethanol inhalation and dietary n-G, n-3, and n-0 fatty acids in the rat: effect on platelet and aortic fatty acid composition. *Alcoholism, Clinical and Experimental Research,* 15(3): 103, 1991.

Fletcher, M.P. & Ziboh, V.A. Effects of dietary supplementation with sicosapentaenoic acid or gamma-linolenic acid on neutrophil phospholipid fatty acid composition and activation responses. *Inflammation,* 11(5): 585-597, 1990.

Griffiths, G., Stobart, A.K., & Stymne, S. Delta 6- and delta 12-desaturase activities and phosphetidic acid formation in microsomal preparations from the developing cotyledons of common borage (*Borago officinalis*). *Biochemical Journal,* 252(3): 611-617, 1988.

Miller, C.C. & Ziboh, V.A. Gammalinolenic acid-enriched diet alters cutaneous eicosenoids. *Biochemical and Biophysical Research Communications,* 151(3): 967-971, 1989.

Miller, C.C., Ziboh, V.A., Wong, T., & Fletcher, M.P. Dietary supplementation with oils rich in (n-3_ and (n-S) fatty acids influences in vivo levels of epidermal lipoxygenase products in guinea pigs. *Journal of Nutrition,* 120(1): 36-44, 1990.

Mills, D.E., Mah, M., Ward, R.P., Morris, B.L., & Flores, J.S. Alteration of baroreflex control of forearm vascular resistance by dietary fatty acids. *American Journal of Physiology,* 259(6, pt. 2): R1151-1171, 1990.

Mills, D.D., Prkachin, K.M., Harvey, K.A., & Ward, R.P. Dietary fatty acid supplementation alters stress reactivity and performance in man. *Journal of Human Hypertension,* 3(2): 111-116, 1989.

Ormarod, L.D., Garad, A., Abelson, M.B., & Kenyon, K.R. Effects of altering the sicosanoid precursor pool on neovascularization and inflammation in the alkali-burned rabbit cornea. *American Journal of Pathology,* 137(5): 1213-1252, 1990.

Pullman-Mocar, S., et al. Alteration of the cellular fatty acid profile and the production of eicosanoids in human monocytes by gamma-linolenic acid. *Arthritis and Rheumatism,* 33(10): 1526-1533, 1990.

Tate, G., et al. Suppression of acute and chronic inflammation by dietary gamma linolenic acid. *Journal of Rheumatology,* 16(6): 729-731, 1989.

Ulmann, L., et al. Effects of age and dietary essential fatty acids on desaturase activities and on fatty acid composition of liver microsomal phospholipids of adult rats. *Lipids,* 28(2): 127-133, 1991.

BOSWELLIN

11th European Congress of Rheumatology, Vol. 5/8-2. Supplement issue, 1987.

Atal, C.K., et al. Salai guggal a new non-steroidal anti-inflammatory agent and its probable mode of action. Recent Advances in Mediators of Inflammation and Anti-inflammatory Agents, Symposium, Nov. 2-4, 1984.

Atal, C.K., Sharma, M.L., Kaul, A., Khajuria, & Singh, G.B. Effect of "Salai guggal"—a new non-steroidal anti-inflammatory drug on leucocyte migration. XV Annual Conference of IPS,

Bhargava, G.G., Negi, J.S., & Ghua, S.R.D. Studies on the chemical components of salai gum. *Indian Forester,* 104: 174-181, 1978.

Gupta, V.N., Yadav, D.S., Jain, M.P., & Atal, C.K. Chemistry and pharmacology of gum resin of *Boswellia serrata* (salai guggal). *Indian Drugs,* 24(5): 221-231, 1987.

Kar, A. & Menon, M.K. Analgesic effect of the gum resin of *Boswellia serrata* roxb. *Life Sciences,* 8(1): 1023-1028, 1969.

Kulkarni, R.R., et al. Treatment of osteoarthritis with a herbomineral formulation: a double-blind, placebo-controlled, cross-over study. *Journal of Ethnopharmacology,* 33(1-2): 91-95, 1991.

Menon, M.K. & Kar, A. Analgesic and psychopharmacological effects of the gum resin of *Boswellia serrata.* *Planta Medica,* 19: 332-341, 1971.

Pardhy, R.S. & Bhattacharya, S.C. Tetracyclic triterpene acids from the resin of *Boswellia serrata* Roxb. *Indian Journal Chem.,* 16(B): 174-175, 1978.

Pardhy, R.S. & Bhattacharya, S.C. Boswellic acid, acetyl-boswellic acid and 11-keta-boswellia acid four pentacyclic triterpene acids from the resin of *Boswellia serrata* Roxb. *Indian Journal Chem.,* 16(B): 176-178, 1978.

Recent advances in mediators of inflammatory agents R.R.I. (Council of Scientific and Industrial Research) Symposium, 1984.

Reddy, G.K., Chandrakasan, G., & Dhar, S.C. Studies on the metabolism of glycosaminoglycalls under the influence of new herbal anti-inflammatory agents. *Biochemical Pharmacology*, 38(2): 3527-3534, 1989.

Safayhi, H., Mack, T., & Ammon, H.P.T. Protection by boswellic acids against galactosamine/endotoxin-induced hepatitis in mice. *Biochemical Pharmacology*, 41(10): 1537-1537, 1991.

Singh, G.B.. & Atal, C.K. Pharmacology of an extract of salai guggul ex-*Boswellia serrata*, a new non-steroidal anti-inflammatory agent. *Agents Actions*, 18: 407-412, 1986.

Zutshi, U., Rao, P.G., Kaur, S., Singh, G.B., & Atal, C.K. Mechanism of cholesterol lowering effect of Salai guggal ex-*Boswelli serrat*. XII Annual Conference of IPS,

BUCKTHORN

Goel, R.K., Des Gupta, G., Ram, S.N., & Panday, V.B. Antiulcerogenic and anti-inflammatory effects of emodin, isolated from *Rhamnus triquerta* wall. *Indian Journal of Experimental Biology*, 29(3): 80-83, 1991.

Goel, R.K., Panday, V.B., Dwivedi, S.P., & Rao, Y.U. Anti-inflammatory and anti-ulcer effects of kaempferol, a flavone, isolated from *Rhamnus procumbens*. *Indian Journal of Experimental Biology*, 26(2): 121-124, 1988.

Gundidza, M. & Sibanda, M. Antimicrobial activities of ziziphus abyssinica and berchemia discolor. *Central African Journal of Medicine*, 37(3): 80-83, 1991.

Ito, Y., Oka, H, & Lee, Y.W. Improved high-speed counter-current chromatograph with three multilayer coils connected in series. II. Separation of various biological samples with a semi-preparative column. *Journal of Chromatography*, 198(1): 169-179, 1991.

Jiao, P.Y. & Fang, J.N. Studies in isolation, purification and structure of NLC-A of *Rhamnus heterophyllus*. *Pharmaceutica Sinica*, 21(5): 353-356, 1989.

Kostrikova, E.V. Experimental study of wound-healing effect of the preparation "Askol" (artificial sea buckthorn oil). *Ortopediia Travmatologita i Protezirovanie*, Jan(1): 32-36, 1989.

Martinez de Villarreal, L., et al. Effects of toxin T-511 from the Karwinskia humboldtiana (buckthorn) plant upon mouse embryos explanted at 11 days. *Toxicon*, 28(1): 119-152, 1990.

Nunes, P.H., Marinho, L.C., Nunes, M.L., & Scares, E.D. Antipyretic activity of an aqueous extract of Zizyphus joazeiro Mart. *Brazilian Journal of Medical and Biological Research*, 20(5): 599-601, 1987.

Terencio, M.C., Sanz, M.J., & Paya, M. A hypotensive procyanidin-glycoside from *Rhamnus lycioides* ssp. lycioides. *Journal or Ethnopharmacology*, 30(2): 205-214, 1990.

Turner, N.J. & Habda, R.J. Contemporary use of bark for medicine by two Salishan native elders of southeast Vancouver Island, Canada. *Journal of Ethnopharmacology*, 29(1): 59-72, 1990.

vand den Dikkenberg, M.I. & Holtkamp, B.M. Alder buckthorn poisoning in horses. *Tijdschrift voor Diergenesskunda*, 112(6): 310-311, 1987.

Zhang, T.Y., Lee, Y.W., Fang, O.C., Xiao, R., & Ito, Y. Preliminary applications of cross-axis synchronous flow-through coil planted centrifuge for large-scale preparative counter-current chromatography. *Journal of Chromatography*, 151: 185-193, 1988.

BUPLEURUM

Amagaya, S., et al. Effects of Shosaikoto, an Oriental herbal medicinal mixture, on age-induced amnesia in rats. *Journal of Ethnopharmacology*, 28:349-356, 1990).

Amagaya, S. & Ogihara Y. Effects of Shosaikoto, an Oriental herbal medicinal mixture, on restraint-stressed mice, *Journal of Ethnopharmacology*, 28:357, 1990.

BURDOCK

Proctor, V.A. & Cunningham, F.E. The chemistry of lysozyme and its use as a food preservative and pharmaceutical. *Critical Review Food Science Nutrition*, 25(1): 359-395, 1988.

Smarda, J. Viroids: molecular infectious agents. *Acta Virologica*, 31(6): 505-521, 1987.

Swanston-Flatt, S.K., et al. Glycaemic affects of traditional European plant treatments for diabetes. Studies in normal and streptozotocin diabetic mice. *Diabetes Research*, 10(2): 69-73, 1989.

BUTCHER'S BROOM

Cahn, J., Herold, M., & Sanault, B. Antiphlogistic and anti-inflammatory activity of F 191. Int. Symp. Non Steroidal Anti-inflammatory Drugs, Milano, 1964.

Cappelli, R., Nicora, M., & Di Perri, T. Use of extract of *Ruscus aculeatus* in vencus disease in the lower limbs. *Drugs under Experimental and Clinical Research*, 11(1): 277-293, 1988.

Capra, C. Studio farmacologico e tossicologico di componenti del *Ruscus aculeatus* L. *Fitoterapia*, 43:99, 1972.

Caujolle, F., Meriel, P., & Stanilas, E. Sur les propriétés pharmacologiques de *Ruscus aculeatus* L. *Ann. Pharm. Franc.*, 11:109, 1953.

Chabanon, R. Expérimentation du Proctolog dans les hémorroides et les fissures anales. *Gaz. Méd de France*, 83:3013, 1976.

Marcelon, G., Verbeuren, T.J., Lauressergues, H., & Vanhoutte, P.M. Effect of *Ruscus aculeatus* on isolated canine cutaneous veins. *Gen. Pharmac.*, 14:103, 1983.

Moscarella, C. Contribution à l'étude pharmacologique du *Ruscus aculeatus* L. (Fragon épineux). Thése de Pharmacie, Toulouse, 1953.

Weindorf, N. & Schultz-Ehrenburg, U. Controlled study of increasing venous tone in primary varicose veins by oral administration of *Ruscus aculeatus* and trimethylhespiridinchalconel. *Zeitschrift fur Haukrankhsiten*, 52(1): 28-38, 1987.

BUTTERCUP

Baker, V. et al. Dissociation of cellular proliferation and c-myo expression by buttercup extract. *American Journal of the Medical Sciences*, 299(5): 283-288, 1989.

Mares, D. Antimicrobial activity of protoanemonin, a lactone from ranunculaceous plants. *Mycopathologia*, 98(3): 133-140, 1987.

CASCARA SAGRADA

Borkje, B., Pederson, R., Lund, G.M., Enehaug, J.S., & Berstad, A. Effectiveness and acceptability of three bowel cleansing regimens. *Scandinavian Journal of Gastroenterology*, 26(2): 162-166, 1991.

de Witte, P. & Lemli, L. The metabolism of anthranoid laxatives. *Hepato-gastrocenterology*, 37(6): 601-605, 1990.

Phillip, J., Schubert, G.E., Thiel, A., & Wolters, U. Preparation for colonoscopy using Golytely—a sure method? Comparative histological and clinical study between lavage and saline laxatives. *Medizinische Klinik*, 85(7): 115-120, 1990.

CAYENNE

Basha, K.M., et al. Capsaicin: A therapeutic option for painful diabetic neuropathy, *Henry Ford Hospital Medical Journal, 39*(2): 138-140, 1991.

De, A.K.Y & Ghosh, J.J. Short and long-term effects of capsaicin on the pulmonary anti-oxidant enzyme system in rats. *Phytotherapy Research, 3*(5), 1989.

Govindarajan, V.S. & Sathyanarayana, M.N. Capsicum—production, technology, chemistry and quality. Part V. Impact on physiology, pharmacology, nutrition, and metabolism; structure, pungency, pain, and desensitization sequences. *Critical Review Food Science Nutrition, 29*(6): 135-171, 1991.

Jancsó, N., Jancsó-Gábor, A., & Szolcsányi, J. Direct evidence for neurogenic inflammation and its prevention by denervation and by pretreatment with capsaicin. *Br. Journal Pharmacol., 31*:138, 1967.

Marabii, S., Ciabatti, P.G., Polli, G., Fusco, B.M., & Geppetti, P. Beneficial effects of intranasal applications of capsaicin in patients with vasomotor rhinitis. *European Archives of Oto-Rhino-laryngology, 218*(4): 181-184, 1991.

Rayner, H.C., Atkins, R.C. & Westerman, R.A. Relief of local stump pain by capsaicin cream. *The Lancet,* 1276-1277, 1989.

Teel, R.W. Effects of capsaicin on rat liver S9-mediated metabolism and DNA binding of aflatoxin. *Nutrition and Cancer, 15*(1): 27-32, 1991.

CHAMOMILE

Fokina, G.I., Frolova, T.V., Roikhel, V.M., & Pogodina, V.V. Experimental phytotherapy of tick-borne encephalitis. *Voprosy Virusologii, 36*(1): 18-21, 1991.

Glowania, H.J., Raulin, C., & Swoboda, M. Effect of chamomile on wound healing—a clinical double-blind study. *Zeitschrift fur Hautkrankheiten, 62*(17): 1262, 1267-1271, 1987.

Maiche, A.G., Grohn, P., & Maki-Hokkonen, H. Effect of chamomile cream and almond ointment on acute radiation skin reaction. *Acta Oncologica, 30*(3): 395-398, 1991.

Subiza, J., et al. Anaphylactic reaction after the ingestion of chamomile tea: a study of cross-reactivity with other composite pollens. *Journal of Allergy and Clinical Immunology, 81*(3): 353359, 1989.

Subiza, J., et al. Allergic conjunctivitis to chamomile tea. *Annals of Allergy, 55*(2): 127-132, 1990.

CHASTEBERRY

Belic, I., Bergant-Dolar, J., Stucin, D., & Stucin, M.A. Biologically active substance from *Vitex agnus-castus. Vestnick Sloven Kemi Drutva,* 5: 63, 1958.

Goerler, K., Dehlke, D., & Soicke, H. Iridoid derivatives from *Vitex agnus castus. Planta Medic, 50*(6): 530-531, 1985.

Gomaa, C.S., El-Moghazy, M.A., Halim, F.A., & El-Sayyad, A.E. Flavonoids, and iridoids from *Vitex agnus castus. Planta Medica, 33*: 277, 1978.

Haller, J. Animal experimentation with the Lipschutz technic on the activity of a phytohormone on gonadotropin function. *Geburtschilfe Frauenheilkund, 18*: 1347, 1958.

Hansel, R. & Winde, E. Constituents of the verbenaceae. 2. Agnuside, a new glycoside from vitex *agnus castus. L. Arzneimittel- Forschung, 9*: 180-190, 1959.

Jochle, W. Menses-inducing drugs. Their role in antique, medieval and renaissance gynaecology and birth control. *Contraception, 10*: 425, 1974.

Perrot, E. & Paris, R.R. *Les plantes medicinales, Part I.* Presses Universitaires De France, Paris, 1971.

Stewart, A. Gerard *agnus castus* in premenstrual tension. Available from Gerard House Ltd., Bournemouth, England, 1987.

Wollenweber, E. & Mann, K. Flavonols from the fruits of *Vitex agnus castus. Planta Medica, 48*: 126-127, 1983.

CHINESE CUCUMBER

Chao, Z. & Liu, J. Chemical constituents of the pericarp of Tricosanthes fosthornii Harmaj. *Journal of Chinese Materiamedica, 16*(2): 97-99, 127, 1991.

Ferrari, P., et al. *Toxicity and activity of purified trichosanthin.* 5(7): 865-870, 1991.

Lee-Huang, S., et al. TAP 29: an anti-human immunodeficiency virus protein from Trichosanthes kirilowii that is nontoxic to intact cells. *Proceedings of the National Academy of Sciences of the United States of America, 88*(15): 6570-6574, 1991.

McGrath, M.S., et al. GLQ 223: An inhibitor of human immuno deficiency virus replication in acutely and chemically infected cells of lymphocyte and mononuclear phagocyte lineage. *Proceedings of National Acadamy Science, 86*: 2844-2848, April 1989.

Schnittman, S.M., et al. The reservoir for HIV-1 in human peripheral blood is a T cell that maintains expression of CD4. *Science, 245*: 305-308, 1989.

Wang, Q.C., et al. Tricosanthin-monoclonal antibody cnojudate specifically cytotoxic to human hepatoma cells in vitro. *Cancer Research, 51*(3): 3353-3355, 1991.

CINCHONA

Abdulrahamn, S., et al. High-performance liquid chromatographic-mass spectrometric assay of high-value compounds for pharmaceutical use from plant cell tissue culture: Cinchona alkaloids. *Journal of Chromatography, 562*(1-2): 719-721, 1991.

Kirk, K. et al. Enhanced choline and Rb+ transport in human erythrocytes infected with the malaria parasite Plasmodium falciparum. *Biochemical Journal, 278*(Pt 2): 521-525, 1991.

Sabcharoen, A. et al. Rec cell and plasma concentrations of combined quinine-quindine and quinine in falciparum malaria. *Annals of Tropical Pediatrics, 11*(4): 315-324, 1991.

CINNAMON

Buch, J.G., Dikshit, R.K. , & Mansuri, S. Effect of certain volatile oils on ejaculated human spermatozoa. *Indian Journal Medical Research, 87*(4): 361-363, 1988.

Conner, D.E. & Beuchat, L.R. Effects of essential oils from plants on growth of food spoilage yeasts. *Journal Food Science, 49*(2): 429-434, 1984.

Fitzpatrick, F.K. Plant substances active against mycobacterium tuberculosis. *Antibiotic Chemother, 4*: 528-, 1954.

Gupta, M. Essential oils: A new source of bee repellents. *Chem India (London), 5*: 161-163, 1987.

Morozumi, S. A new antifungal agent in cinnamon. *Shinkin To Shinkinsho, 19*: 172-180, 1978.

Namba, T., et al. Studies on development of immunomodulating drugs (11) effect of Ayurvedic medicines on blastogenesis of lymphocytes from mice. *Shoyakugaku Zasshi, 43*(3): 250-255, 1989.

Noding, A., Stoa, K.F., & Nordal, A. Investigation of the estrogenic effect of extracts of Ceylon cinnamon. *Norsk Farm Selskap, 12*: 68-73, 1950.

Raharivelomanana, P.J., Terrom, G.P., Bianchini, J.P., & Coulanges, P. Study of the antimicrobial action of various oil extracts from madagascan plants. 11. The aluraceae. *Arch Institute Pasteur Madagascar*, 56(1): 261-271, 1989.

Sivaswamy, S.W., Balachandran, B., Balanehru, S., & Sivaramakrishnan, V.W. *Indian Journal Exp Biology*, 29(8): 730-737, 1991.

Sugaya, A., Tsuda, T., Sugaya, E., Usami, M., & Takamura, K. Local anaesthetic action of the Chinese medicine saiko-keishi-to. *Planta Medica*, 37: 274-276, 1979.

Sugaya, E., et al. Inhibitory effect of a mixture of herbal drugs (TJ-960, SK) on pentylenetetrazol-induced convulsions in el mice. *Epilepsy Research*, 2(5): 337-339, 1988.

Ungsurungsie, M. Paovalo, C., & Noonai, A. Mutagencity of extracts from Ceylon cinnamon in the rec assay. *Food Chem Toxicology*, 22(2): 109-112, 1984.

CITRUS

Clegg, R.J., Middleton, B., Bell, G.D., & White, D.A. Inhibition of hepatic cholesterol synthesis by monoterpenes administered in vivo. *Biochem Pharmacol*, 29: 2125-2127, 1980.

Elegbede, J., Elson, C. Tanner, M., Qureshi, A., & Gould, M. Regression of rat primary mammary tumors following dietary d-limonene. *Journal of the National Cancer Institute*, 76: 323-325, 1986.

Elson, C., Maltzman, T., Boston, J., Tanner, M., & Gould, M. Anti-carcinogenic activity of d-limonene during the initiation and promotion/progression stages of DMBA-induced rat mammary carcinogenesis. *Carcinogenesis*, 9: 331-332, 1988.

Evans, D., Miller, D., Jacobsen, K., & Bush, P. Modulation of immune responses in mice by d-limonene. *Journal of Toxicological and Environmental Health*, 20: 51-66, 1987.

Igimi, J., Hisatsugu, T., & Nishimura, M. The use of d-limonene preparation as a dissolving agent of gallstones. *Amer J Dig Dis*, 21:926-, 1976.

Maltzman, T., Tanner, M., Elson, C., & Gould, M. Anticarcinogenic activity of specific orange peel oil monoterpenes. *Federation Proceedings*, 45: 970, 1986.

Wattenberg, L. Inhibition of neoplasia by minor dietary components. *Cancer Research*, 43(supplement): 2448s-2453s, 1983.

CLOVES

Al-Khayat, M.A. & Blank, G. Phenolic spice components sporostatic to bacillus subtilis. *Journal Food Sci.*, 50(4): 971-980, 1985.

Buch, J.G., Dikshit, R.K., & Mansuri, S.M. Spermicidal effects of certain volatile oils on human spermatozoa in vitro. *Journal Androl.*, 6(2): Abstr-M41, 1985.

Buch, J.G., Dikshit, R.K., & Mansuri, S.M. Effect of certain volatile oils on ejaculated human spermatozoa. *Indian Journal Med. Res.*, 87(4): 361-363, 1988.

Burapanont, P., Siriwongpairat, P., & Leartskulpiriya, M. Preparation and evaluation of cough pills. *Undergraduate Special Project Report 1984*: 30pp-, 1984.

Caceres, A., Giron, L.M., Alvarado, S.R., & Torres, M.F. Screening of antimicrobial activity of plants popularly used in Guatemala for the treatment of dermatomucosal diseases. *Journal Ethnopharmacol.*, 20(3): 223-237, 1987.

Conner, D.E. & Beuchat, L.R. Effects of essential oils from plants on growth of food spoilage yeasts. *Journal Food Sci.*, 49(2): 429-434, 1984.

Dabral, P.K. & Sharma, R.K. Evaluation of the role of rumalaya and geriforte in chronic arthritis—A preliminary study. *Probe*, 22(2): 120-127, 1983.

Dhawan, B.N., Patnaik, G.K., Rastogi, R.P., Singh, K.K., & Tandon, J.S. Screening of Indian plants for biological activity, VI. *Indian Journal Exp. Biol.*, 15: 208-, 1977.

Giron, L.M., Aguilar, G.A., Caceres, A., Arroyo, G.L. Anticandidal activity of plants used for the treatment of vaginitis in Guatemala and clinical trial of solanum nigrescens preparation. *Journal Ethnopharmacol.*, 22(3): 307-313, 1988.

Guerin, J.C. & Reveillere, H.P. Antifungal activity of plant extracts used in therapy. II. Study of 40 plant extracts against 9 fungi species. *Ann. Pharm. Fr.*, 43(1): 77-81, 1985.

Gupta, M. Essential oils: A new source of bee repellents. *Chem. Ind. (London) 1987*, 5: 161-163, 1987.

Iwasaki, M., Ishikawa, C., Maesuura, Y., Ohhashi, E., & Harada, R. Antioxidants of allspice and clove. *Sagami Joshi Daigaku Kiyo*, 48: 1-6, 1984.

Janssen, A.M., Chin, N.L.J., Scheffer, J.J.C., & Baerheim-Svendsen, A. Screening for antimicrobial activity of some essential oils by the agar overlay technique. *Pharm. Weekbl (Sci. Ed.)*, 8(6): 289-292, 1986.

Janzen, D.H., Juster, H.B., & Bell, E.A. Toxicity of secondary compounds to the seed-eating larvae of the bruchid beetle callosobruchus maculatus. *Phytochemistry*, 16: 223-227, 1977.

Kramer, R.E. Antioxidants in clove. *Journal American Oil Chem. Soc.*, 62(1): 111-113, 1985.

Maruzzella, J.C., Scrandis, D., Scrandis, J.B., & Grabon, G. Action of odoriferous organic chemicals and essential oils on wood-destroying fungi. *Plant Dis. Rept.*, 44: 789-, 1960.

Namba, T., Tsunezuka, M., Bae, K.H., & Hattori, M. Studies on dental caries prevention by traditional Chinese medicines Part I. Screening of crude drugs for antibacterial action against streptococcus mutans. *Shoyakugaku Zasshi*, 35(4): 295-302, 1981.

Namba, T., et al. Studies on dental caries prevention by traditional Chinese medicines (Part IV) screening of crude drugs for anti-plaque action and effects of artemisia capillaris spikes on adherence of streptococcus mutans to smooth surfaces and synthesis of glucan. *Shoyakugaku Zasshi*, 38(3): 253-263, 1984.

Nes, I.F., Skjelkvale, R., Olsvik, O., & Berdal, B.P. The effect of natural spices and oleoresins on lactobacillus plantarum and staphylococcus aureus. *Microb. Assoc. Interact. Food Proc. Int. Iums-ICFMH Sym. 12th 1983 1984*: 435-440, 1984.

Reiter, M. & Brandt, W. Relaxant effects on tracheal and ileal smooth muscles of the guinea pig. *Arzneim-Forsch*, 35(1): 408-414, 1985.

Saito, Y., Kimura, Y., & Sakamoto, T. The antioxidant effects of petroleum ether soluble and insoluble fractions from spices. *Eiyo To Shokuryo Vryo*, 29: 505-510, 1976.

Salem, F.S. Evaluation of clove oil and some of its derivatives as trichomonacidal agents. *Journal Drug Res (Egypt)*, 12: 115-119, 1980.

Seetharam, K.A. & Pasricha, J.S. Condiments and contact dermatitis of the finger-tips. *Indian Journal Dermatol. Venereol Leprol*, 53(6): 325-328, 1987.

Shukia, B., Khanna, N.K., & Godhwani, J.L. Effect of brahmi rasayan on the central nervous system. *Journal Ethnopharmacol.*, 21(1): 65-74, 1987.

Singh, B.G. & Agrawal, S.C. Efficacy of odoriferous organic compounds on the growth of keratinophilic fungi. *Curr. Sci.*, 57(14): 807-809, 1988.

Soytong, K., Rakvidhvasastra, V., Sommartya, T. Effect of some medicinal plants on growth of fungi and potential in plant disease control. *Abstr. 11th Conference of Science and Technology, Thailand. Kasetsart University, Bangkok, Thailand. 24th-26th October, 1985*: 361-, 1985.

Srivastava, K.C. & Justesen, U. Inhibition of platelet aggregation and reduced formation of thromboxane and lipoxygenase products in platelets by oil of cloves. *Prostaglandins Leukotrienes Med.*, 29(1): 11-18, 1987.

Stager, R. New studies on the effect of plant odors of ants. *Mitt. Schweiz. Antomol. Ges.*, 15: S67-, 1933.

Takechi, M. & Tanaka, Y. Purification and characterization of antiviral substance from the bud of syzygium aromatica. *Planta Med.*, 42: 69-74, 1981.

To-A-Nun, C., Sommart, T., & Rakvidhyasastra, V. Effect of some medicinal plants and spices on growth of aspergillus. *Abstr. 11th Conference of Science and Technology, Thailand. Kasetsart University, Bangkok, Thailand. 24th-26th October, 1985*: 364-365, 1985.

Tu, H.Y. Pharmaceuticals for peptic ulcer. *Patent-Japan Kokai Tokkyo Koho-79 76, 815*: 3pp-, 1979.

Ungsurungsie, M., Suthienkul, O., & Paovalo, C. Mutagenicity screening of popular Thai spices. *Food Chem. Toxicol.*, 20: 527-530, 1982.

Urata, M. Antitrichophyton agents containing natural phytoncides. *Patent-Japan Kokai Tokkyo Koho-63 30, 324*: 4pp-, 1988.

Wagner, H., Wierer, M., & Bauer, R. Screening of essential oils and phenolic compounds for in vitro- inhibition of prostaglandin biosynthesis. *Planta Med. 1986*, 6: 549-B, 1986.

Watanabe, F., Nozaka, T., Tadaki, S.I., & Morimoto, I. Desmutagenicity of clove extracts on TRP-P-2-induced mutagenesis in salmonella typhimurium TA 98. *Shoyakugaku Zasshi*, 43(4): 324-330, 1989.

Wesley-Hadzija, B. & Bohing, P. Influences of some essential oils on the central nervous system of fish. *Ann. Pharm. Fr.*, 14: 283-, 1956.

COLTSFOOT

Fu, J.X. Measurement of MEFV in 66 cases of asthma in the convalescent stage and after treatment with Chinese herbs. *Chinese Journal of Modern Developments in Traditional Medicine*, 9(11): 658-659, 644, 1989.

Li, Y.P. & Wang, Y.M. Evaluation of tussilagone: a cardiovascular-respiratory stimulant isolated from Chinese herbal medicine. *General Pharmacology*, 19(2): 261-263, 1988.

Wang, C.d. Chemical studies of flower buds of *Tussilago farfara* L. *Yao Hsueh Pao*, 24(12): 913-916, 1989.

COMFREY

Awang, D.V.C. Comfrey. *Canadian Pharmacology Journal*, 120: 110-104, 1987.

Awang, D.V.C. Comfrey update. *HerbalGram*, 25: 20-23, 1991.

Gafar, M., Dumiktriu, H., Dumitriu, S., & Guti, L. Apiphytotherapetic original preparations in the treatment of chronic marginal parodontopathies. A clinical and microbiological study. *Revista de Chirugie, Oncologie, Radiologie, Orl, Oftalmologie, Stomatolgie, Seriia*, 36(2): 91-98, 1989.

Huizing, H.J., Gadella, T.W., & Kliphuis, E. Chemotoaxonomical investigations of the *Symphatum officinale* polyploid complex and *S. asperum* (Boraginaceac): The Pyrrolizidine alkaloids. *Plant Systematics and Evolution*, 140: 279-292, 1982.

Mattocks, A.R. Toxicity of Pyrrolizidine alkaloids, *Nature*, 217: 724, 1968.

Smith, L.W. & Culvenor, C.C.J. The alkaloids of *Symphatum x uplandicum* (Russian Comfrey). *Journal Natural Products*, 44: 129-152, 1981.

ECHINACEA

Anonymous. *Journal of the National Cancer Institute*, 81(2): 162-164, 1989.

Bauer, R., Jurcic, K., Puhlmann, J., & Wagner, H. Immunological in vivo examinations of echinacea extracts. *Arzneim-Forsch*, 38(2): 276-281, 1988.

Coeugniet, E.G. & Elek, E. Immunomodulation with *Viscum album* and *Echinacea purpurea* extracts. *Onkologie*, 10(3): 27-33, 1987.

Hartwell, J.L. Plants used against cancer. A survey. *Lloydia*, 32: 247-296, 1969; 33: 97-194; 288-392, 1970.

Hewett, A.C. *Echinacea purpurea, echinacea angustifolia, echafolta. Dental Rev.*, 20: 1218-1230, 1906.

Kabelik, J. The echinacea: Possibly an important medicinal plant? *Ziva*, 13(1): 4-5, 1965.

Lersch, C., et al. Stimulation of the immune response in outpatients with hepatocellular carcinomas by low doses of cyclophosphamide (LDCY), echinacea purpurea extracts (Échinacin) and thymostimulin. *Archiv fur Geschwulstforschung*, 60(5): 379-383, 1990.

Luettig, B., et al. Macrophage activation by the polysaccharide arabinogalactan isolated from plant cell cultures of *Echinacea purpurea*. *Journal of the National Cancer Institute*, 81(9): 669-675, 1989.

Roesler, J., et al. Application of purified polysaccharides from cell cultures of the plant *Echinacea purpurea* to mice mediates protection against systemic infections with Listeria monocytogenes and Candida albicans. *International Journal of Immunopharmacology*, 19(1): 27-37, 1991.

Schumacher, A. & Friedberg, K.D. The effect of *Echinacea angustifolia* on non-specific cellular immunity in the mouse. *Arzneim-Forschung*, 41(2): 141-147, 1991.

Stimpel, M., Proksch, A., Wagner, H., & Lohmann-Matthes, M.L. Macrophage activation and induction of macrophage cytotoxicity by purified polysaccharide fractions from the plant echinacea purpurea. *Inf Immun*, 46(3): 845-849, 1984.

Tragni, et al. Anti-inflammatory activity of *Echinacea angustifolia* fractions separated on the basis of molecular weight. *Pharmacological Research Communications, Suppl 5*: 87-90, 1988.

Tubaro, A., et al. Anti-inflammatory activity of a polysaccharidic fraction of *Echinacea angustifolia*. *Journal of Pharmacy and Pharmacology*, 39(7): 567-569, 1987.

Voaden, D.J. & Jacobson, M. Tumor inhibitors. 3. Identification and synthesis of an oncolytic hydrocarbon from American coneflower roots. *J Med Chem*, 15: 619-, 1972.

Wacker, A. & Hilbig, W. Virus-inhibition by *Echinacea purpurea*. *Planta Medica*, 33: 89-, 1978.

Wagner, H., et al. Immunologically active polysaccharides from tissue cultures of *Echinacea purpurea*. Proc 34th Annual Congress on Medicinal Plant Research-Hamburg, Sept 22-27, 1986: -, 1986.

Wagner, H., Zenk, M.H., & Ott, H. Polysaccharides derived from echinacea plants as immunostimulants. Patent-Ger Offen-3, 541,945 : 10pp-, 1988.

ELDER
Shibuya, N., et al. A comparative study of bark lectins from three elderberry (*Sambucus*) species. *Journal of Biochemistry*, 105(6): 1099-1103, 1989.

EPHEDRA
Arch, J. R. S., Ainsworth, A. T., & Cawthorne, M. A. Thermogenic and anorectic effects of ephedrine and congener in mice and rats. *Life Sci.*, 30:1817, 1982.

Astrup, A., et al. Enhanced thermogenic responsiveness during chronic ephedrine treatment in man. *Am. J. Clin. Nutr.*, 42:83, 1985.

Dulloo, A.G. & Miller, D.S. Obesity—a disorder of the sympathetic nervous system. *World Rev. Nutr. Diet*, 50:1, 1987.

Dulloo, A.G. and Miller, D.S. Reversal in obesity in the genetically obese fa/fa Zucker rat with an ephedrine/Methylzanthine (caffeine) thermogenic mixture. *J. Nutrition*, 117:383-389, 1987.

Jecuier, E. & Schultz, Y. New evidence for a thermogenic defect in human obesity. *Int. J. Obesity*, 9(Suppl 2):1, 1985.

Kalix, P. The pharmacology of psychoactive alkaloids from ephedra and catha. *Journal of Ethnopharmacology*, 32(1-3): 201-208, 1991.

Katzeff, H.L., et al. Metabolic studies in human obesity during overnutrition and undernutrition: Thermogenic and hormonal responses to norepinephrine. *Metabolism*, 35:166, 1988.

Lansberg, L., Saville, M.E., & Young J.B. Sympathoadrenal system and regulation of thermogenesis. *Am. J. Physio.*, 247:181, 1984.

Morgan, J.B., York, D.A., Wasilewska, A., et al. A study of the thermogenic responses to a meal and to a sympathomimetic drug (ephedrine) in relation to energy balance in man. *Br. J. Nutr.*, 47:21, 1982.

Pasquali, R., Cesari, M.P., Melchionda, N., Stefanini, C., Raitano, A., & Labo, G. Does ephedrine promote weight loss in low-energy-adapted obese women? *International Journal of Obesity*, 11:163-168, 1987.

Roth, R.P., et al. Nasal decongestant activity of pseudoephedrine. *Annals of OTOL*, 86, 1977.

EUCALYPTUS
Cai, Z., Li, X., & Xu, X. Determination of eucalyptole in eucalyptus oil by gas chromatography. *Journal of Chinese Materiamedica*, 15(5): 298-299, 319, 1990.

Hong, C.Z. & Shellock, F.G. Effects of a topically applied counterirritant (Eucalyptamint) on cutaneous blood flow and on skin and muscle temperatures. A placebo-controlled study. *American Journal of Physical Medicine and Rehabilitation*, 70(1): 29-33, 1991.

Swanston-Flatt, S.K., Day, C., Bailey, C.J., & Flatt, P.R. Traditional plant treatments for diabetes. Studies in normal and streptozotopin diabetic mice. *Diabetaolgoia*, 33(8): 162-164, 1990.

Takasaki, M., et al. Inhibitors of skin-tumor promotion. VIII. Inhibitory effects of euglobals and their related compounds on Epstein-Barr virus activation. *Chemical and Pharmaceutical Bulletin*, 38(10): 2737-2739, 1990.

FENNEL
Abdul-Ghani, A.S. & Amin, R. The vascular action of aqueous extracts of *Foeniculum vulgare* leaves. *Journal of Ethnopharmacology*, 24(2-3): 213-218, 1988.

FENUGREEK
Madar, Z., Abel, R., Samiah, S., & Arad, J. Glucose-lowering effect of fenugreek in non-insulin dependent diabetics. *European Journal of Clinical Nutrition*, 42(1): 51-54, 1988.

Sambaiah, K. & Srinivasan, K. Influence of spices and spice principles on hepatic mixed function oxygenase system in rats. *Indian Journal of Biochemistry and Biophysics*, 26(4): 254-258, 1989.

Sauvaire, Y., et al. Implication of steroid saponins and sapogenins in the hypocholesterolemic effect of fenugreek. *Lipids*, 26(3): 191-197, 1991.

Sharma, R.D., Raghuram, T.C., & Rao, N.S. Effect of fenugreek seeds on blood glucose and serum lipids in type I diabetes. *European Journal of Clinical Nutrition*, 44(4): 301-306, 1990.

FEVERFEW
Hayes, N.A. & Foreman, J.C. The activity of compounds extracted from feverfew on histamine release from rat mast cells. *Journal of Pharmacy and Pharmacology*, 39(6): 466-470, 1987.

Hobbs, C. The modern rediscovery of feverfew. *HerbalGram*, 20: 36, 1989.

Hobbs, C. Feverfew. *HerbalGram*, 20: 27-35, 1989.

Johnson, E.S., et al. Efficacy of feverfew as prophylactic treatment of migraine. *British Medical Journal*, 291: 569, 1985.

Johnson, E.S., et al. Investigation of possible genotoxic effects of feverfew in migraine patients. *Human Toxicology*, 6: 533, 1987.

Loesche, W., et al. Effects of an extract of feverfew (*Tanacetum parthenium*) on arachiodonic acid metabolism in human blood platelets. *Biomedica Biochmice Acta*, 47(10-11): S241-243, 1988.

Murphy, J.J., Heptinstall, S., & Mitchell, J.R. Randomized double-blind placebo-controlled trial of feverfew in migraine prevention. *Lancet*, 2(8604): 189-192, 1988.

Voyno-Yasenetskaya, T.A., et al. Effects of an extract of feverfew on endothelial cell integrity and on cAMP in rabbit perfused aorta. *J. Pharm. Pharmacol* 40: 501-501, 1988.

FO-TI
Chung Shan Medical College. *Kanpo no rinsho oyo* (The Clinical Applications of Chinese Herbal Formulas), Tokyo, I-chih-yao shuppansha / Dental and Pharmaceutical Press, 1976.

Hsu, H. *Chung yao tsai chih yen chiu* (Study of Chinese Medicinal Plants), Taipei: Hsin i-yao chu-pan-she / Modern Drug Press, 1980.

Huang, H.C., Chu, S.H., & Chao, P.D. Vasorelaxants from Chinese herbs, emodin and scoparoine, possess immunosuppressive properties. *European Journal of Pharmacology*, 198(2-3): 211-213, 1991.

Kam, J.K. Mutagenic activity of Ho Shao Wu (*Polygonum Multiflorum* thunb), *American Journal of Chinese Medicine*, 9(3):213-215, 1981.

Muddathir, A.K., et al. Anthelmintic properties of *Polygonum glabrum*. *Journal of Pharmacy and Pharmacology*, 39(4): 296-300, 1987.

Singh, B., Pandey, V.B., Joshi, V.K., & Gambhir, S.S. Anti-inflammatory studies on *Polygonum glabrum. Journal of Ethnopharmacology, 19*(3): 255-267, 1987.

FOXGLOVE

Marullax, P.D. Digitalis: is there a future for this classical ethnopharmacological remedy? *Journal of Ethnopharmacology, 32*(1-3): 111-115, 1991.

GARLIC

Amla, V., Verma, S.L., Sharma, T.R., Guptu, O.P., & Atal, C.K. Clinical study of *Allium cepa* Linn in patients of brochial asthma. *Ind. J. Pharmacol., 13*:63, 1980.

Barone, F. & Tansey, M. Isolation, purification, identification, synthesis, and kinetics of activity of the anticandidal component of *Allium sativum*, and a hypothesis for its mode of action. Mycologia *69*: 793-825, 1977.

Belman, S. Inhibition of soybean lipoxygenase by onion and garlic oil constituents. *Proc. Am. Assoc. Cancer Res., 26*: 131, 1985.

Belman, S. Onion and garlic oils and tumour promotion. *Carcinogenesis, 4*: 1063-1065, 1983.

Bilyk, A., Cooper, P., & Sapers, G. Varietal differences in distribution of quercetin and kaempferol in onion (*Allium cepa*) tissue. *Journal of Agricultural Food Chemistry, 32*: 274-285, 1984.

Bordia, A. & Verma, S. Effect of garlic feeding on regression of experimental atherosclerosis in rabbits. *Artery, 7*: 428-436, 1980.

Bordia, A., et al. The effect of active principle of garlic and onion on blood lipids and experimental atherosclerosis in rabbits and their comparison with clofibrate. *Journal of the Association of Physicians of India, 25*: 509-521, 1977.

Chi, M. Effects of garlic products in lipid metabolism in cholesterol-fed rats. *Proceedings of the Society for Experimental Biology and Medicine, 171*: 174-178, 1982.

Dabas, Y., Rao, V., Saxena, O., & Sharma, V. Efficacy of therapy against infectious genital tract disorders in bovine. *Indian Journal of Animal Science, 53*: 81-89, 1983.

Fenwich, G.. & Hanley, A. The genus *Allium*-Part 2. *CRC Critical Reviews in Food Science and Nutrition, 22*: 273-341, 1985.

Srivastiva. K.C. Effect of onion and ginger consumption on platelet thromboxane production in humans. *Prostaglandins, Leukotrienes and Essential Fatty Acids, 35*:183-185, 1989.

Subrahmanyan, V., Sreenivasamurthy, V., & Krishnamurthy, S.M. The effect of garlic on certain intestinal bacteria. *Food Science, 7*: 223-230, 1958.

Vanderhoek, J.Y. Inhibition of fatty acid oxygenases by onion and garlic oils. *Biochem. Pharmacol., 29*: 3169-3173, 1980.

Vanderhoek, J.Y., Makheia, A.N., & Bailey, J.M. Inhibition of fatty acid oxygenases by onion and garlic oils: Evidence for the mechanism by which these oils inhibit platelet aggregation. *Biochemical Pharmacology, 29*:3169-3173, 1980.

Wagner, H., Wierer, M., & Fessler, B. Effects of garlic constituents on arachidonate metabolism. *Planta Medica, 53*, 1987.

Yamada, Y. & Azuma, K. Evaluation of the in vitro antifungal activity of allicin. *Antimicrobial Agents and Chemotherapy, 11*: 743-749, 1977.

GENTIAN

Schaufelberger, D. & Hostettmann, K. Chemistry and pharmacology of *Gentiana lactea. Planta Medica, 54*(3): 219-221, 1988.

Yuan, Z.Z. & Feng, J.C. Observations on the treatment of systemic lupuc erythematous with a Gentiana macrophylla complex table and a minimal dose of prednisone. *Journal of Modern Developments in Traditional Medicine, 9*(3): 156-157, 133-134, 1989.

GINGER

Fischer-Rasmussen, W., Kjaer, S.K., Dahl, C., & Asping, U. Ginger treatment of hyperemesis gravidarum. *European Journal of Obstetrics, Gynecology, and Reproductive Biology, 38*(1): 19-24, 1991.

Srivastiva. K.C. Effect of onion and ginger consumption on platelet thromboxane production in humans. *Prostaglandins, Leukotrienes and Essential Fatty Acids, 35*:183-185, 1989.

Vane, J.R. Nature, 231:232, 1971.

Yamahara, J., *et al.*, The anti-ulcer effect in rats of ginger constituents. *Journal of Ethnopharmacology, 23*:299-304, 1988.

GINKGO

Barth, S.A., Inselmann, G., Engemann, R., & Heidermann, H.T. Influences of *Ginkgo biloba* on cyclosporin A induced lipid peroxidation in human liver microsomes in comparison to vitamin E, glutathione and N-acetylcysteine.

Braquet, P. & Hosford, D. Ethnopharmacology and the development of natural PAF antagonists a therapeutic agents. *Journal of Ethnopharmacology, 32*(1-3): 135-139, 1991.

Chung, K. F., et al. Effect of a ginkgolide mixture (BN 52063) in antagonizing skin and platelet responses to platelet activating factor in man. *The Lancet*, January 31, 1987.

Massoni, G., Piovella, C., & Fratti, L. Effects microcirculatoires de la *Ginkgo biloba* chez les personnes agées. *Gioren. Geront., 20*:444, 1972.

Peter, H. Vasoactivity of *Ginkgo biloba* preparation. 4th Conf. Hung. Ther. Invert. Pharmacol. Soc. Pharmacol. Hung. (Edited by Dumbovitch, B.), 177, 1968.

Rai, G.S., Shovlin, C., & Wesnes, K.A. A double-blind, placebo controlled study of *Ginkgo biloba* extract ("tanakan") in elderly outpatients with mild to moderate memory impairment. *Current Medical Research and Opinion, 12*(6): 350-355, 1991.

Sikora, R., et al. *Ginkgo biloba* extract in the therapy of erectile dysfunction. *Journal of Urology, 141*:188A, 1989.

Warot, D., et al. Comparative effects of *Ginkgo biloba* extracts on psychomotor performances and memory in healthy subjects. *Therapie, 46*(1): 33-36, 1991.

GINSENGS

The drug that builds Russians. *New Scientist*, August 21, 1980.

Bohn, B., Nebe, C.T., & Birr, C. Flow-cytometric studies with *Eleutherococcus senticosus* extracts as an immunomodulatory agent. *Arzneimittel-Forschung, 37*(10): 1193-1196, 1987.

Domashenko, O.N. & Sotnik, I.P. Evaluation of the cationic-lysomal test in patients with pneumonia against a background of therapy. *Laboratornoe Delo*, (5): 15-17, 1989.

Dörling, E. Do ginsenosides influence performance? *Notabene Medici, 10*(5):241-246, 1980.

Elden, H. R. Ginsenosides—new uses for an old root. *Drug and Cosmetic Industry*, pp. 36-40, April 1990.

Forgo, I. & Schimert, G. The duration of effect of the standardized Ginseng extract G115® in healthy competitive athletes. *Notabene Medici*, 15(9):636-640, 1985.

Forgo, I. On the question of influencing the performance of sportsmen. *Aerztliche Praxis*, 33(44):1784-1786, 1981.

Kim, H., Jang, C., & Lee, M. Antinarcotic effects of the standardized ginseng extract G115 on morphine. *Planta Medica*, 56:158, 1990.

McCaleb, R. Ginseng conference report. *Herbalgram*, No. 16, pp. 8-12, Spring 1988.

Itoh, T., Zang, Y. F., Murai, S., & Saito, H. Effects of *Panax ginseng* on the vertical and horizontal motor activities and on brain monoamine-related substances in mice. *Planta Medica*, 55:429, 1989.

Takaku, T., Kameda, K., Matsuura, Y., Sekiya, K., & Okuda, H. Studies on insulin-like substances in Korean red ginseng. *Planta Medica*, 56:27, 1990.

GOLDENSEAL

Boyd, L.J. The pharmacology of the homeopathic drugs. *J. Amer Inst Homeopathy*, 21: 312-323, 1920.

D'Amico, M.L. Investigation of the presence of substances having antibiotic action in higher plants. *Fitoterapia*, 21: 77-, 1950.

Hay, G. & Willuhn, G. Antiviral activity of aqueous extracts from medicinal plants in tissue cultures. *Drug Res*, 28(1): 1-7, 1978.

GOTU KOLA

Arpaia, M.R., et al. Effects of *Centella asiatica* extract on mucopolysaccharide metabolism in subjects with varicose veins. *International Journal of Clinical Pharmacology Research*, 10(4): 229-233, 1990.

Baltina, L.A., et al. Synthesis and antiphlogistic activity of protected glycopeptides of glycyrrhizic acid. *Pharm. Chem. J.*, 226:460-462, 1989.

Belcaro, G.V., Grimaldi, R., & Guidi, G. Improvement of capillary permeability in patients with venous hypertension after treatment with TTFCA. *Angiology*, 41(7): 588, 1990.

Belcaro, G.V., Rulo, A., & Grimaldi, R. Capillary filtration and ankle edema in patients with venous hypertension treated with TTFCA. *Angiology*, 41(1): 12-18, 1990.

Finney, R.S.H., Somers, C.F., & Wilkinson, J.H. Pharmacological properties of glycyrrhetinic acid—a new anti-inflammatory drug. *J. Pharm. Pharmacol.*, 10:687, 1958.

Fujita, H., Sakurai, T., Yoshida, M., & Toyoshima, S. Anti-inflammatory effects of glycyrrhizinic acid. *Oyo Yakuri*, 19:481-484, 1980.

Gijon, J. R. & Murcia, C. R. Estudio farmacologico comparativo de la actividad anti-inflammatoria local del acido glicirretinico con la de la cortisona. *An. Real Acad. Farm.*, 26:5, 1960.

Grimaldi, R., et al. Pharamcokinetics of the total triterpenic fraction of *Centella asiatica* after single and multiple administration to healthy volunteers. A new assay for asiatic acid. *Journal of Ethnopharmacology*, 28(2): 235-241, 1990.

Maquart, F.X., et al. Stimulation of collagen synthesis in fibroblast cultures by a triterpene extracted from *Centella asiatica. Connective Tissue Research*, 24(2): 107-120, 1990.

Montecchio, G.P., et al. Centella Asiatica Triterpenic Fraction (CATTF) reduces the number of circulating endothelial cells in subjects with post phlebitic syndrome. *Haematologica*, 76(3): 256-259, 1991.

Pointel, J.P., et al. Titrated extract of *Centella asiatica* (TECA) in the treatment of venous insufficiency of the lower limbs. *Angiology*, 38(1 Pt 1): 46-50, 1987.

Sugishita, E., Amagaya, S., & Ogihara, Y. Studies on the combination of glycyrrhizae radix in shakuyakukanzo-to. *J. Pharmacobio Dyn*, 7:427-435, 1984.

GREEN TEA

Ali, M., Afzal, M., Gubler, C.J., and Burka, J.F. A potent thromboxane formation inhibitor in green tea leaves. *Prostaglandins Leukotrienes and Essential Fatty Acids*, 40(4): 281-283, 1990.

Anonymous, Tea-totaling mice gain cancer protection. *Science News*, August 31, 1991, p. 133.

Bokuchava, M., Skoveleva, N.I., and Sanderson, G.W. The biochemistry and technology of tea manufacture. *CRC Critical Reviews in Food Science and Nutrition*, 12(4): 303-370, 1980.

Conney, A.H. Induction of microsomal enzymes by foreign chemicals and carcinogenesis by polycyclic aromatic hydrocarbons. G.H.A. Clowes Memorial Lecture, *Cancer Research*, 42: 4875-4917, 1982.

Cooke, R. Studies: Green tea may prevent cancer. *Newsday*, August 27, 1991.

Demirer, T., Icli, F., Uzunalimoglu, O., and Kucuk, O. Diet and stomach cancer incidence. A case-control study in Turkey. *Cancer*, 65(10): 2344-2348, 1990.

Ding, L.A. Inhibition effect of epicatechin on phenobarbitol-induced proliferation precancerous liver cells. *Chinese Journal of Pathology*, 19(4): 261-263, 1990.

Guo, B.Y. and Wan, H.B. Rapid determination of caffeine in green tea by gas-liquid chromatography with nitrogen-phosphorous-selective detection. *Journal of Chromatography*, 505(2): 435-437, 1990.

Hara, Y., et al. Antitumor action of the green tea extract. *Proc. Annual Meeting Japanese Society Cancer Research*: 993, 1984.

Hattori, M., et al. Effect of tea polyphenols on glucan synthesis by glucosyltransferase from Streptococcus mutans. *Chemical and Pharmaceutical Bulletin*, 38(3): 717-720, 1990.

Higashi, A., et al. A case-control study of ulcerative colitis. *Japanese Journal of Hygiene*, 45(6): 1035-1043, 1991.

Huang, et al. Inhibition of the mutagenicity of bay-region diol-epoxides of polycyclic aromatic hydrocarbons by tannic acid, hydroxylated anthaquinones and hydroxylated cinnamic acid derivatives. *Carcinogenesis*, 6: 237-242, 1985.

Imanishi, H., et al. Tea tannin components modify the induction of sister-chromatic exchanges and chromosome aberrations in mutagen-treated cultured mammalian cells and mice. *Mutation Research*, 259(1): 79-87, 1991.

Kaiser, H.E. Cancer-promoting effects of phenols in tea. *Cancer*, 20: 614, 1967.

Kubota, K., et al. Effect of green tea on iron absorption in elderly patients with iron deficiency anemial. *Japanese Journal of Geriatrics*, 27(5): 555-558, 1990.

Kursanov, A.L., et al. Biological effects of tea tannins. *Biokhim Chain. Proizvod*, 6, 1950, p. 170.

Lee, H.H., et al. Epidemiologic characteristics and multiple risk factors of stomach cancer in Taiwan. *Anticancer Research*, 10(4): 875-881, 1990.

Li, Y, Yan, R.Q., Qin, G.Z., Qin, L.L., and Duan, X.X. Reliability of a short-term test for hepatocarcinogenesis induced by aflatoxin B1. *Iarc Scientific Publications*, (105): 431-433, 1991.

Liu, X.L. Genotoxicity of fried fish extract, MeIQ and inhibition by green tea antioxidant. *Chinese Journal of Oncology*, 12(3): 170-173, 1990.

Mgaloblishvili, E.K., in *Therapeutic Effects of the Green Tea Infusion*, Izdatelstvo Medgiz, Batumi, 1967, p. 23.

Mgaloblishvili, E.K. and Tsutsunava, A.I. Healthful properties of the green tea infusion. *Bulletin USSR Research Institute Tea Subtrop. Cult.*, 1(26): 64, 1971.

Morton, J. Further association of plant tannins and human cancer. *Q.J. Crude Drug Research*, 12: 1829, 1972.

Nomura, A.M., Kolonel, L.N., Hankin, J.H., and Yoshizawa, C.N. Dietary factors in cancer of the lower urinary tract. *International Journal of Cancer*, 48(2): 199-205, 1991.

Oguni, I., Nasu, K., and Nomua, T. Epidemiological and physiological studies on the antitumor activity of the fresh green tea leaf. *Proceeding of International Tea-Quality-Human Health Symposium*, Nov. 4-9, 1987. Hanzhou, China Abstracts p. 120.

Ruch, R.J., Cheng, S., and Klaunig, J.E. Prevention of cytotoxity and inhibition of intercellular communication by antioxidant catechins isolated from Chinese green tea. *Carcinogens*, 10(6), 1989, pp. 1003-1008.

Sagesaka-Mitane, Y., Miwa, M., and Okada, S. Platelet aggregation inhibitors in hot water extract of green tea. *Chemical and Pharmaceutical Bulletin*, 38(3): 7909-793, 1990.

Stagg, G.V. and Millin, D.J. The nutritional and therapeutic value of tea. *Journal Sci. Food Agric.*, 26, 1975, p. 1439.

Taramoto, K., et al. Neutron activation analysis of manganese contents in ordinary hospital meals. *Osaka City Medical Journal*, 36(1): 53-59, 1990.

Tewes, F.J., Koo, L.C., Meisgen, T.J., and Rylander, R. Lung cancer risk and mutagenicity of tea. *Environmental Research*, 52(1): 23-33, 1990.

Wang, H. and Wu, Y. Inhibitory effect of Chinese tea on N-nitrosation in vitro and in vivo. *Iarc Scientific Publications*, (105): 546-549, 1991.

Wang, W. and Chen, W.W. Antioxidative activity studies on the meaning of same original of herbal drug and food. *Chinese Journal of Modern Developments in Traditional Medicine*, 11(3): 159-161, 1991.

Wang, Z.Y., Agarwal, R., Bickers, D.R. and Mukhtar, H. Protection against ultraviolet B radiation-induced photocarcinogenesis in hairless mice by green tea polyphenols. *Carcinogens*, 12(8): 1527-1530, 1991.

Wang, Z.Y. et al. Antimutagenic activity of green tea polyphenols. *Mutation Research*, 223: 273-285, 1989.

Wang, Z.Y., Khan, W.A., Bickers, D.R. and Mukhtar, H. Protection against polycyclic aromatic hydrocarbon-induced skin tumor initiation in mice by green tea polyphenols. *Carcinogens*, 10(2): 411-415, 1989.

Wang, Z.Y., Mukul, D., Bickers, D.R. and Mukhtar, H. Interaction of epicatechins derived from green tea with rat hepatic cytochrome P-450. *Drug Metabolism and Disposition*, 16(1): 98-103, 1988.

Yamaguchi, Y, Hayashi, M., Yamazoe, H., and Kunitomo, M. Preventive effects of green tea extract on lipid abnormalities in serum, liver and aorta of mice fed a atherogenic diet. *Nippon Yakurigaku Zasshi*, 97(6): 329-337, 1991.

Yan, Y.S. Effect of Chinese green tea extracts on the human gastric carcinoma cell in vitro. *Chinese Journal of Preventive Medicine*, 24(2): 80-82, 1990.

Zhao, B.L., Li, X.J., He, R.G., Cheng, S.J., & Xin, W.J. Scavenging effect of extracts of green tea and natural antioxidants on active oxygen radicals. *Cell Biophysics*, 14(2): 175-185, 1989.

GUARANA

Bydlowski, S.P., Yunker, R.L., & Subbiah, M.T. A novel property of an aqueous guarana extract (*Paullinia cupana*): inhibition of platelet aggregation in vitro and in vivo. *Brazilian Journal of Medical and Biological Research*, 21(3): 535-538, 1988.

GUAR GUM

Miettinen, T.A. & Tarpila, S. Serum lipids and cholesterol metabolism during guar gum and plantago ovata and high fibre treatments. *Clinical Chimica Acta*, 183(3): 253-262, 1989.

Tonstad, S. Dietary supplementation in the treatment of hyperlipidemia. *Tidsskrift for den Norske Laegegorening*, 111(28): 3398-4000, 1991.

GUGGAL

Agarwal, R.C., et al. Clinical trial of gugulipid a—new hypolipidemic agent of plant origin in primary hyperlipidemia. *Indian Journal Med. Res.*: 626, 1986.

Bombardelli, E., et al. *Commiphora mukul* extracts: A reinvestigation on chemical constituents and biological activity. Unpublished Manuscript, Presented at the 32nd Annual Meeting of the American Society Pharmacognosy, Chicago, Illinois, July 1991.

Bordia, A. & Chuttani, S.K. Effect of gum guggulu on fibrinolysis and platelet adhesiveness in coronary heart disease. *Indian Journal Med. Res.*, 70: 992-996, 1979.

Bordia, A. & Bansal, H.C. Essential oil of garlic in prevention of atherosclerosis, *Lancet*, 2: 1491, 1973.

Bordia, A., et al. Effect of the essential oil (active principle) of garlic on serum cholesterol, plasma fibrinogen, whole blood, coagulation time and fibrinolytic activity in alimentary lipaemia, *Journal Assoc. Phys. India*, 22: 267, 1974.

Chopra, R.N., Chopra, I,C., Handa, K.L., & Kapur, L.D. *Indigenous Drugs of India*, 2nd. ed. Academic Publishers, Calcutta, 1958, reprint 1982.

Chopra, R.N., Chopra, I.C., & Verma, B.S. *Supplement to glossary of Indian medicinal plants*. Publication and Information Directorate (CSIR), New Delhi, 1969.

Conant, R. Gum guggul: a protective herb from India. *Let's Live*: 68. June 1991.

Das, D., Sharma, R.C., & Arora, R.B. Antihyperlipidaemic activity of fraction A of *Commiphora mukul* in monkeys. *Indian Journal Pharm.*, 5: 283, 1973.

DellaLoggia, R. Sosa, S., Tubaro, A., & Bombardelli, E. Anti-inflammatory activity of *Commiphora mukul* extracts. Unpublished Manuscript, Presented at the 32nd Annual Meeting of the American Society Pharmacognosy, Chicago, Illinois, July 1991.

Dev, S. A modern look at an age-old Ayurvedic drug—guggulu. *Science Age*: 13, July 1987.

Dhar, M.L., Dhar, M.M., Dhawan, B.N., Mehrotra, B.N., & Ray, C. Screening of Indian plants for biological activity. I, *Indian Journal Exp. Biology, 6*: 232, 1968.

Dwarakanath, C. & Satyavati, G.V. Research in some of the concepts of Ayurveda and application of modern chemistry and experimental pharmacology therefore. *Ayurveda Pradeepika, 1*: 69, 1970.

Gujral, M.L., Sareen, K., Tangri, K.K., Amma, M.K.P., & Roy, A.K. Anti-arthritic and anti-inflammatory activity of gum guggal (*Balsamodendron mukul* Hook). *Indian Journal Physiol. Pharmacol.,. 4*: 267, 1960.

Jain, R.C., Vyas, C.R., & Mahatma, O.P. Hypoglycemic action of onions and garlic, *Lancet, 2*: 1491, 1973.

Khanna, D.S., Agarwal, O.P., Gupta, S.K. & Arora, R.B. A biochemical approach to antiatherosclerotic action of *Commiphora mukul*: an Indian indigenous drug in Indian domestic pigs (*Sus scrofa*), *Indian Journal Med. Res., 57*: 900, 1969.

Malhotra, S.C., Ahuja, M.M.S., & Sundaram, K.R. Long term clinical studies on the hypolipidaemic effect of *Commiphora mukul* (Guggulu) and Clofibrate. *Indian Journal Med. Res., 65*(3): 390-395, 1977.

Menon, M.K. & Kar, A. Analgesic and psychopharmacological effects of the gum resin of *Boswellia serrata*, *Planta Medica, 19*: 333, 1971.

Mester, L., Mester, M., & Nityanand, S. Inhibition of platelet aggregation by "Guggulu" steroids. *Hippokrates Verlag GmgH, 37*: 367-369, 1979.

Nadharni, A.K. *Dr. K.M. Nadharni's Indian Materia Medica*, revised ed. Popular Book Deport, Bombay, 1954.

Patil, V.D., Nayak, U.R., & Dev, S. Chemistry of Ayurvedic crude drugs—1. Guggulu (resin from *Commiphora mukul*)—1: steroidal constituents.

Sastry, V.V.S. Experimental and clinical studies on the effect of the oleogum resin of *Commophora mukul* Engl. on thrombotic phenomena associated with hyperlipaemia (Snehavyapat), Thesis, D. Ay, M. Banaras Hindu University, Varanasi, 1967.

Satyavati, G.V., Dwarakanath, C., & Tripathi, S.N. Experimental studies on the hypocholesterolemic effect of *Commiphora mukul* Engl. (Guggul). *Indian Journal Med. Res., 57*(10): 1950-1962, 1969.

Satyavati, G.V. Effect of an indigenous drug on disorders of lipid metabolism with special reference to atherosclerosis and obesity (medaroga). Thesis, D. Ay. M. Banaras Hindu University, Varanasi, 1966.

Satyavati, G.V. Pathogenesis of atherosclerosis: an analogy between ancient and modern concepts.

Shankar, R. Herbal hope for the heart. *Sci. Exp. of Ind. Exp.*: 3, January 26, 1988.

Tripathi, S.N., Shastri, V.V.S., & Satyavati, G.V. (Achayra) Experimental and clinical studies on the effect Guggulu (*Commiphora mukul*) in hyperlipaemia and thrombosis. *Journal Res. Indian Med., 2*: 10, 1968.

Tripathi, Y.B., Malhotra, O.P., & Tripathi, S.N. Thyroid stimulating action of z-guggulsterone obtained from *Commiphora mukul*. *Planta Medica*: 22-24, February 1984.

HAWTHORN
Ammon, H.P.R. & Handel, M. Cratageus, toxicology and pharmacology, Part I. Toxicology. *Planta Med, 43*: 105-120, 1981.

Ammon, H.P.R. & Handel, M. Cratageus, toxicology and pharmacology, Part II. pharmacodynamics. *Planta Med, 43*: 313-322, 1981.

Ammon, H.P.R. & Handel, M. Cratageus, toxicology and pharmacology, Part III. pharmacodynamics and pharmacokinetics, *Planta Med, 43*: 209-239, 1981.

He, G. Effect of the prevention and treatment of atherosclerosis of a mixture of Hawthorn and Motherwort. *Journal of Modern Development in Traditional Medicine, 10*(6): 361, 326, 1990.

Hobbs, C. & Foster, S. Hawthorn, a literature review. *HerbalGram, 22*: 19-33, 1990.

Meier, B. Plant vs. synthetic medicines. *Schweiz Apothek-Zeit, 19*: 472-477, 1989.

Occhiuto, F., et al. Study comparing the cardiovascular activity of shoots, leaves and flowers of C. laevigata L. II. Effect of extracts and pure isolated active principles on the isolated rabbit heart. *Plantes Med. Phytoher, 20*: 52-63, 1986.

Zeylstra, H. Cratageus, *New Herbal Practitioner, 9*: 53-61, 1983.

HENNA
Sharma, V.K. Tuberculostatic activity of henna (*Lawsonia inermis Linn*). *Tubercle, 71*(4): 293-295, 1990.

HORSE CHESTNUT
Kunz, K., Schaffler, K., Biber, A., & Wauschkuhn, C.H. Bioavailability of beta-aescin after oral administration of two preparations containing aesculus extract to healthy volunteers.

Lehtole, T. & Huhtikengas, A. Radioimmunoassay of aescine, a mixture of triterpene glycosides. *Journal of Immunoassay, 11*(1): 17-30, 1990.

Magliulo, E., Carco, F. P., Gorini, S., & Barigazzi, G. M. Ricerche in vivo ed in vitro sull'azione antiflogistica dell'escina. *Arch. Sc. Med., 125*:207, 1968.

Manca, P. & Passarelli, E. Aspetti farmacologici dell'escina principio attivo dell'aesculus hyppocastanum. *Clin. Terap., 32*:297, 1965.

Siering, H. Die permeabilität von Zellmembranen, für lonen unter dem Einfluss von Aescin. *Arzneim. Forsch, 12*:376, 1962.

Senatore, F., Mscisz, A., Mrugasiewicz, K., & Gorecki, P. Steroidal constituents and anti-inflammatory activity of the horse chestnut bark. *Bollettino—Societa Italiana Biolgia Sperimentale, 65*(2): 137-141, 1989.

IPECAC
Hodgkinson, D.W., Jellett, L.B., & Ashby, R.H. A review of the management of oral drug overdose in the Accident and Emergency Department of the Royal Brisbane Hospital. *Archives of Emergency Medicine, 8*(1): 8-16, 1991.

Kornberg, A.E. & Dolgin, J. Pediatric ingestions: charcoal alone versus ipecac and charcoal. *Annals of Emergency Medicine, 20*(6): 648-651, 1991.

Tennebein, M., Wiseman, N., & Yatscoff, R.W. Gastronomy and whole bowel irritation in iron poisoning. *Pediatric Emergency Care, 7*(5): 286-288, 1991.

IVY
Elias, R., et al. Antimutagenic activity of some saponins isolated from *Calendula officinalis L., C. arvensis L.* and *Hedera helix L. Mutagenesis, 5*(4): 327-331, 1990.

Majester-Savornin, B., et al. Saponins of the ivy plant, *Hedera helix*, and their leishmanicidic activity. *Planta Medica*, 57(3): 260-262, 1991.

JUNIPER

Swanston-Flatt, S.K., Day, C., Bailey, C.J., & Flatt, P.R. Traditional plant treatments for diabetes. Studies in normal and streptozotopin diabetic mice. *Diabetaolgoia*, 33(8): 162-164, 1990.

KAVA

Cheng, D., et al. Identification by methane chemical ionization gas chromatography/mass spectrometry of the products obtained by steam distillation and aqueous acid extraction of commercial Piper methysticum. *Biomedical and Environmental Mass Spectrometry*, 17(5): 371-376, 1988.

Duffield, A.M., et al. Identification of some human urinary metabolites of the intoxicating beverage kava. *Journal of Chromatography*, 475: 273-81, 1989.

Duffield, P.H., Jamieson, D.D., & Duffield, A.M. Effect of aqueous and lipid-soluble extracts of kava on the conditioned avoidance response in rats. *Archives Internationales de Pharmacodynamie et de Therapie*, 301: 81-90, 1989.

Jamieson, D.D., Duffield, P.H., Cheng, D., & Duffield, A.M. Comparison of the central nervous system activity of the aqueous and lipid extract of kava. *Archives Internationales de Pharmacodynamie et de Therapie*, 301: 66-80, 1989.

Ruze, P. Kava-induced dermopathy: a niacin deficiency? *Lancet*, 335(8703): 1442-1445, 1990.

LAVENDER

Gamez, M.J., Jimenez, J., Navarro, C., & Zarzuelo, A. Study of the essential oil of *Lavandula dentata L. Pharmazie*, 45(1): 69-70, 1990.

Gamez, M.J., et al. Hypoglycemic activity in various species of the genus Lavandula. Part 1: *Lavandula stoeches L.* and *Lavandula multifida L. Pharmazie*, 42(10): 706-707, 1987.

Gamez, M.J., et al. Hypoglycemic activity n various species of the genus Lavandula. Part 2: *Lavandula dentata* and *Lavandula latifolia. Pharmazie*, 43(6): 441-442, 1988.

Shubine, L.P., Siurin, S.A., & Savchenko, V.M. Inhalations of essential oils in the combined treatment of patients with chronic bronchitis. *Vrachebnoe Delo*, (5): 66-67, 1990.

LEMONGRASS

da-Silva, V.A., et al. Nuerobehavioral study of the effect of beta-myrcene on rodents. *Brazilian Journal of Medical and Biological Research*, 24(8): 827-831, 1991.

Elson, C.E., et al. Impact of lemongrass oil, an essential oil, on serum cholesterol. *Lipids*, 24(8): 677-679, 1989.

Kauderer, B., Zamith, H., Paumgartten, F.J., & Speit, G. Evaluation of the mutagenicity of beta-myrcene in mammalian cells in vitro. *Environmental and Molecular Mutagenesis*, 18(1): 28-34, 1991.

Lorenzetti, B.B., et al. Myrcene mimics the peripheral analgesic activity of lemongrass tea. *Journal of Ethnopharmacology*, 34(1): 43-48, 1991.

Onawunmi, G.O. In vitro studies on the antibacterial activity of phenoxyethanol in combination with lemon grass oil. *Pharmazie*, 43(1): 42-44, 1988.

Rao, V.s., Menezes, A.M., & Viana, G.S. Effect of myrcene on nociceptiuon in mice. *Journal of Pharmacy and Pharmacology*, 42(12): 877-878, 1990.

LICORICE

Abe, N., Ebina, T., & Ishida, N. Interferon induction by glycyrrhizin and glycyrrhetinic acid in mice. *Microbiology and Immunology*, 26: 535, 1982.

Agarwal, R., Wang, Z.Y., & Mukhtar, H. Inhibition of mouse skin tumor-initiating activity of DMBA by chronic oral feeding of glycyrrhizin in drinking water. *Nutrition and Cancer*, 15(3-4): 187-193, 1991.

Baba, M. & Shigeta, S. Antiviral activity of glycyrrhizin against varicella-zoster virus in vitro. *Antiviral Research*, 7: 99-107, 1987.

Borst, J.G.G., ten Holt, S.P., de Vries, L.A., & Molhuysen, J.A. Synergistic action of liquorice and cortisone in Addison's and Simmonds's disease. *Lancet*, 1: 657-668, 1953.

Baker, M.E. & Fanestil, D.D. Licorice, computer-based analyses of dehydrogenase sequences, and the regulation of steroid and prostaglandin action. *Molecular and Cellular Endocrinology*, 78(1-2): C99-102, 1991.

Baltina, L.A., et al. Synthesis and antiphlogistic activity of protected glycopeptides of glycyrrhizic acid. *Pharm. Chem. J.*, 226:460-462, 1989.

Finney, R.S.H., Somers, C.F., & Wilkinson, J.H. Pharmacological properties of glycyrrhetinic acid—a new anti-inflammatory drug. *J. Pharm. Pharmacol.*, 10:687, 1958.

Fujisawa, K., Watanabe, Y., & Kimura, K. Therapeutic approach to chronic active hepatitis with glycyrrhizin. *Asian Medical Journal*, 23: 745-756, 1981.

Fujita, H., Sakurai, T., Yoshida, M., & Toyoshima, S. Anti-inflammatory effects of glycyrrhizinic acid. *Oyo Yakuri*, 19:481-484, 1980.

Gijon, J. R. & Murcia, C. R. Estudio farmacologico comparativo de la actividad anti-inflammatoria local del acido glicirretinico con la de la cortisona. *An. Real Acad. Farm.*, 26:5, 1960.

Hatano, T., et al. Phenolic constituents of licorice. IV. Correlation of phenolic constituents and licorice specimens from various sources and inhibitory effects of licorice extracts on xanthine oxidase and monoamine oxidase. *Journal of the Pharmaceutical Society of Japan*, 111(6): 311-321, 1991.

Kiso, Y., Tohkin, M., & Hikino, H. Assay method for anti-hepatotoxic activity using carbon tetrachloride induced cytotoxicity in primary cultured hepatocytes. *Planta Medica*, 49: 222-225, 1983.

Kitagawa, K., Nishino, H., & Iwashima, A. Inhibition of the specific binding of 12-0-tetradecacanoylphorbol-13-acetate to mouse epidermal membrane fractions by glycyrrhetic acid. *Oncology*, 43: 127-130, 1986.

Kraus, S.D. The anti-oestrogenic action of glycyrrhetic acid. *Experimental Medicine and Surgery*, 27: 411-420, 1969.

Segal, R., Pisanty, S., Wormser, R., Azaz, E., & Sela, M.N. Anticarcinogenic activity of liquorice and glycyrrhizin I: Inhibition of in vitro plaque formation by *Streptococcus mutans. Journal of Pharmaceutical Sciences*, 74: 79-81, 1985.

Sugishita, E., Amagaya, S., & Ogihara, Y. Studies on the combination of glycyrrhizae radix in shakuyakukanzo-to. *J. Pharmacobio Dyn*, 7: 427-435, 1984.

Tanaka, S., Kuwai, Y., & Tabata, M. Isolation of monoamine oxidase inhibitors from *Glycyrrhiza uralensis* roots and the structure-activity relationship. *Planta Medica*: 5-7, 1987.

Teelucksingh, S., et al. Potentiation of hydrocortisone activity in skin by Glycyrrhetinic acid. *The Lancet, 335*: 1060-1063, 1990.

LOBELIA

Sopranzi, N., De Feo, G., Mazzanti, G., & Braghiroli, L. The biological and electrophysiological parameters in the rat chronically treated with *Lobelia inflata L. Clinica Terapeutica, 137*(4): 265-268, 1991.

MADDER

Westerndorf, J., et al. The genotoxicity of lucidin, a natural component of *Rubia tinctorum L.*, and lucidinethylether, a component of ethanolic Rubia extracts. *Cell Biology and Toxicology, 4*(2): 225-239, 1988.

Poginsky, B. et al. Evaluation of DNA-binding activity of hydroxyanthraquinones occurring in *Rubia tinctorum L. Carcinogenesis, 12*(7): 1265-1271, 1991.

MAGNOLIA

Gui, J.F., Zhang, G.D., & Song, W.Z. Reversed phase ion-pair HPLC determination of quaternary ammonium alkaloids in the traditional Chinese drug Hou-po (*Magnolia officinalis*). *Pharmaceutica Sinica, 23*(6): 383-387, 1988.

Konoshima, T., et al. Studies on inhibitors of skin tumor promotion, IX. Neolignans from *Magnolia officinalis. Journal of Natural Products, 54*(3): 816-822, 1991.

Teng, C.M., et al. EDRF-release and Ca+(+)-channel blockade by magnolol, an antiplatelet agent isolated from Chinese herb Magnolia officinalis, in rat thoracic aorta. *Life Sciences, 47*(13): 1153-1161.

MANDRAKE

Beutner, K.R. & von Krogh, G. Current status of podophyllotoxin for the treatment of genital warts. *Seminars in Dermatology, 9*(2): 148-151, 1990.

Emboden, W. The sacred journey in dynastic Egypt: shamanistic trance in the context of the narcotic water lily and the mandrake. *Journal of Psychoactive Drugs, 21*(1): 61-75, 1989.

Larsen, A., Petersson, I., & Svensson, B. Podophyllum derivatives (CPH 82) compared with placebo in the treatment of rheumatoid arthritis. *British Journal of Rheumatology, 28*(2): 124-127, 1989.

MARIGOLD

Chemli, R., et al. *Calendula officinalis L.* Impact of saponins on toxicity, hemolytic effect, and anti-inflammatory activity. *Journal de Pharmacie de Belgique. 45*(1): 12-16, 1990.

Elias, R., et al. Antimutagenic activity of some saponins isolated from *Calendula officinalis L., C. arvensis L.* and *Hedera helix L. Mutagenesis, 5*(4): 327-331, 1990.

Krivenki, V.V., Potebnia, G.P., & Loiko, V.V. Experience in treating digestive organ diseases with medicinal plants. *Vrachebnoe Delo*, (3): 76-78, 1989.

Szakiel, A. & Kasprzyk, Z. Distribution of oleanolic acid glycosides in vacuoles and cell walls isolated from protoplasts and cells of *Calendula officinalis* leaves. *Steroids, 53*(3-5): 501-511, 1989.

MARSHMALLOW

Schultz, H. & Albroscheit, G. High-performance liquid chromatographic characterization of some medical plant extracts used in cosmetic formulas. *Journal of Chromatography, 442*: 353-361, 1988.

MATHAKÉ

Collier, W.A. & Van De Piji, L. The antibiotic action plants, especially the higher plants, with results from Indonesian plants. *Chron Nat, 105*: 8-, 1949.

Haddon, A.C. Reports of the Cambridge anthropological expedition to Torres Straits. Cambridge at the University Press, Cambridge England *Book 6*: 107-, 1908.

Huxtable, R.J. Herbs along the western Mexican-American border. *Proc West Pharmacol Soc, 26*: 185-191, 1983.

Quisumbing, E. Medicinal plants of the Philippines. JMC Press, Inc. Quezon City, Philippines, 1978.

Tiwari, A.K., Gode, J.D., & Dubey, G.P. Effect of *Terminalia arjuna* on lipid profiles of rabbits fed hypercholesterolemic diet. *International Journal Crude Drug Research, 28*(1): 43-47, 1990.

MATÉ

Anonymous, *Nutrition Today, 24*(6): 4, Nov.-Dec. 1989.

Acheson, K.J., Zahorska-Markiewicz, B., Pittet, P., Anantharaman, K., & Jequier, E. Caffeine and coffee: Their influence on metabolic rate and substrate utilization in normal weight and obese individuals. *American Journal Clin. Nutr., 33*: 989-997, 1980.

Astrup, A., Toubro, S., Cannon, S., Hein, P., Breum, L., & Madsen, J. Caffeine: A double-blind, placebo-controlled study of its thermogenic, metabolic, and cardiovascular effects in healthy volunteers. *American Journal Clin. Nutr., 51*: 759-767, 1990.

Bønaa, K., Arnesen, E., Thelle, D.S., & Førde, O.H. Coffee and cholesterol: Is it all in the brewing? The Tromsø study. *Br. Med. Journal, 297*: 1103-1104, 1988.

Bukowiecki, L.J., Lupien, J., Folléa, N., & Jahjah, L. Effects of sucrose, caffeine, and cola beverages on obesity, cold resistance, and adipose tissue cellularity. *American Journal Physiol., 244*: R500-507, 1983.

Cheraskin, E., Ringsdorf, W.M., Setyaadmadja, A.T.S.H., & Barrett, R.A. Effect of caffeine versus placebo supplementation on blood-glucose concentration. *Lancet, 2*: 1299-1300, 1967.

Dulloo, A.G., Geissler, G.A., Horton, T., Collins, A., & Miller, D.S. Normal caffeine consumption: Influence on thermogenic and daily energy expenditure in lean and postobese human volunteers. *American Journal Clin. Nutr., 49*: 44-50, 1989.

Fredholm, B.B. Gastrointestinal and metabolic effects of methylxanthines. In Dews, P. B., ed., *The methylxanthine beverages and foods: Chemistry, consumption, and health effects*. New York: A.R. Liss Press, 1984, pp. 331-354.

Jung, R.T., Shetty, P.S., James, W.P.T., Barrand, M.A., & Callingham, B.A. Caffeine: Its effect on catecholamines and metabolism in lean and obese subjects. *Clin. Sci., 60*: 527-535, 1981.

Malchow-Møller, A., Larsen, S., Hey H., Stokholm, K.H., Juhl, E., & Quaade, F. Ephedrine as an anorectic: The story of the "Elsinore pill." *International Journal Obes., 5*: 183-187, 1981.

Whitsett, T.L., Manion, C.V., & Christensen, H.D. Cardiovascular effects of coffee and caffeine. *American Journal Cardiol., 53*: 918-922, 1984.

MEADOW SAFFRON

Dustin, P. The centennial of the discovery of the antimitotic properties of colchicine. *Revue Medicale de Bruxelles, 10*(9): 385-390, 1989.

Muzaffar, A., Brossi, A., Lin, C.M., & Hamel, E. Antitubulin effects of derivatives of 3-demethylthiocolchicine, methylthio ethers of natural colchicinoids, and thicketones derived from thiocolchicine. Comparison with colchicinoids. *Journal of Medicinal Chemistry, 33*(2): 567-571, 1990.

MILK THISTLE
Campos, R., Garrido, A., Guerra, R. & Valenzuela, A. Silybin dihemisuccinate protects against glutathione depletion and lipid peroxidation induced by acetaminophen on rat liver. *Planta Medic, 55*: 417-419, 1989.

Chander, R., Kapoor, N.K., & Dhawan, B.N. Hepatoprotective activity of silymarin against hepatic damage in Mastomys natalensis infected with Plasmodium berghei. *Indian Journal of Medical Research, 90*: 472-477, 1989.

Ferenci, P, et al. Randomized controlled trial of silymarin treatment in patients with cirrhosis of the liver. *Journal of Hepatology, 9*(1): 105-113, 1989.

Kalmar, L., et al. Silibinin (Legalon-70) enhances the motility of human neutrophila immobilized by formyl-tripeptide, calcium ionophore, lymphokine and by normal human serum. *Agents and Actions, 29*(3-4), 239-246, 1990.

Mereish, K.A., Bunner, D.L., Regland, D.R., & Creasia, D.A. Protection against microcystin-LR-induced hepatotoxicity by Silymarin: biochemistry, histopathology, and lethality. *Pharmaceutical Research, 8*(2): 273-277, 1991.

Valenzuela, A., Aspillaga, M., Vial, S., & Guerra, R. Selectivity of silymarin on the increase of the glutathione content in different tissues of the rat. *Planta Medica, 55*(5): 420-422, 1989.

MISTLETOE
Mannel, D.N., et al. Induction of tumor necrosis factor expression by a Tectin from *Viscum album*. *Cancer Immunology and Immunotherapy, 33*(3): 177-182, 1991.

Schultze, J.L., Stettin, A., & Berg, P.A. Demonstration of specifically sensitized lymphocytes in patients treated with an aqueous mistletoe extract (*Viscum album L.*). *Klinische Wochenschrift, 69*(9): 397-403, 1991.

Yoshida, T., et al. Enhancement of the cytotoxicity of mistletoe lectin-1 (ML-1) by high pH or perturbation in Golgi functions. *Pharmazie, 46*(5): 349-351, 1991.

MOTHERWORT
He, G. Effect of the prevention and treatment of atherosclerosis of a mixture of Hawthorn and Motherwort. *Journal of Modern Development in Traditional Medicine, 10*(6): 361, 326, 1990.

Kuant, P.G., Zou, X.F., Shang, F.Y., & Lang, S.Y. Motherwort and cerebral ischemia. *Journal of Traditional Chinese Medicine, 8*(1): 37-40, 1988.

Nagasaw, H., et al. Effects of motherwort (*Leonurus sibiricus L.*) on preneoplastic and neoplastic mammary gland growth in multiparous GR/A mice. *Anticancer Research, 10*(4): 1019-1023, 1990.

Zou, Q.Z., et al. Effect of motherwort on blood hyperviscosity. *American Journal of Chinese Medicine, 17*(1-2): 65-70, 1989.

PARSLEY
Christomanos, A.A. Apiolom viride as an abortifacient: Animal experiments. *Klin Wochenschr, 6*: 1859-1860, 1927.

Christomanos, A.A. The pharmacology of apiol and some of its allies. *Naunyn-Schmiederbergs Arch Exp Pathol Pharmakol, 123*: 252-258, 1927.

Joachimoglu, G. Apiolum viride as an abortifacient. *Dtsch Med Wochenschr, 52*: 2079-2080, 1926.

Meyer, K., Kohler, A., Kauss, H. Biosynthesis of ferulic acid esters of plant cell wall polysaccharides in endomembranes from parsley cells. *Febs Letters, 290*(1-2): 209-212, 1991.

Schmitt, D., Pakusch, A.E., & Matern, U. Molecular cloning, induction, and taxonomic distribution of caffeoyl-CoA 3-0-methyltransferase, an enzyme involved in disease resistance. *Journal of Biological Chemistry, 266*(26): 17416-17423, 1991.

PASSIONFLOWER
Li, Q.M., et al. Mass spectral characterization of C-glycosidic flavonoids isolated from a medicinal plant (*Passiflora incarnata*). *Journal of Chromatography, 562*(1-2), 435-446, 1991.

PAU D'ARCO
Austin, F.G. Schistosoma mansoni chemoprophylaxis with dietary lapachol. *The American Journal of Tropical Medicine and Hygiene, 23*(3): 412-415, 1974.

Avirutnant, W. & Pongpan, A. The antimicrobial activity of some Thai flowers and plants. *Mahidol Univ. J. Pharm. Sci., 10*(3): 81-86, 1983.

Barros, G.S.G., Matos, F.J.A., Vieira, J.E.V., Sousa, M.P., & Medeiros, M.C. Pharmacological screening of some Brazilian plants. *J. Pharm Pharmacol, 22*: 116-, 1970.

Da Consolacao, F., Linardi, M., De Oliveira, M.M. & Sampaio, M.R.P. A lapachol derivative active against mouse lymphocytic leukemia P-388. *J Med Chem, 18*: 1159-, 1975.

Di Carlo, F.J., Haynes, L.J., Sliver, N.J., & Phillips, G.E. Reticuloendothelial system stimulants of botanical origin. *J. Reticuloendothelial Soc., 1*: 224-, 1964.

Dominguez, X.A. & Alcorn, J.B. Screening of medicinal plants used by Huastec Mayans of northeastern Mexico. *J. Ethnopharmacol., 13*(2): 139-156, 1985.

Ferreira De Santana, C., Goncalves De Lima, O., D'Albuquerque, I.L., Lacerda, A.L., & Martins, D.G. The antitumor and toxic properties of substances extracted from the wood of *Tabebuia avellanedae*. *Rev Inst Antibiot Univ Fed Pernambuco Recife, 81*: 89-94, 1968.

Forgacs, P., Jacquemin, H., Moretti, C., Provost, J., & Touche, A. Phytochemical and biological activity studies on 18 plants from French Guyana. *Plant Med. Phytother, 17*(1): 22-32, 1983.

Heal, R.E., Rogers, E.F., Wallace, R.T., & Starnes, O. A survey of plants of insecticidal activity. *Lloydia, 13*: 89-162, 1950.

Kingston, D.G.I. & Rao, M.M. Isolation structure elucidation and synthesis of two new cytotoxic napthoquinones from *Tabebuia cassinoides*. *Planta Medica, 39*: 230-231, 1980.

Oga, S. & Sekino, T. Toxicity and antiinflammatory activity of *Tabebuia avellanedae* extracts. *Rev. Fac. Farm Bioqium Univ. Sau Paulo, 7*(1): 47-53, 1969.

Ogunlana, E.O. & Ramstad, E. Investigations into the antibacterial activities of local plants. *Planta Med, 27*: 354-, 1975.

Rao, M.M. & Kingston, D.G.I. Plant anticancer agent. XII. Isolation and structure elucidation of new cytotoxic quinones from *Tabebuia cassinoides*. *J. Nat. Prod., 45*: 600-604, 1982.

Spencer, C.F., et al. Survey of plants for antimalarial activity. *Lloydia, 10*: 145-174, 1947.

Wagner, H., Kreher, B., & Jurcic, K. Immunological investigations of naphthaquinone containing plant extracts, isolated quinones and other cytostatic compounds in cellular immunosystems. *Planta Medica, 6*: 550-A, 1986.

PENNYROYAL

Gordon, W.P., et al. The metabolism of the abortifacient terpene, (R)-(+)-pulegone, to a proximate toxin, menthofuran. *Drug Metabolism and Disposition: the Biological Fate of Chemicals*, 15(5): 589-594, 1987.

PERIWINKLE, TROPICAL

De Bruyn, et al. Modification of *Catharanthus roseus* alkaloids: a lactone derived from 17-deacetylvinblastine. *Planta Medica*, 55(4): 364-365, 1989.

Facchini, P.J., Neumann, A.W., & DiCosmo, F. Adhesion of suspension-cultured *Catharanthus roseus* cells to surfaces: effect of pH, ionic strength, and cation valency. *Biomaterials*, 10(5): 318-324, 1989.

Naaranlahti, T., et al. Isolation of Catharanthus alkaloids by solid-phase extraction and semipreparative HPLC. *Journal of Chromatographic Science*, 28(4): 173-174, 1990.

Naaranlahti, T., et al. Electrochemical detection of indole alkaloids of *Catharanthus roseus* in high-performance liquid chromatography. *Analyst*, 114(10): 1229-1231, 1989.

PINEAPPLE

Batkin, S., Taussig, S., & Szekerczes, J. Modulation of pulmonary metastasis (Lewis lung carcinoma) by bromelain, an extract of the pineapple stem (*Ananas comosus*) [letter]. *Cancer Investigation*, 6(2): 241-242, 1988.

Rowan, A.D., Buttle, D.J., & Barrett, A.J. The cysteine proteinases of the pineapple plant. *Biochemical Journal*, 266(3): 869-875, 1990.

Rowan, A.D., et al. Debridement of experimental full-thickness skin burns of rats with enzyme fractions derived from pineapple stem. *Burns*, 16(4): 243-246, 1990.

Taussig, S.J. & Batkin, S. Bromelain, the enzyme complex of pineapple (*Ananas comosus*) and its clinical application. An update. *Journal of Ethnopharmacology*, 22(2): 191-203, 1988.

Noble, R.L. The discovery of the vinca alkaloids—chemotherapeutic agents against cancer. *Biochemistry and Cell Biology*, 68(12): 1344-1351, 1990.

POMEGRANATE

Ferrara, L., et al. Identification of the root of *Punica granatum* in galenic preparations using TLC. *Bollettino—Societa Italiana Biolgia Sperimentale*, 65(5): 385-390, 1989.

Segura, J.J., Morales-Ramos, L.H., Verde-Star, J., & Guerra, D. Growth inhibition of Entamoeba histolytica and E. invadens produced by pomegranate root (*Punica granatum L.*). *Arhivos de Investigacion Medica*, 21(3): 235-239, 1990.

PSYLLIUM

Anderson, et al. Cholesterol-lowering effects of psyllium hydrophilic mucilloid for hypercholesterolemic men. *Archives of Internal Medicine*, 148(2): 292-296, 1988.

Bell, L.P., Hectorn, K.J., Reynolds, H., Balm, T.K., & Hunninghake, D.B. Cholesterol-lowering effects of psyllium hydrophilic mucilloid. Adjunct therapy to a prudent diet for patients with mild to moderate hypercholesterolemia.

Bell, L.P., Hectorn, K.J., Reynolds, H., & Hunninghake, D.B. Cholesterol-lowering effects of soluble-fiber cereals as part of a prudent diet for patients with mild to moderate hypercholesterolemia. *American Journal of Clinical Nutrition*, 52(6): 1020-1026, 1990.

Davidson, L.J., Belknap, D.C., & Flournoy, D.J. Flow characteristics of enteral feeding with psyllium hydrophilic muciloid added. *Heart and Lung*, 20(4): 404-408, 1991.

Friedman, E., Lightdale, C., & Winawer, S. Effects of psyllium fiber and short-chain organic acids derived from fiber breakdown on colonic epithelial cells from high-risk patients. *Cancer Letters*, 43(1-2): 121-124, 1988.

Hallert, C., Kaldma, M., & Petersson, B.G. Ispaghula husk may relieve gastrointestinal symptoms in ulcerative colitis in remission. *Scandinavian Journal of Gastroenterology*, 26(7): 747-750, 1991.

Haskell, W. L., et al. Role of water-soluble dietary fiber in teh management of elevated plasma cholesterol in healthy subjects. *American Journal of Cardiology*, 69(5): 433-439, 1992.

Heather, D.J., Howell, L., Montana, M., Howell, M., & Hill, R. Effect of a bulk-forming cathartic on diarrhea in tube-fed patients. *Heart and Lung*, 20(4): 409-413, 1991.

James, J.M., Cooke, S.K., Barnett, A., & Sampson, H.A. Anaphylactic reactions to a psyllium-containing cereal. *Journal of Allergy and Clinical Immunology*, 88(3 Pt. 1): 402-8, 1991.

Levin, E.G., et al. Comparison of psyllium hydrophilic mucilloid and cellulose as adjuncts to a prudent diet in the treatment of mild to moderate hypercholesterolemia. *Archives of Internal Medicine*, 150(9): 1822-1827, 1990.

Lipsky, H., Gloger, M., & Frishman, W.H. Dietary fiber for reducing blood cholesterol. *Journal of Clinical Pharmacology*, 30(8): 699-703, 1990.

Miettinen, T.A. & Tarpila, S. Serum lipids and cholesterol metabolism during guar gum and plantago ovata and high fibre treatments. *Clinical Chimica Acta*, 183(3): 253-262, 1989.

Misra, S.P., Thorat, V.K., Sachdev, G.K., & Anand, B.S. Long-term treatment of irritable bowel syndrome: results of a randomized controlled trial. *Quarterly Journal of Medicine*, 73(270): 931-939, 1989.

Neal, G.W. & Balm, T.K. Synergistic effects of psyllium in the dietary treatment of hypercholesterolemia. *Southern Medical Journal*, 83(10): 1131-1137, 1990.

Pape, D. Improvement in blood lipids and lipoproteins by simple nutritional modification, exemplified by a high-fiber modified so-called "heart diet" of a West German clinic: the therapeutic gain due to expanding and high fiber foods. *Vasa. Supplementum*, 33: 247-249, 1991.

Pastors, J.G., Blaisdell, P.W., Balm, T.K., Asplin, C.M., & Pohl, S.L. Psyllium fiber reduces rise in postprandial glucose and insulin concentrations in patients with non-insulin-dependnet diabetes. *American Journal of Clinical Nutrition*, 53(6): 1431-1435, 1991.

Stewart, R.B., Hale, W.E., Moore, M.T., May, F.E., & Marks, R.G. Effect of psyllium hydrophilic mucilloid on serum cholesterol in the elderly. *Digestive Diseases and Sciences*, 36(3): 329-334, 1991.

Sussman, G.L. & Dorian, W. Psyllium anaphylaxis. *Allergy Proceedings*, 11(5): 241-242, 1990.

Turley, D.d., Daggy, B.P., & Dietschy, J.M. Cholesterol-lowering action of psyllium mucilloid inthe hamsters: sites and possible mechanism of action. *Metabolism: Clinical and Experimental*, 40(10): 1063-1073, 1991.

Wolever, T.M., et al. Effect of method of administration of psyllium on glycemic resonse and carbohydrate digestibility. *Journal of the American College of Nutrition*, 10(4): 364-371, 1991.

RASPBERRY, RED

Alonso, R., Cadavid, I., & Calleja, J.M. A preliminary study of hypoglycemic activity of *Rubus fruticosus*. *Planta Med. Suppl.*, 40: 102-106, 1980.

Bamford, D.S., Percival, R.C., & Tothill, A.U. Raspberry leaf tea: A new aspect to an old problem. *Brit. J. Pharmacol, 40:* 161P-, 1970.

Burn, J.H. & Withell, E.R. A principle in raspberry leaves which relaxes uterine muscle. *Lancet, 2:* 1-, 1941.

Kim, M.S., Lee, N.G., Lee, J.H., Byun, S.J., & Kim, Y.C. Immunopotentiating activity of water extracts of some crude drugs. *Korean J. Pharmacog., 19*(3): 193-200, 1988.

Konowalchuk, J. & Speirs, J.I. Antiviral activity of fruit extracts. *J. Food Sci, 41:* 1013-, 1976.

Kurzepa, S. & Samojlik, E. Studies on the effects of extracts from plants of the family rosaceae on gonadotropin and thyrotropin in the rat. *Endokrinol Pol., 14:* 143-. 1963.

May, G. & Willuhn, G. Antiviral activity of aqueous extracts from medicinal plants in tissue cultures. *Arzneim-Forsch, 28*(1): 1-7, 1978.

Ribeiro, R.A., et al. Acute diuretic effects in conscious rats produced by some medicinal plants used in the state of Sao Paulo, Brazil. *J. Ethnopharmacol, 24*(1): 19-29, 1988.

Yang, L.L., Sheu, F.M., Yen, K.Y., & Tung, T.C. Study of interferon inducer in Taiwan fold medicines. *Asian J. Pharm. Suppl. 6*(8): 121-, 1986.

RED CLOVER

Cassady, J.M., et al. Use of a mammalian cell culture benzo(a)pyrene metabolism assay for the detection of potential anticarcinogens from natural products: inhibition of metabolism by biochanin A., an osiflavone from *Trifolium pratense L. Cancer Research, 48*(22): 6257-6261, 1988.

Chae, Y.H., et al. Effects of synthetic and naturally occurring flavonoids on benzo[a]pyrene metabolism by hepatic microsomes prepared from rats treated with cytochrome P-450 inducers. *Cancer Letters, 60*(1): 15-24, 1991.

REISHI MUSHROOM

Cheng, H.H., et al. The anti-tumor effect of cultivated *Ganoderma lucidum* extract. *Journal of the Chinese Oncology Society, 1*(3): 12-16, 1982.

Gong, Z. & Lin, Z.B. The pharmacological study of lingzhi (*Ganoderma lucidum*) and the research of therapeutical principle of "fuzheng guben" in traditional Chinese medicine. *Pei-Ching I Hsueh Yuan Hsueh Pao, 13:* 6-10, 1981.

Kubo, M., Matsuda, H., Nogami, M., Arichi, S., & Takahashi, T. Studies on *Ganoderma lucidum*. IV. Effects on the disseminated intravascular coagulation. *Yakugaku Zasshi, 103*(8): 871-877, 1983.

Lee, S.Y. & Rhee, H.M. Cardiovascular effects of mycelium extract of *Ganoderma lucidum*: inhibition of sympathetic outflow as a mechanism of its hypotensive action. *Chemical and Pharmaceutical Bulletin, 38*(5): 1359-1364, 1990.

Nogami, M., Tsuji, Y., Kubo, M., Takahashi, M., Kimura, H., & Matsuike, Y. Studies on *Ganoderma lucidum*. VI. Anti-allergic effect.(i). *Yakugaku Zasshi, 106*(7): 594-599, 1986.

Nogami, M., Kubo, M., Kimura, H., & Takahashi, M. Studies on *Ganoderma lucidum*. V. Inhibitory activity on the release of histamine from the isolated mast cells. *Shoyakugaku Zasshi, 40*(2): 241-243., 1986.

Nogami, M., Ito, M., Kubo, M., Takahashi, M., Kimura, H., & Matsuike, Y. Studies on *Ganoderma lucidum*. VII. Anti-allergic effects. (2). *Yakugaku Zasshi, 106*(7): 600-604, 1986.

Shimizu, A., Yano, T., Saito, Y., & Inada, Y. Isolation of an inhibitor of platelet aggregation from a fungus, *Ganoderma lucidum. Chem Pharm Bull, 33*(7): 3012-3015, 1985.

Shin, H.W., Kim, H. W., Choi, E.C., Toh, S.H., & Kim, K.B. Studies on inorganic composition and immunopotentiating activity of *Ganoderma lucidum* in Korea. *Korean J Pharmacog, 16*(4): 181-190, 1985.

Sone, Y., Okuda, R., Wada, N., Kishida, E., & Misaki, A. Structures and antitumor activities of the polysaccarides isolated from fruiting body and the growing culture of mycelium of *Ganoderma lucidum. Agr Biol Chem, 49*(9): 2641-2653, 1985.

Tao, J. & Feng, K.V. Experimental and clinical studies on inhibitory effect of *Ganoderma lucidum* on platelet aggregation. *Journal of Tongji Medical University, 10*(4): 24-243, 1990.

Wilson, J.W. & Plunkett, O.A. The fungus diseases of man. Berkeley, University of California, 1965.

RHUBARB

Cyong, J., et al. Anti-bacteroides fragilis substance from rhubarb. *Journal of Ethnopharmacology, 19*(3): 279-283, 1987.

Umeda, M., Amagaya, S., & Ogihara, Y. Effects of certain herbal medicines on the biotransformation of arachidonic acid: a new pharmacological testing method using serum. *Journal of Ethnopharmacology, 23*(1): 91-98, 1988.

Zhou, H. & Jiao, D. 312 cases of gastric and duodenal ulcer bleeding treated with 3 kinds of alcoholic extract rhubarb tablets. *Journal of Modern Developments in Traditional Medicine, 10*(3): 150-151, 131-132, 1990.

ROSEMARY

Singletary, K.W. & Nelshopen, J.M. Inhibitioin of 7,12-dimethylbenz[a]anthracene (DMBA)-induced mammary tumorigensis and of in vivo formation of mammary DMBA-DNA adducts by rosemary extract. *Cancer Letters, 60*(2): 169-175, 1991.

Zhao, B.L., Li, X.J., He, R.G., Cheng, S.J., & Xin, W.J. Scavenging effect of extracts of green tea and natural antioxidants on active oxygen radicals. *Cell Biophysics, 14*(2): 175-185, 1989.

SAFFLOWER

Adelstein, R., Ferguson, L.D., & Rogers, K.A. Effects of dietary N-3 fatty acid supplementation on lipoproteins and intimal foam cell accumulation in the casein-fed rabbit. *Clinical and Investigative Medicine, 15*(1): 71-81, 1992.

Huang, Y.S., et al. Effect of maternal dietary fats with variable n-3/n-6 ratios on tissue fatty acid composition in suckling mice. *Lipids, 27*(2): 104-110, 1992.

Li, D. & Randerath, K. Modulation of DNA modifcation (I-compound) levels in rat liver and kidney by dietary carbohydrate, protein, fat, vitamin, and mineral content. *Mutation Research, 275*(1): 47-56, 1992.

Mills, D.E., et al. Attenuation of cyclosporine-induced hypertension by dietary fatty acids in the borderline hypertensive rat. *Transplantatio, 53*(3): 649-654, 1992.

Okuyama, H. Minimum requirements of n-3 and n-6 essential fatty acids for the function of the central nervous system and for the prevention of chronic diseases. *Proceedings of the Society for Experimental Biology and Medicine, 200*(2): 174-176, 1992.

Vajreswari, A. & Narayanareddy, K. Effect of dietary fats on erythrocyte membrane lipid composition and membrane-bound enzyme activities. *Metabolism: Clinical and Experimental, 41*(4): 352-358, 1992.

Venkatraman, J.T., Toohey, T., & Clandinin, M.T. Does a threshold for the effect of dietary omega-3 fatty acids on the fatty acid composition of nuclear envelope phospholipids exist? *Lipids, 27*(2): 94-97, 1992.

SAFFRON

Nair, S.C., Salomi, M.J., Panikkar, B., & Panikkar, K.R. Modulatory effects of *Crocus sativus* and *Nigella sativa* extracts on cisplatin-induced toxicity in mice. *Journal of Ethnopharmacology, 31*(1): 75-83, 1991.

Salomi, M.J., Nair, S.C., & Panikkar, K.R. Inhibitory effects of *Nigella sativa* and saffron (*Crocus sativus*) on chemical carcinogenesis in mice. *Nutrition and Cancer, 16*(1): 67-72, 1991.

SAGE

Lee, C., et al. Miltirone, a central benzodiazepine receptor partial agonist from a Chinese medicinal herb *Salvia Militiorrhiza. Neuroscience Letters, 127*: 237-241, 1991.

ST. JOHN'S WORT

Aizenman, B.E. Antibiotic preparations from *Hypericum perforatum. Mikrobiol Zh, 31*: 128-133, 1969.

Derbentseva, N.A. & Rabinovich, A.S. Isolation, purification, and study of some physicochemical properties of novoimanin. In Solov'eva, A.I. (Ed.), *Novoimanin Ego Lech Svoistva*, Kiev, 1968.

Gurevich, A.I., et al. Hyperiforin, an antibiotic from *Hypericum perforatum. Antibiotiki, 16*: 51-52, 1971.

Hobbs, C. St. John's Wort, *Hypericum perforatum L.*: A review. *HerbalGram, 18/19*: 24-33, 1989.

Meruelo, D., et al. Therapeutic agents with dramatic antiretroviral activity and little toxicity at effective doses: Aromatic polycyclic diones hypericin and pseudohypericin. *Proceedings of the National Academy of Sciences, 85*: 5230-5234, 1988.

Muldner, Von H. & Zoller, M. Antidepressive wirkung eines auf den wirkstoffkomplex hypericin standardisierten hypericum-extraktes. *Arzneim-Forsch, 34*: 918, 1984.

Negrash, A.K. & Pochinok, P.Y. Comparative studies of chemotherapetuic and pharmacological properties of antimicrobial preparations from common St. John's Wort. *Fitonotsidy Mater Soveshch*: 198-200, 1969.

Okpanyi, S., Lidzba, H., Scholl, B.C., & Miltenburger, H.G. Genotoxicity of a standardized Hypericum extract. *Arzheimittel-Forschung, 40*(8): 851-855, 1990.

Sajic, J. Ointment for the treatment of burns. *Ger. Offen* 2,406,452 (CL. A61K), August 21, 1975.

Suzuki, O., et al. Inhibition of monoamine oxidase by hypericin. *Planta Medica, 50*: 272-274, 1874.

SASSAFRAS

Grande, G.A. & Dannewitz, S.R. Symptomatic sassafras oil ingestion. *Veterinary and Human Toxicology, 29*(6): 447, 1987.

Pereira, E.F., et al. Anti-inflammatory properties of new bioisosteres of indomethacin synthesized from safrole which are sulindac analogues. *Brazilian Journal of Medical and Biological Research, 22*(11): 1415-1419, 1989.

SAW PALMETTO

Champault, G., et al. Actualite therapeutique: traitement meeical de l'adenome prostatique. *Annals Urological, 6*: 407-410, 1984.

Griffiths, D.J. & Abrams, H. The assessment of prostatic obstruction from urodynamic measurement and from residual urine. *British Journal of Urology, 51*: 129-134, 1979.

Hinman, F. & Cox, C.E. Residual urine volume in normal male subjects. *the Journal of Urology, 97*: 641-645, 1967.

Murray, M.T. Herbal treatment for liposterolic extract of *Serenoa repens* in the treatment of bening prostatic hyperplasmia (BPH). *Phyto-Pharmica Review, 1*(5): 1988.

Tasca, A., et al. Trattamanto della sintomatologia ostruttive d'adenoma prostatico con estratto di serenoa repents. *Minerva Urologica e Nefrologica, 37*: 87-91, 1985.

SCHIZANDRA

Ahumada, F., et al. Studies on the effect of *Schizandra chinensis* extract on horses submitted to exercise and maximum effort. *Phytotherapy Research, 3*(5):175-179, 1989.

Chang, I. H., Kim. J. H., & Han, D. S. Toxicological evaluation of medicinal plants used for herbal drugs (4). Acute toxicity and antitumor activities. *Korean J. Pharmacog, 13*(2):62-69, 1983.

Chen, Y. Y., Shu, Z., & Li, L. N. Studies of *Fructus shizanorae*. IV. Isolation and determination of the active compounds (in lowering high SGPT levels) of *Schizandra chinensis. Chung-Kuo K. O. Hsueh, 19*:276-, 1976.

Hancke, J. L., Wikman, G., & Hernandez, D. E. Antidepressant activity of selected natural products. *Planta Med., 1986*(6):542-543, 1986.

Hendrich, S. & Bjeldanes, L. F. Effects of dietary cabbage, brussels sprouts, illicium verum, *Schizandra chinensis* and alfalfa on the benzopyrene metabolic system in mouse liver. *Food Chem. Toxicol., 21*(4):479-486, 1983.

Hendrich, S. & Bjeldanes, L. F. Effects of dietary *Schizandra chinensis*, brussels sprouts and illicium verum extracts on carcinogen metabolism systems in mouse liver. *Food Chem. Toxicol., 24*(9):903-912, 1989.

Hernandez, O. E., Hancke, J. L., & Wikman, G. Evaluation of the anti-ulcer and antisecretory activity of extracts of aralia elata root and *Schizandra chinensis* fruit in the rat. *J. Ethnopharmacol., 23*(1):109-114, 1988.

Hikino, H., Kiso, Y., Taguchi, H., & Ikeya, Y. Antihepatotoxic actions of lignoids from *Schizandra chinensis* fruits. *Planta Med., 50*(3):213-218, 1984.

Kim, M. S., Lee, M. G., Lee, J. H., Byun, S. J., & Kim, Y. C. Immunopotentiating activity of water extracts of some crude drugs. *Korean J. Pharmacolog, 19*(3):193-200, 1988.

Koda, A., Nishiyori, T., Nagai, H., Matsuura, N., & Tsuchiya, H. Anti-allergic actions of crude drugs and blended Chinese traditional medicines. Effects on Type I and Type IV allergic reactions. *Nippon Yakurigaku Zasshi, 80*:31-41, 1982.

Liu, G. T., Wang, G. F., Wei, H. L., Bao, T. T., & Song, Z. Y. A comparison of the protective actions of biphenyl dimethyl-dicarboxylate trans-stilbene, alcoholic extracts of fructus schizanorae and ganoderma against experimental liver injury in mice. *Yag Hsueh Hsueh Pao, 14*:598-604, 1979.

Liu, G. T. & Wei, H. L. Protection by fructus schizanorae against acetaminophen hepatotoxicity in mice. *Yao Hsueh Hsueh Pao, 22*(9):650-654, 1987.

Nishiyori, T., Matsuura, N., Nagai, H., & Koda, A. Anti-allergic action of Chinese drugs. *Jap. J. Pharmacol. Suppl., 31*:115-, 1981.

Pao, T.T., Liu, K.I., Hsu, K.F., & Sung, C.Y. Studies on schizandra fruit. I. Its effect on increased SGPT levels in animals caused by hepatotoxic chemical agents. *Natl. Med. J. China, 54*:275-, 1974.

Shin, K. H. and Woo, W. S. A survey of the response of medicinal plants on drug metabolism. *Korean J. Pharmacog, 11*:109-122, 1980.

Shipochliev, T. & Ilieva, S. Pharmacologic study of Bulgarian *Schizandra chinensis. Farmatseyacsofia, 17*(3):56-, 1967.

Volicer, L., Srahka, M., Jankumi, Capek, R., Smetana, R., & Ditteova, V. Some pharmacological effects of *Schizandra chinensis*. *Arch. Int. Pharmacodyn Ther.*, *163*:249-, 1966.

Wahlström, M. *Adaptogens*, Utgivare, Goteborg, 1987.

Woo, W. S., Shin, K. H., Kih, I. C., & Lee, C. K. A survey of the response of Korean medicinal plants on drug metabolism. *Arch. Pharm. Res.*, *1*:13-19, 1978.

Yin, H. Z. A report of 200 cases of neurosis treated by "shen wei he ji" (decoction of ginseng, schisandra fruit and others). *Zhejiang-Zhongyi Zazhi*, *17*(9):411-, 1982.

Yu, J. & Chen, K. J. Clinical observations of AIDS treated with herbal formulas. *Int. J. Oriental Med.*, *14*(4):189-193, 1989.

SCULLCAP

Lu, Z. Clinical comparative study of intravenous piperacillin sodium or injection of scutellaria compound in patients with pulmonary infection. *Journal of Modern Developments in Traditional Medicine*, *10*(7): 413-415, 1990.

SEAWEEDS

Barchi, J.J., et al. Identification of a cytoxin from *Tolypothrix byssoidea* as Tubercidin. *Phytochemistry*, *22*: 2851-2852, 1983.

Chang, J. & Lewis, A.J. Prostaglandins and cyclooxygenase inhibitors, in Immune-modulation agents and their mechanisms, E.L. Fenischel and M.A. Chirigos (Eds.) Marcel Dekker, New York, 1984.

Chida, K. & Yamamoto, I. Antitumor activity of a crude fucoidan fraction prepared from the roots of kelp (*laminaria* species). *Kitasato Arch. of Exp. Med.*, *60*(1-2): 33-39, 1987.

Fukuyama, K., Wakabayashi, S., Matsubara, H., & Rogers, L.J. Tertiary structure of oxidized flavodoxin from an eukaryotic red alga *Chondrus crispus* at 2.35-A resolution. Localization of charged residues and implication for interaction with electron transfer partners. *Journal of Biological Chemistry*, *265*(26): 15804-15812, 1990.

Gustafson, K.R., et al. AIDS-antiviral sulfolipids from cyanobacteria (blue-green algae). *Journal of the National Cancer Institute*, *81*(16): 1989.

Hoppe, H.A., Levring, T., & Tanaka, Y. (eds.). *Marine algae in pharmaceutical science*. Walter de Gruyter, Berlin, New York, 1979,

Maruyama, H., Nakajima, J., & Yamamoto, I. A study on the anticoagulant and fibrinolytic activities of a crude fucoidan from the edible brown seaweed *laminaria religiosa*, with special reference to its inhibitory effect on the growth of a sarcoma-180 ascites cells subcutaneously implanted into mice. *Kitasato Arch. of Exp. Med.*, *60*(3), 105-121, 1987.

Miyazawa, Y., Murayama, T., Ooya, N., Wang, L.F., Tung, Y.C., & Yamaguchi, N. Immunomodulation by a unicellular green algae (*chlorella pyrenoidosa*) in tumor-bearing mice. *J. Ethnopharmacol*, *24*(2-3): 135-146, 1988.

Teas, J. The dietary intake of *laminaria*, a brown seaweed and breast cancer prevention. *Nutrition and Cancer 4*: 217-22, 1983.

Vane, J.R. *Nature 231*: 232, 1971.

Watanabe, S., and Fujita, T. Immune adjuvants as antitumor agents from marine algae. Patent-Japan Kokai Tokkyo Koho-61 197,525: 3pp-, 1986.

Yamamoto, I. Takahashi, M., Tamura, E., & Maruyama, H. Antitumor activity of crude extracts from edible marine algae against L-1210 leukemia. *Botanica Marina*, *XXV*: 455-457, 1982.

Yamamoto, I. Takahashi, M., Tamura, E., Maruyama, H., & Mori, H. Antitumor activity of edible marine algae: Effect of crude fucoidan fractions prepared from edible brown seaweeds against L-1210 leukemia. *Hydrobiologia*, *116/117*: 145-148, 1984.

Zhukova, G.E., Novokhatskii, A.S., & Telitchenko, M.M. Inactivation of some RNA-contained viruses with green and blue-green algae. *Vestn Mosk Univ Biol Pochvoved*, *27*(4): 108-, 1972.

SENNA

Elujoba, A.A., Ajulo, O.O., & Iweibo, G.O. Chemical and biological analyses of Nigerian Cassia species for laxative activity. *Journal Pharm Biomed Anal*, *7*(12): 1453-1457, 1989.

SHIITAKE MUSHROOM

Iizuka, C. Antiviral substance. Patent-Fr Demande Fr-2, 485,373: 30pp-, 1980.

Imaki, M., et al. Study on digestibility and energy availability of daily food intake (Part 1 Shiitake mushrom). *Japanese Journal of Hygiene*, *16*(1): 905-912, 1991.

Kabir, Y., Yamaguchi, M., & Kimura, S. Effect of shiitake (*Lentinus edodes*) and maitake (*Grigola frondosa*) mushrooms on blood pressure and plasma lipids of spontaneously hypertensive rats. *Journal of Nutritional Science and Vitaminology*, *33*(5): 341-346, 1987.

Kamm, Y.J., Folgering, H.T., van den Bogart, H.G., & Cox, A. Provocation tests in extrinsic allergic alveolitis in mushroom workers. *Netherlands Journal of Medicine*, *38*(1-2): 59-61, 1991.

Maeda, Y.Y. & Chihara, G. The effects of neonatal thymectomy on the antitumor activity of lentinan. *Int J Cancer*, *11*: 153-161, 1973.

Mizoguchi, Y., et al. Protection of liver cells against experimental damage by extract of cultured *Lentinus edodes mycelia* (LEM). *Gastroenterologia Japonica*, *22*(4): 459-464, 1987.

Mizoguchi, Y., et al. Effects of extract of cultured *Lentinus edodes mycelia* (LEM) on polyclonal antibody response induced by pokeweed mitogen. *Gastroenterologia Japonica*, *22*(5): 627-632, 1987.

Nanba, H. & Kuroda, H. Antitumor mechanisms of orally administered shiitake fruit bodies. *Chem Pharm Bull*, *35*(6): 2459-2464, 1987.

Nanba, H., Mori, K., Toyomasu, T., & Kuroda, H. Antitumor action of shiitake (*Lentinus edodes*) fruit bodies orally administered to mice. *Chemical and Pharmaceutical Bulletin*, *35*(6): 2453-2458, 1987.

Sugano, N., Choji, Y., Hibino, Y., Yasumura, S., & Maeda, H. Anticarcinogenic action of an alcohol-insoluble fraction (lapi) from culture medium of lentinus edodes mycelia. *Cancer Lett*, *27*(1): 1-6, 1985.

Sugano, N., Hibino, Y., Choji, Y., & Maeda, H. Anticarcinogenic action of water-soluble and alcohol-insoluble fractions from culture medium of lentinus edodes mycelia. *Cancer Lett*, *17*(2): 109-114, 1982.

Suzuki, F., Koide, T., Tsunoda, A., & Ishida, N. Mushroom extract as an interferon inducer. I. Biological and physico-chemical properties of spore extracts of lentinus edodes.

Takatsu, M., Tabuchi, M., Sofue, S., & Minami, J. Anticancer substances produced by basidiomycetes. Patent-Japan Kokai-75 12(293): -, 1975.

Tarvainen, K., et al. Allergy and toxicodermia from shiitake mushrooms. *Journal of the American Academy of Dermatology, 24*(1): 61-66, 1991.

Tochikura, T.S., Nakashima, H., Ohashi, Y., & Yamamoto, N. Inhibition (in vitro) of replication and of the cytopathic effect of the human immunodeficiency virus by an extract of culture medium of lentinus edodes mycelia. *Med Microbiol Immunol, 177*(5): 235-244, 1988.

SOAPWORT
Cazzola, M., et al. Cytotoxic activity of an anti-transferrin receptor immunotoxin on normal and leukemic human hematopoietic progenitors. *Cancer Research, 51*(2): 536-541, 1991.

Gasperi-Campani, A., et al. Inhibition of growth of breast cancer cells in vitro by the ribosome-inactivating protein saporin 6. *Anticancer Research, 11*(2): 1007-1111, 1991.

Tecce, R., et al. Production and characterization of two immunotoxins specific for M5b ANLL leukaemia. *International Journal of Cancer, 49*(2): 310-316, 1991.

Tochikura, T.S., Nakashima, H., Ohashi, Y., & Yamamoto, N. Inhibition (in vitro) of replication and of the cytopathic effect of human immunodeficiency virus by an extract of the culture medium of *Lentinus edodes mycelia. Medical Microbiology and Immunology, 177*(S): 235-244, 1988.

SQUIRTING CUCUMBER
Yesilada, E., Tanaka, S., Sezik, E., & Tabata, M. Isolation of an anti-inflammatory principle from the fruit juice of *Ecballium elaterium. Journal of Natural Products, 51*(3): 504-508, 1988.

SWEET FERN
Mannan, A., Khan, R.A., & Asif, M. Pharmacodynamic studies on *Polypodium vulgare* (Linn.). *Indian Journal of Experimental Biology, 27*(6): 556-560, 1989.

SWEET FLAG
Panchal, G.M., Venkatakrishna-Bhatt, H., Doctor, R.B., & Vajpayee, S. Pharmacology of *Acorus calumus L. Indian Journal of Experimental Biology, 27*(6): 5612-567, 1989.

Vohora, S.B., Shah, S.A., & Dandiya, P.C. Central nervous system studies on an ethanol extract of *Acorus calamus* rhizomes.

TANSY
Hethelyi, E., Tetenyi, P., Dabi, E., & Danos, B. The role of mass spectrometry in medicinal plant research. *Biomedical and Environmental Mass Spectrometry, 14*(1): 627-632, 1987.

TURMERIC
Ammon, H.P. & Wahl, M.A. Pharmacology of *Curcuma longa. Planta Medica, 57*(1): 1-7, 1991.

Chandra, D. & Gupta, S. S. Anti-inflammatory and anti-arthritic activity of volatile oil of *Curcuma longa* (haldi). *Indian J. Med. Res., 60*, 1972.

Donatus, I.A., Sardjoko, & Vermeulen, N.P. Cytotoxic and cytoprotective activities of curcumin. Effects on paracetamol-induced cytotoxicity, lipid peroxidation and glutathione. *Biochemical Pharmacology, 39*(12): 1869-1875.

Kulkarni, R.R., et al. Treatment of osteoarthritis with a herbomineral formulation: a double-blind, placebo-controlled, cross-over study. *Journal of Ethnopharmacology, 33*(1-2): 91-95, 1991.

Nagabhushan, M. & Bhide, S. V. Antimutagenicity and anticarcinogenicity of turmeric (*Curcuma longa*). *Journal of Nutrition, Growth and Cancer, 4*:83-89, 1987.

Polassa, K., Sesikaran, B., Krishna, T.P., & Krishnasawan, K. Turmeric (*Curcuma longa*)-induced reduction in urinary mutagens. *Food and Chemical Toxicology, 29*(10): 699-706, 1991.

Rafatullah, S., et al. Evaluation of turmeric (*Curcuma longa*) for gastric and duodenal antiulcer activity in rats. *Journal of Ethnopharmacology, 29*(1): 25-34, 1990.

Shalini, V.K. & Srinivas, L. Fuel smoke condensate induced DNA damage in human lymphocytes and protection by turmeric (*Curcuma longa*). *Molecular and Cellular Biology, 95*(1): 21-30, 1990.

Tønnesen, H. H. Studies on curcumin and curcuminoids. XIII. Catalytic effect of curcumin on the peroxidation of linoleic acid by 15-lipoxygenase. *International Journal of Pharmaceutics, 50*:67-69, 1989.

VALERIAN
Fehri, B. *Valeriana officinalis* and *Cratasgus oxyacantha*: toxicity from repeated administration and pharmacologic investigations. *Journal de Pharmacie de Belgique, 16*(3): 165-176, 1991.

Houghton, P.J. The biological activity of Valerian and related plants. *Journal of Ethnopharmacology, 22*(2): 121-142, 1989.

Kohnen, R. & Oswald, W.D. The effects of valerian, propranolol, and their combination on activation, performance, and mood of healthy volunteers under social stress conditions. *Pharmacopsychiatry, 21*(6): 117-118, 1989.

Lindahl, D. & Landwall, L. Double blind study of a valerian preparation. *Pharmacology, Biochemistry and Behavior, 32*(1): 1065-1066, 1989.

Molodoshnikova, L.M. Medicinal valerian. *Feldsher i Akusherka, 53*(1): 11-16, 1989.

Narimanov, A.A. & Gavriliuk, B.K. The synergism of the action of gamma radiation and cardiovascular preparations on lymphoid cells in culture. *Radiobiolgiia, 29*(2): 189-191, 1989.

WALL GERMANDER
Tariq, M., et al. Anti-inflammatory activity of *Teucrium polium. International Journal of Tissue Reactions, 11*(1): 185-189, 1989.

WATER LILY
Emboden, W. The sacred journey in dynastic Egypt: shamanistic trance in the context of the narcotic water lily and the mandrake. *Journal of Psychoactive Drugs, 21*(1): 61-75, 1989.

Gomorti, J.M., Cohen, D., Eyd, A., & Pomerans, S. Water lily sign in CT of cerebral hydatid disease: a case report. *Neuroadiology, 30*(1): 358, 1989.

Lee, D.H., Garvin, D.K., & Wimpee, C.F. Molecular evolutionary history of ancient aquatic angiosperms. *Proceedings of the National Academy of Sciences of the United States of America, 88*(2): 10119-10123, 1991.

Swanston-Flatt, S.K., Day, C., Bailey, C.J., & Flatt, P.R. Traditional plant treatments for diabetes. Studies in normal and streptozotopin diabetic mice. *Diabetaolgoia, 33*(8): 162-164, 1990.

WHITE OAK
Basden, K.W. & Dalvi, R.R. Determination of total phenolics on acorns from different species of oak trees in conjunction with acorn poisoning in cattle. *Veterinary and Human Toxicology, 29*(1): 305-306, 1987.

Ipsen, H. & Hansen, O.C. The NH2-terminal amino acid sequence of the immunochemically partial identical major allergens of Alder (*Alnus glutinosa*) Aln g I, Birch (*Betula verrucosa*) Bet v I, hornbeam (*Carpinus betulus*) Car b I and Oak (*Quercus alba*) Que a I pollen. *Molecular Immunologfy, 28*(1): 1279-1288, 1991.

Loria, R.C., Wilson, P., & Wedner, H.J. Identification of potential allergens in white oak (*Quercus alba*) pollen by immunoblotting. *Journal of Allergy and Clinical Immunology, 81*(1): 9-18, 1989.

WINTERGREEN
Boakes, R.A., Rossi-Arnaud, C., & Garcia-Hoz, V. Early experience and reinforcer quality in delayed flavour—food learning in the rat. *Appetite, 9*(3): 191-206, 1987.

Cauthen, W.L. & Hester, W.H. Accidental ingestion of oil of wintergreen. *Journal of Family Practice, 29*(5): 880-881, 1989.

WORMWOOD
Chawira, A.N., Warhurst, D.C., Robinson, B.L., & Peters, W. The effect of combination of qinghacau (artemisinin) with standard antimalarial drugs in the suppressive treatment of malaria in mice. *Transactions of the Royal Society of Tropical Medicine and Hygiene, 81*(1): 551-558, 1987.

Elford, B.C., Roberts, M.F., Phillipson, J.d., & Wilson, R.J. Potentiation of the antimalarial activity of qinghaceu by methoxylated flavones. *Transactions of the Royal Society of Tropical Medicine and Hygiene, 81*(3): 131-136, 1987.

elSohly, H.N., Croom, E.M., & elSohly, M.A. Analysis of the antimalarial sesquiterpene artemisinin in *Artemisia annua* by high-performance liquid chromatography (HPLC) with postcolumn derivatization and ultraviolet detection. *Pharmaceutical Research, 1*(3): 258-260, 1987.

Lang, X. & Ye, S.T. An investigation on in vivo allergenicity of *Artemisia annua* leaves and stems. *Asian Pacific Journal of Allergy and Immunology, 5*(2): 125-128, 1987.

Lwin, M., Maun, C., & Aye, K.H. Trial of antimalarial potential of extracts of *Artemisia annua* grown in Myanmar. *Transactions of the Royal Society of Tropical Medicine and Hygiene, 85*(1): 119, 1991.

Phillipson, J.D. & Wright, C.W. Can ethnopharmacology contribute to the development of antimalarial agents? *Journal of Ethnopharmacology, 32*(1-3): 155-165, 1991.

Ramay, B. Botany of Artemisia. *Allergie at Immunoligia, 19*(6): 250, 252, 1987.

Tawfid, A.F., Bishop, S.J., Ayalp, A., & el-Feraly, F.S. Effects of artemisinin, dihydroanemisinin and arteather on immune responses of normal mice. *International Journal of Immunopharmacology, 12*(1): 385-389, 1990.

Woerdenbag, H.J., Lugt, C.B., & Pras, N. *Artemisia annua* L.: a source of novel antimalarial drugs. *Pharmaceutisch Weekblead, 12*(5): 169-181, 1990.

Zhao, K.C. & Song, Z.Y. The pharmacokinetics of dihydroqinghasa given orally to rabbits and dogs. *Pharmaceutica Sinica, 25*(2): 17-119, 1990.

YAM, WILD
Huai, Z.P., Ding, Z.Z., He, S.A., & Sheng, C.G. Research on correlation between climactic factors and diosgenin content in Doswcorea zingiberensia Wright. *Pharmaceutical Sinica, 21*(9): 702-706, 1989.

Liu, Y.T. & Liu, S.O. Factors influencing the production of Chinese yam (*Dioscorea batatas Decne*). *Bulletin of Chinese Materia Medica, 12*(10): 15-17, 51, 53, 1987.

Sagara, K., Ojima, M., Suto, K., & Yoshida, T. Quantitative determination of aliointoin in Dioscrorea rhizome and an Oriental pharmaceutical preparation, hachimi-gan, by high-performance liquid chromatography [letter]. *Planta Medica, 55*(1): 93, 1989.

YARROW
De Pasquale, R., et al. Effect of cadmium on germination, growth and active principles contents of *Achillea millefolium* L. *Pharmacological Research Communications, Suppl 5*: 115-119, 1988.

Hausen, B.M., Brauer, J., Weglewski, J., & Rucker, S. alpha-Peroxyachifolid and other new sensitizing sesquiterpene lactones from yarrow (*Achillea millefolium L.*, compositae). *Contact Dermatitis, 21*(1): 271-280, 1991.

Krivenko, V.V., Potebnia, G.P., & Loiko, V.V. Experience in treating digestive organ diseases with medicinal plants. *Vrachebnoe Delo*, (3): 76-79, 1989.

Lamaisoin, J.L. & Carnat, A.P. Study of azulen in 3 subspecies of *Achillea millefolium L. Annales Pharmaceutiques Francaises, 16*(2): 139-143, 1988.

Schultz, H. & Albroscheit, G. High-performance liquid chromatographic characterization o some medical plant extracts used in cosmetic formulas. *Journal of Chromatography, 112*: 353-361, 1988.

YELLOW DOCK
Reig, R., et al. Fatal poisoning by *Rumex crispus* (curled dock): pathological findings and applications of scanning electron microscopy. *Veterinary and Human Toxicology, 32*(5): 169-170, 1990.

YERBA SANTA
Liu, Y.L., Ho, D.K., & Cassady, J.M. Isolation of potential cancer chemopreventive agents from *Eriodictyon californicum. Journal of Natural Products, 55*(3): 357-363, 1992.

CHAPTER 6

COSMETIC HERBS

Natural products have been utilized since antiquity to enhance human beauty. Whether for ornamentation, ritual, religious, or simply personal enhancement, nearly every culture has recorded usage of plant extracts, earth dyes, aromatic oils, in unique and individual ways. In fact, the discovery and use of natural "cosmetics" and natural "medicines" might have more in common than we thought, and may well have developed concurrently.

Coinciding with the development of synthetic drugs that followed the end of World War II, cosmetics underwent a similar transformation. As more and more of our natural pharmacopeia was replaced with synthetic drugs, so too were natural beauty aids discarded in favor of more "modern," high-tech synthetic products. Development was concentrated on synthetic cosmetics and this trend has continued to the present day. However, in the 1960s, with the emphasis on more natural lifestyles, there came a surge in demand for a new group of perfumes, soaps, fragrances, oral care products, and other cosmetics that were free of synthetic components.

This interest led to the birth of new companies dedicated to the manufacture of cosmetics and other beauty aids free of the petrochemicals, artificial colors, and other adulterants that dominate mainstream cosmetic manufacturing.

A particular field in natural products dealing with the healing effects of essential oils is called *aromatherapy*. Developed by the French perfumer and chemist Gathefossé, the French physician Jean Valnet later collaborated with the biochemist Marguerite Maury to develop a complete system of skin care and rejuvenation.

It is important to note that there are laws imposed on the manufacture of foods, drugs, and cosmetics that require certain preservatives be added to protect the consumer. Also all labels must be written to conform with the CTFA (Cosmetic Toiletries & Fragrances Association) guidelines. Consequently, it may appear to a consumer who is purchasing a natural product that "on investigation of the ingredient label," there are synthetic-appearing items listed that give the impression of being synthetics, when in fact they are natural substances.

Some examples of these synthetic-sounding ingredients that are actually natural products include:

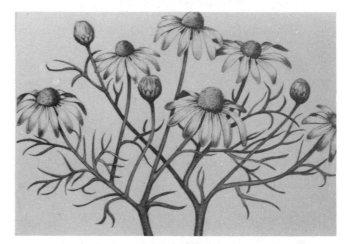

Chamomile

Acetic Acid: A component of acetylated alcohol. It is an acid that is generally derived from vinegar. It is present in apples, grapes, oranges, peaches, pineapple, strawberries, and many other plants. It is used in skin care products as a vehicle for other ingredients because it causes no known allergic reactions and resembles the sterols normally found on human skin.

Acrylic Acid: This unsaturated liquid acid comes from red and green algae.

Azulene: Distilled from Chamomile flowers or from Yarrow.

Butyladipate: An emollient and pH adjusting agent derived from beets!

Caprylic/Capric Glyceride: This oily liquid is derived from palm kernel or coconut oil.

Cetyl Alcohol: Found in coconut, palm kernel, and other vegetable oils. It is a constituent of most plant waxes. It is a natural emollient.

Cocamidopropyl Betain: Derived from the salts of coconut oil.

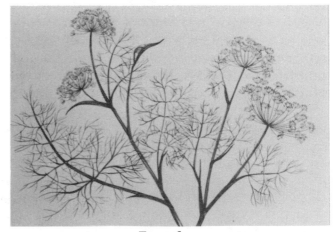

Fennel

Decyl Oleate: Derived from olive oil.

Glyceryl Oleate: A stabilizer and emollient derived from olive oil.

Glyceryl Stearate: An emulsifier derived from palm kernel or soy oil.

Imidazolidinyl Urea: Used to preserve cosmetics against bacterial contamination and to prolong shelf life.

Isopropyl Alcohol: Derived from petrochemicals—it is *not* a natural product.

Lysozyme: A basic protein that is an effective bactericide.

Perhydrosqualene: An emollicnt that comes from bran, olive, and wheat germ oils.

Phytosterol: Derived from soybeans, this is an emollient and emulsion stabilizer.

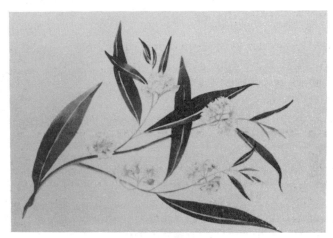

Eucalyptus

As you can see from the above examples, reading labels can become an extremely confusing business. Substances that sound synthetic may, in fact, be natural products with standardized names. Additionally, Food and Drug Administration (FDA) requirements may demand that certain synthetic ingredients *must* be added to the product. The manufacturer must use the substance in order to conform to FDA requirements.

A good rule of thumb is to trust a manufacturer who emphasizes *cruelty-free* products. Such manufacturers have made an effort to avoid using any ingredients (natural or synthetic) where significant animal trials have taken place. Since synthetics are generally tested on animals while natural products often have been used for centuries by humans, these manufacturers tend to use natural ingredients, adding synthetics only when the law demands.

Other important labelling clues: **organically grown botanicals, botanical ingredients free of irradiation, grown without pesticides,** and **containers** that are **biodegradable.** Each of these attributes indicate that the manufacture is committed to providing a quality, natural product.

The information provided in the above list will aid in understanding ingredients on the label and so help better determine the true content of cosmetics. What follows is a list of natural ingredients contained in products used for hair, skin, teeth, eyes, feet, and body.

Always remember: simpler is better.

ALOE VERA

Used since the time of the ancient Egyptians to treat burns; it moistens and softens the skin. Soothes minor irritations of gum and mouth lining. Please be aware that the leaves need to be processed correctly so the irritants are sufficiently removed.

ANEMONE

Soothing; used to treat skin problems.

ANGELICA

Antiseptic, antibacterial, and bacteriostatic; used externally to treat infections, skin fungus, and to assist with wound healing.

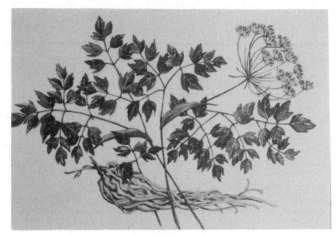

Angelica

AVOCADO OIL

Emollient and anti-bacterial.

BALM

As the name states, it soothes the skin.

BASIL

Antiseptic; used as a skin toner and cleanser.

BEESWAX

Used in skin emulsions as a thickening agent and emollient; unbleached beeswax is better to use since it has much lower pH levels.

BEETS

An emollient and pH adjusting agent; it is the source of the ingredient Butyladipate.

BELLADONNA

At one time, it was used as a cosmetic dye and to dilate the pupils of the eyes; it is still used as a dye.

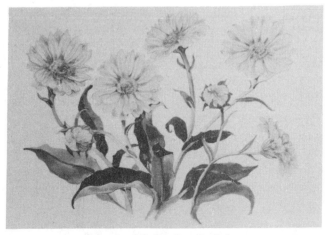

Marigold (Calendula)

BENZOIN

From the resin of the tree *Styrax benzoin*; antiseptic, deodorizing, and soothing to irritated skin. It is used as a natural preservative in many cream and ointment recipes.

BERGAMOT

From the peel of the green, bitter-orange, it is antiseptic, astringent, and has been used as an anti-perspirant. Bergamot oil is added to black tea to make "Earl Grey" tea. Bergamot oil is used widely in many external skin and hair applications. It tans the skin and increases its sensitivity to light. Caution should therefore be used when sunbathing.

BIRCH, BLACK

Very astringent; it is found in body and foot creams and toners, and in some natural dandruff preparations.

BLACKBERRY

Astringent and tonic; used in skin preparations.

BLESSED THISTLE

Astringent; used in skin care products to tone the skin.

BLOODROOT

Anti-plaque; also traditionally used as a natural red dye coloring.

BOSWELLIN

Oil is distilled from the resin; used in Egypt for corpse preservation, it's current use in natural products cosmetics is as an aid to treat wrinkles, raw or chapped skin, and as a fragrance factor.

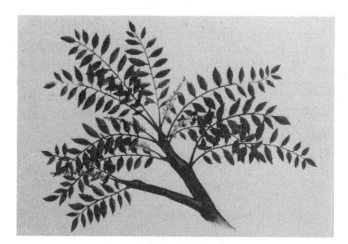

Boswellin

BURDOCK

Used to slow the secretion of oil.

CAJEPUT

It is antiseptic, antimicrobial, and it is thought to be an external anodyne. This oil is mainly found in hair preparations dealing with scalp infection, dandruff, and/or hair loss. It is irritating to sensitive skin.

CALENDULA (MARIGOLD)

Anti-septic and anti-inflammatory; oil and a blossom extract are used for skin conditions and to tone delicate skin.

CAMPHOR
Very strong external medicine employed to heal bruises, burns, and wounds.

CARROT SEED OIL
Contains carotene, and stimulates cell renewal. It has been added to wrinkle creams and facial oils. Most often mixed with almond oil, it will dye the skin due to the carotene content.

CASTOR OIL
Emollient; often used as a base and to bind ingredients together.

CEDARWOOD
Antiseptic and astringent; used in hair care for dandruff and to eliminate greasy hair. Externally it is used to treat a variety of skin conditions. Due to its manly fragrance, it is very popular as an additive to men's products. As it is soothing to the skin, it is found in aftershave lotions in particular.

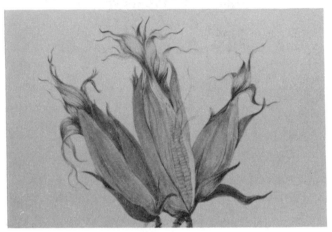
Corn

CHAMOMILE
An anti-inflammatory used in skin treatments. Useful against infections. When Chamomile tea is mixed with lemon, it is an effective highlight rinse for light-colored hair. The ingredient Azulene is usually distilled from Chamomile.

CITRONELLA
Possesses fungicidal, anti-bacterial, and insect repellent properties; used for skin fungus and infections. Citronella has been added to bath soaps and preparations.

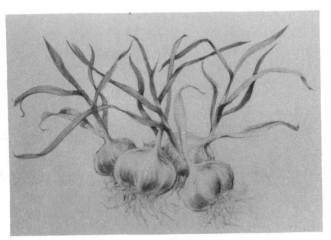
Garlic

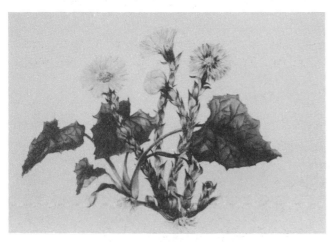
Coltsfoot

CLOVE

Antiseptic and pain-relieving, it is used externally to treat warts, callouses, infected wounds, and insect stings. Men's cosmetics and fragrances seem to favor Clove as an agreeable scent.

COLTSFOOT

High mucilage content; used for soothing skin.

COMFREY

Renowned for its wound-healing properties, Comfrey is found in skin-care products, particularly those treating rough and irritated skin and eczema, as well as hemorrhoid preparations.

CORN

An oil derived from the germ of the seeds is a skin softener.

CUCUMBER

Astringent, tonic, and refreshing, cucumber has been used for centuries to freshen and tone facial skin.

CYPRESS

The expressed distilled oil is astringent and deodorizing. It is also an insect repellent and, like Clove, is favored as fragrance for men's cosmetic preparations.

DEVIL'S CLAW

Anti-inflammatory; used in skin products.

DOGWOOD

The young branches are sometimes stripped of their bark and used to clean teeth.

ECHINACEA

Helps treat sensitive or inflamed gums.

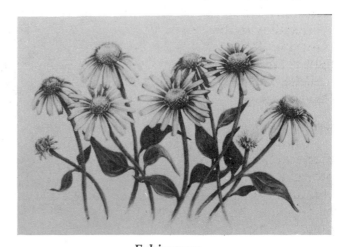
Echinacea

EUCALYPTUS

It is very strong and can irritate the skin. Diluted in oil, it has been used as an insect repellent; stronger preparations are applied topically to herpes blisters.

EYEBRIGHT

Used to treat eye irritations.

FENNEL

Extract of fennel seeds are used to formulate many natural toothpastes, as the seeds are beneficial for gums; it also helps heal mouth infections. It has a pleasing taste.

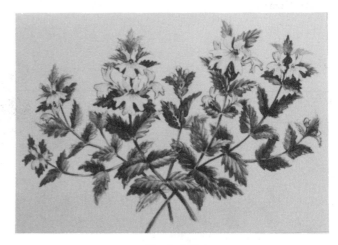

Eyebright

FLAX

Anti-inflammatory, demulcent, and emollient; the source of linseed.

FO-TI

The Chinese drink a tea of this herb to prevent gray hair.

GARLIC

Strongly antiseptic and fungicidal, oil of garlic is used to treat warts as well as calluses and corns on the feet.

GINSENG

Panax ginseng (Korean Ginseng) is used to heal and soften skin.

GOLDENSEAL

Antibacterial; it is used extensively in many female douche preparations. This herb is also found in many products for tooth and gum health and maintenance.

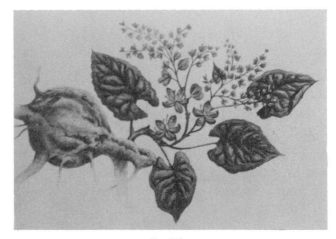

Fo-Ti

GROUNDSEL
Used in herbal medicine to stop bleeding gums.

GUAR GUM
Used as a thickener and emulsifier.

HENNA
Used as a hair dye since antiquity; imparts a reddish tint to the hair.

HORSETAIL
Taken internally, the silica content strengthens hair, nails, and teeth; externally it is used for skin conditions.

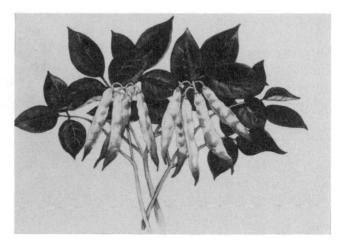

Guar Gum

JASMINE
Has a soothing effect on sensitive skin; utilized mainly as a fragrance for bath oils.

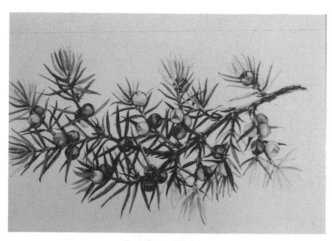

Juniper Berry

JUNIPER BERRY
Anti-bacterial, astringent, and toning; the oil is used in conjunction with other herbs to provide a refreshing facial steam bath.

LADY'S MANTLE
Used for skin conditions and for skin care in general.

LAVENDER
There are two distinctly separate Lavenders, English and French; they have altogether different fragrances. Both scents are used in various cosmetic and bath preparations. Lavender oil is antibacterial and antiseptic. Some external skin care products include this for warts and eczema as well as athlete's foot.

LEMON

Astringent, antibacterial, and antiseptic; it is somewhat irritating, but has been found useful in the treatment of acne. It is included in many sun-tanning preparations as it enhances skin light sensitivity.

LEMONGRASS

Deodorizing and refreshing; this oil has a delightful, totally unique fragrance and in bath oil can be very stimulating.

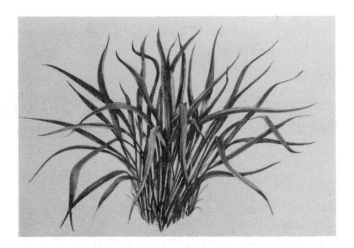

Lemongrass

LEMON BALM

Used for sunburn relief, skin allergies, and as an insect repellent; it is very strong, so only highly diluted preparations are available. Some success treating herpes blisters has been reported.

LICORICE

Soothes minor irritations of the gum and mouth lining; flavor and aroma; breath freshener.

LINDEN

Extracts from the blossoms are used to soothe irritated skin.

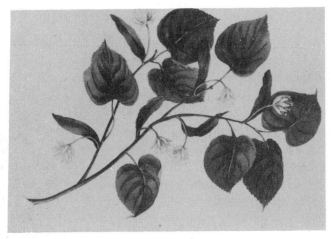

Linden

MADDER

Used as a facial to remove freckles.

MARSHMALLOW

The tea is useful as a rinse for oily hair and to add luster.

MAIDENHAIR FERN

Some herbalists reported that a dandruff remedy consisting of the ashes of this fern combined with vinegar and olive oil, was applied to the scalp.

MUSTARD

The oil expressed from the seeds is combined with a massage oil (to dilute the strength of the mustard oil, which can be quite irritating) and applied externally for the relief of muscle aches and pains due to injury or infirmity.

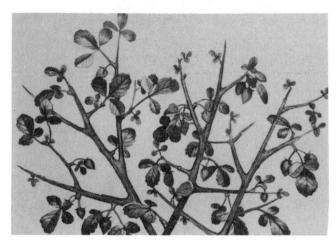

Myrrh

MYRRH

One of the ancient Egyptian components of embalming agents, the oil is extracted from the resin of the plant. Today it is found in many natural preparations such as skin care products that treat fungus infections and eczema as well as wrinkles and rough skin; toothpastes and mouth washes as an aid for bad breath and gum disease. Additionally, the exotic fragrance is a pleasing addition for those wishing a strong fragrance.

NETTLE

Astringent; used in hair products and facials.

ORANGE BLOSSOMS

The oil is non-irritating and is used as a fragrance as well as for chapped skin and acne (mixed with avocado oil). It is found in many bath preparations.

ORANGE BLOSSOM WATER

Astringent and refreshing; it is added to many facial preparations and is a component of an herbal facial steam formula.

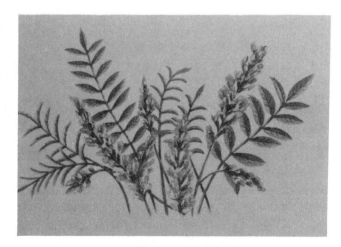

Licorice

PANSY
Used in skin care products.

PATCHOULI OIL
Used in perfumes for its own odor as well as its ability to preserve the scent of other fragrances.

PEPPERMINT
Cooling and stimulating for the skin; also used as a breath freshener.

QUASSIA
The bark is sometimes included in hair products.

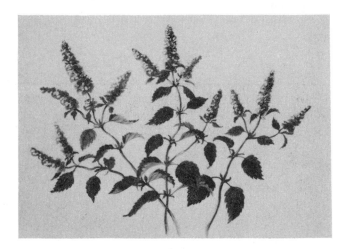

Peppermint

RESTHARROW
Emollient; used for itching and eczema.

ROSE
Astringent; Rose water soothes irritated skin.

SAGE
Used in dandruff shampoo preparations and for gum disease.

SESAME OIL
Emollient; used in skin care products and in sunscreens.

SLIPPERY ELM BARK
Softens and lubricates the skin; non-greasy and therefore added to more subtle cosmetics as an emollient.

SQUIRTING CUCUMBER
Ecballine, a compound derived from the fruits, is used in treating baldness as well as a cure against scalp diseases.

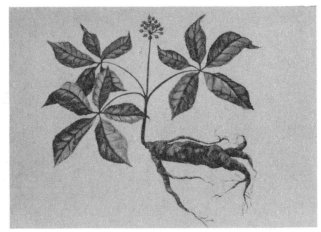

Korean Ginseng

TEA TREE
Antiseptic and anti-fungal, Tea Tree oil distilled from the leaves is used in salves, ointments, lotions, hair care and oral care products.

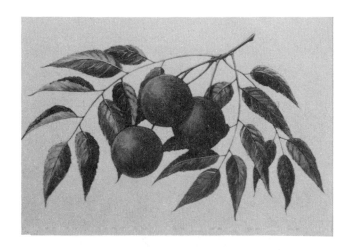

Black Walnut

WALNUT
Used to sooth the skin and reduce enlarged pores.

WITCH HAZEL
Astringent; used in liniments for body aches and pains; also a common ingredient in face creams and lotions.

WORMWOOD
Anti-parasitic when taken internally, Wormwood is a topical anesthetic for local irritations such as poison ivy and sunburn.

YARROW
Heals wounds and cleans oily skin; along with Chamomile, it is the source of the ingredient Azulene.

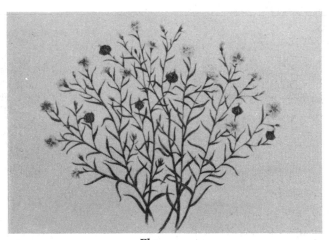

Flax

Herbal Recipes

Bunion Balsam

1. Aloe Powder   1/4 tsp.
   Soothing; promotes healing

2. Myrrh Powder   5/12 tsps.
   Astringent, healing (a little less)

3. Vitamin E Oil   4 oz.

Mix well in a bottle, let stand for a few days, occasionally shaking the mixture, then strain off the clear liquid, discarding the sediment.

Directions
Apply to bunions with a brush morning and night.

This recipe is well-tried and very effective preparation for bunions and inflamed joints.

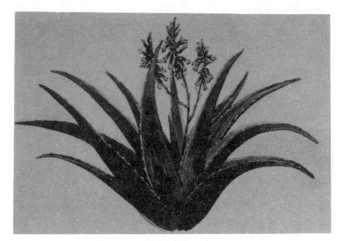
Aloe Vera

Dandruff Hair Wash

1. Quassia Bark   2 tsp.

2. Soap Bark   12 tsp.
   Forms lather

3. Red Oak Bark   2 tsp.
   Astringent

4. Black Walnut Leaves   1½ tsp.
   Astringent

5. Black Birch Leaves   1½ tsp.
   Astringent

Mix well and divide into 20 doses, using herbs especially cut for tea.

Directions
Boil one dose in a pint of water slowly for about 5 minutes, then strain and use the liquid while still warm as a shampoo before retiring, washing and brushing the scalp thoroughly with the decoction. When nearly dry, massage the scalp well with the Scalp Massage Oil, working it in well with the fingertips, moving the skin in a circular movement and then loosening the scalp by pulling the hair. Hair coming out by this procedure would fall out anyway. It is the new hair that will stay and be healthy and strong. Use the shampoo twice a week.

Scalp Massage Oil

1. Castor Oil   1 oz.
   Oil base

2. Oil of Burdock Root   2$\frac{1}{2}$ oz.

3. Liquid Petrolatum $\frac{1}{2}$ oz.
   Softens skin

4. Oil of English Lavender 15 drops
   Scent

5. Alkanet Root Extract $\frac{1}{2}$ grain
   Astringent; coloring agent

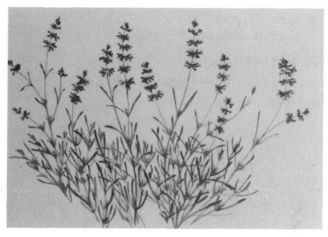

Lavender

Mix well and rub into scalp as directed in the instructions for Dandruff Hair Wash. Loss of hair is mostly due to an unhealthy condition of the scalp, brought on by parasites of either plant or animal origin, or to inactivity of the sebaceous glands and poor circulation. Dandruff Hair Wash and *Scalp Massage Oil* will give good results in all these disturbances if the instructions are carefully followed. They tend to clean the scalp, help the circulation of the blood, invigorate the hair follicles, and keep the scalp in a sanitary condition. If used faithfully for a while, they will tend to stop falling out of the hair and stimulate the growth of new hair. Very often the loss of hair is also due to nervous disturbances; in such cases the nervous system should be treated at the same time in order to get best results.

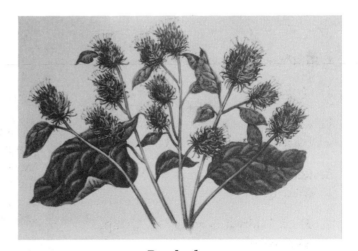

Burdock

For Poison Oak and Poison Ivy

1. Grindelia   7 tsp.
   Beneficial in poison oak, poison ivy and other skin irritations

2. Wormwood Herb   2 tsp.
   Topical anesthetic in local irritations

3. Soap Bark   5 tsp.
   Makes a lather

4. Slippery Elm Bark   4 tsp.
   Softens and lubricates skin

5. Wild Sage   2 tsp.
   Astringent; relieves inflammation

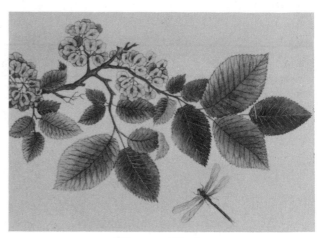

Slippery Elm

Mix well and divide into ten doses.

Directions
Add one dose to a pint of boiling water, boil slowly for about 10 minutes, let stand until cool, then strain. Apply cold to affected parts on saturated linens. Continue the application until the swelling is down and the itching has ceased.

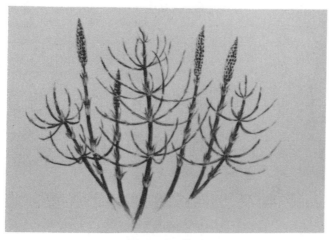

Horsettail

For Gargle and Mouthwash

1. Wild Sage Leaves   10 tsp.
   Expectorant; relieves inflammation

2. Marsh Rosemary   10 tsp.
   Astringent

3. Comfrey Root   2 tsp.
   An aromatic stimulant

4. Goldenseal   1 tsp.
   Anti-bacterial

Mix well and divide into 10 doses, using herbs especially cut for tea.

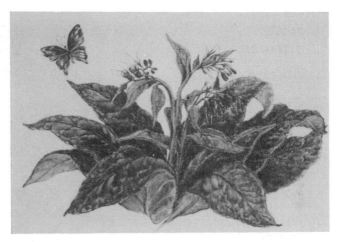

Comfrey

Directions
Add one dose to a pint of boiling water, boil slowly for 5 minutes, let stand for about 10 minutes, then strain and add 1 tablespoon of table salt to the decoction. Use as a gargle and mouthwash every 2 to 3 hours, until the inflammation and swelling have subsided. If the decoction is found too astringent, it may be diluted with water.

For canker sores may be used externally.

The astringent and antiseptic properties of this recipe make it a very valuable remedy, not only in sore throat, but also in spongy, diseased, gum states.

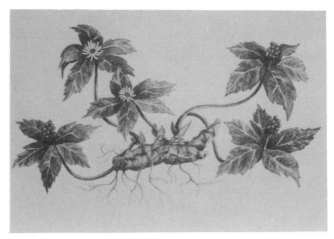

Goldenseal

Herbs for Foot Bath

1. Wild Sage   2 tsp.
   Relieves inflammation

2. Red Oak Bark   6 Tbsp.

3. Soap Bark   2 Tbsp.
   Makes a lather

4. Marshmallow   2 Tbsp.
   Tones skin

Mix well, using herbs especially cut for tea.

Directions
Take 3 tablespoonfuls of the mixed herbs and 2 tablespoonfuls of borax (to soften the water) and place in water of sufficient quantity to make a foot bath. Boil slowly for about 5 minutes, then strain and soak the feet in the decoction for about 10 minutes.

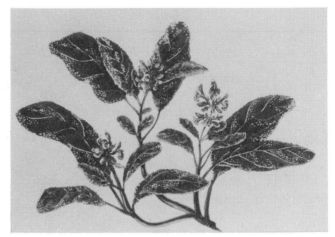

Sage

Deodorizing Lotion

1. Soap Bark   1 tsp.
   Makes a soapy lather

2. Red Oak Bark   2 tsp.

3. Distilled Water   8 Tbsp.

Slowly boil the Soap Bark and Red Oak Bark (items no. 1 and no. 2) in the Distilled Water (item no. 3) for about 5 minutes. Add sufficient distilled water to make four ounces.

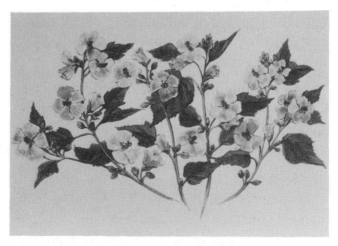

Marshmallow

CHAPTER 7

GLOSSARY

ABORTIFACIENT
A drug that causes abortion.

ADAPTOGEN
An agent that causes adaptive reactions; adaptogenic drugs appear to increase SNIR (State of Non-specifically Increased Resistance) in the human body, protecting against diverse stresses.

ADSORBENT
A drug used to produce absorption of exudates or diseased tissues.

ALKALOID
An alkaline principle of organic origin; any nitrogenous base, especially one of vegetable origin having a toxic effect.

ALTERATIVE
Agent which tends gradually to alter a condition.

AMENORRHEA
Absence of or suppression of menstruation.

AMINO ACID
One of a large group of organic compounds marked by presence of both an amino and a carbosyl radical. They are the building blocks from which proteins are constructed and they are the end products of protein digestion.

ANABOLIC
The conversion of simple substances into more complex compounds; usually considered "constructive" metabolism.

ANALGESIC
Medicine used to allay pain.

ANEMIA
A disorder characterized by a decrease in hemoglobin in the blood to levels below the normal range.

ANODYNE
Any medicine which allays pain.

ANESTHETIC
Medicine used to produce anesthesia or unconsciousness.

ANTACID
Medicines used to neutralize acid in the stomach and intestines.

ANTHELMINTICS (VERMIFUGES)
Medicines capable of destroying or expelling worms that inhabit the intestinal canal.

ANTHOCYANINS
A group of pigments that cause flowers and plants to be reddish purple in color.

ANTHRAQUINONE
Glycoside that acts as a laxative.

ANTIOXIDANT
Diminishes the effects of harmful "free-radical" compounds.

ANTIPHLOGISTIC
An agent that tends to relieve inflammation.

ANTIPYRETIC
Medicine that reduces the bodily temperature in fevers.

ANTISCORBUTIC
A remedy for or conteractant to scurvy.

ANTISEPTIC
Substance which prevents infection decay; tending to inhibit the growth and reproduction of microorganisms.

ANTISPASMODIC
Medicine that relieves nervous irritability and minor spasms.

APERIENT
An extremely mild, weak laxative.

APHRODISIAC
Substance used to increase sexual power or excitement.

AROMATIC
Used chiefly to expel gas from stomach and intestines. Also employed to make other medicines, less agreeable in taste and smell, more palatable, due to the fragrant smells and tastes of the aromatics.

ASTRINGENT
Tightens and contracts skin and/or mucous membranes. Externally as lotions and gargles, internally to check diarrhea.

ATONIC MENORRHAGIA
Weakness due to heavy menstrual bleeding.

AYURVEDIC MEDICINE
The "science of the lifespan," a system of healing developed and practiced in India.

BACTERIA
Small unicellular microorganisms of the class Schizomyates.

BIOFLAVONOID
Colored flavones found in many fruits; essential for absorption and metabolism of ascorbic acid; needed for maintenance of collagen and capillary walls.

BLOOD PRESSURE
The pressure exerted by the blood on the walls of the arteries.

CALMATIVE
Simply a calming agent, not necessarily sedative.

CAPILLARY FRAGILITY
Weakness of the capillaries (tiny blood vessels where blood and tissue cells exchange substances).

CARBOHYDRATE
Group of organic compounds, including sugar, starch, cellulose, and gum.

CARCINOGENIC
Substance that can induce cancer.

CARDIOTONIC
Substance that tones the hearts.

CARMINATIVE
Substance which removes gases from the gastrointestinal tract.

CATARRHAL
Inflammation of the air passages of the nose and trachea.

CATHARTIC

(1) Laxative and Aperient—*Mild* promotion of evacuation of the bowels by action on alimentary canal. (2) Purgative—Induces copious evacuation of the bowels, generally used to treat stubborn constipation in adults.

CATHETER

Flexible, hollow tube that is inserted into a vessel of the body to instill or remove fluids.

CHI'I

"Life-force," "inner energy," and other undefinable (to Westerners) health manifestations known to traditional Chinese medicine.

CHOLAGOGUE

Agents that increase the flow of bile into the intestines.

CHOLESTEROL

Fat-soluble steroid alcohol found in animals fats, oils, and egg yolk; continuously synthesized in the body, mainly in the liver.

COLLAGEN

A protein that can be prepared from connective tissue and from which gelatin can be made.

CORDIAL

A refreshing medicine which is held to revive the "spirits," being cheering, invigorating, and exhilarating.

CORTISONE

A glucocorticoid (may also be prepared synthetically) often prescribed as an anti-inflammatory.

COUMARIN

An anticoagulant.

CYTOTOXIN

Substance that has a toxic effect on certain organs, tissues, and cells; produced by injection of foreign cells.

DECOCTION

A preparation made by boiling the plant material in water.

DEMULCENT

Those medicines, used *internally,* that possess soothing, mucilaginous properties, shielding surfaces and/or mucous membranes from irritating substances.

DEPURATIVE

Agents that purify or cleanse, generally: "depurate a wound" or "depurate a fluid."

DEXTRAN-SULFATE
Created when dextran is boiled with chlorosulfonic acid; used in Japan to reduce blood clotting; may be anti-viral

DIAPHORETIC
Agent which increases perspiration. Commonly used as an aid for relief of common cold, administered hot, before bedtime.

DIURETIC
Medicine which increases urination, often combined with demulcents.

"DOCTRINE OF SIGNATURES"
An ancient medical theory that "like cures like."

DYSPEPSIA
Uncomfortable digestion.

EMETIC
A medicine that provokes vomiting.

EMMENAGOGUE
A substance with medicinal properties designed to assist and promote the menstrual discharges.

EMOLLIENT
Generally of oily or mucilaginous nature, used *externally* for its softening, supple, or soothing qualities.

ENEMA
Injection of solution into the rectum and colon for cleansing or therapeutic purposes.

ESTROGENIC
Substance causing estrus.

EXPECTORANT
Medicine that promotes the discharge of matter from the lungs, whether it be mucus, pus, or any other morbid accumulation.

FEBRIFUGE
Any medicine that mitigates or dispels fever.

FOLLICLE STIMULATING HORMONE (FSH)
Secreted by anterior pituitary gland, stimulates growth and maturation of Graafian follicles in the ovary and promotes spermatogenesis in the male.

GLACATAGOGUE
Increasing the flow of milk.

GAMMA GLOBULIN
Protein found in blood, concentration related to ability to resist infection.

GLUTATHIONE
Takes up and gives off hydrogen; important in cellular respiration.

GLYCOPROTEIN
A compound in which a protein is joined with a carbohydrate nonprotein.

GLYCOSIDE
Carbohydrate that yields a sugar and non-sugar on hydrolysis.

HDL
High-density lipoprotein: protein that may stabilize low-density lipoprotein; also important in transporting cholesterol and other lipids.

HEMOSTATIC
Medicine that arrests hemorrhages.

HEPATIC
Agent that promotes the action of the liver and the flow of bile.

HISTAMINE
A compound, found in all cells, where tissue is damaged associated with allergies and other inflammatory reactions.

HYDRAGOGUE
Purgative, causing watery evacuations.

HYDROCORTISONE
A cortisone derivative used in the treatment of rheumatoid arthritis.

HYPERTENSIVE
Agent that increases blood pressure.

HYPOGLYCEMIA
Low blood sugar.

HYPNOTIC
An agent producing sleep.

HYPOTENSIVE
An agent that causes low blood pressure

IMMUNOSTIMULANT
An agent that stimulates immune responses.

INFUSION
A preparation made by steeping the plant material in hot water.

INTERFERON
An antiviral glycoprotein.

LAXATIVE
Increases the peristaltic motion of the bowels, without purging or producing a fluid discharge. Never to be used when pregnant.

LDL
Low-density lipoprotein: protein containing more cholesterol and triglycerides than protein.

LITHOTROPIC
An agent that dissolves stones in the urinary organs.

NARCOTIC
A hypnotic, inducing stupor.

NEPHRITIC
An agent useful in kidney complaints.

NERVINE
Having a soothing influence and quieting the nerves without numbing them.

PANACEA
A "cure-all."

PECTORAL
A medicine adapted to cure or relieve complaints of the breast and lungs.

PHOTOTOXIC
An agent that makes the skin more susceptible to damage by ultraviolet light.

POLYSACCHARIDE
A complex carbohydrate.

PROPHYLACTIC
Medicine that prevents the development of disease.

PURGATIVE
Agent which induces copious evacuation of the bowels. Generally used only for stubborn cases, such as chronic constipation among adults. *Never to be used when pregnant.*

REFRIGERANTS
Cooling beverages.

RELAXANTS
Relaxing muscle fiber and alleviating spasm, allaying nervous irritation due to excitement, strain, or fatigue.

RUBEFACIENT

External application which produces redness of the skin, by virtue of drawing the blood and fluids toward the skin's surface; helpful in treatment of boils and blisters.

SAPONIN

A complex glycoside that forms a soapy lather in water.

SEDATIVE

Allays irritability or nerve action and induces a state of calmness.

SOPORIFIC

Medicine that causes sleep.

STIMULANT

Any agent temporarily increasing activity of cardiac, bronchial, gastric, cerebral, intestinal, nervous, motor, vasomotor, respiratory, or secretory organs.

STOMACHIC

A stimulant to the stomach.

SUDORIFIC

Causes copious perspiration.

TANNIN

An astringent phenolic plant constituent.

THROMBOSIS

Clots in the bloodstream that block the blood vessel.

TONIC

Medicine that permanently increases the systemic tone by stimulating nutrition.

VERMICIDE

A medicine that kills intestinal worms.

VERMIFUGE

See ANTHELMINTICS.

VOLATILE OIL (ESSENTIAL OIL)

A mixture of hydrocarbons that are less soluble in water than alcohol or fat.

VULNERARY

Application for external wounds.

CHAPTER 8

TABLES

Introduction

The following tables offer a quick overview of some convenient categories, as follows:

Table 1

SOME NATIVE AMERICAN HERBS*

Common Name	Latin Name	Function(s)
Angelica	*Angelica* (various species)	• aids asthmatics • helps in recuperation from illness • manages fevers • for night sweats
Arbor Vitae (Tree of life)	*Thuja occidentalis*	• for bronchial conditions • urinary infections • psoriasis • vaginal infections & warts
Bayberry (Warberry)	*Myrica cerifera*	• detoxifies inflamed bowels • reduces excessive menstrual bleeding • as a douche • a gargle for sore throat • on wounds & ulcers
Bearberry (Uva Ursi)	*Arctostaphylos uva-ursi*	• for urinary infections
Boneset	*Eupatorium perfoliatum*	• combats colds & flu • relieves mild pain • reduces fever
Cascara Sagrada	*Rhamnus purshiana*	• best laxative
Cohosh, Blue (Squaw Root)	*Caulophyllum thalictroides*	• treats menstrual irregularities; relieves menstrual pain
Corn Silk	*Zea mays*	• diuretic • urinary infections
Damiana	*Turnera aphrodisiaca*	• aphrodisiac • mild laxative • fights depression
Echinacea	*Echinacea angustifolia*	• antibacterial; nonspecific immune stimulation; • antitumor effects
Ginseng, American	*Panax quinquefolius*	• adaptogenic • fights stress • improves energy
Goldenseal	*Hydrastis canadensis*	• antibiotic • antiviral • for gastric & urinary infections
Oak (Bark)	*Quercus* spp.	• kills parasites • astringent (for bruises & wounds)

SOME NATIVE AMERICAN HERBS (continued)

Common Name	Latin Name	Function(s)
Passionflower	*Passiflora incarnata*	• the queen of herbal sedatives • to aid in insomnia, anxiety, & for "hyperactive" children
Poplar Buds (Balm of Gilead)	*Populus gileadensis*	• respiratory infections, especially bronchitis • stimulates circulation
Saw Palmetto	*Serenoa repens*	• reduces swollen prostate • for urinary infection • mild sedative
Scullcap	*Scutellaria laterifolia*	• sedative • for epilepsy • for nervous exhaustion
Wild Cherry (bark)	*Prunus serotina*	• for coughs • mild sedative action
Wintergreen (Teaberry)	*Gaultheria procumbens*	• for rheumatoid arthritis • for aches & pains • mild stimulant
Witch Hazel	*Hamamelis virginiana*	• astringent • hemmorhoids • for bruises & wounds
Yerba Santa	*Eriodictyon californicum*	• for asthma • for colds • as a mouthwash

* See *Earth Medicine - Earth Foods* by M. A. Weiner for a more complete list. (Ballantine Books, 1991)

Table 2
HERBS FOR MEN

Common Name	Latin Name	Function(s)
Astragalus	*Astragalus membranaceous*	• stimulates immunity • anti-cancer • anti-fatigue
Damiana	*Turnera aphrodisiaca* (and other species)	• aphrodisiac • may overcome impotence • fights depression
Echinacea	*Echinacea angustifolia*	• diminishes herpes sores • immuno-stimulant • antiviral • antitumor
Ginseng, American	*Panax* (various species)	• reverses radiation damage • protects liver • balances energies • aids in diabetes • improves performance • anti-stress
Ginseng, Siberian	*Eleutherococcus senticosus*	• combats fatigue, depression, & anxiety • anti-stress • improves memory
Ginkgo	*Ginkgo biloba*	• improves memory • treats impotence • improves circulation • inhibits bacteria & fungi
Green Tea	various species	Polyphenols: • are antiviral, antioxidant • enhance immunity • destroy bacteria • reduce cancer risk • lower serum cholesterol • act (like aspirin) to keep blood from excessive clumping
Guar Gum	*Cyanopsis tetragonoloba*	• laxative • decreases serum cholesterol • weight control • aids in diabetes
Mathaké	*Terminalia catappa*	• kills *candida* (yeast infections) • weakens flu virus • protects mucous membranes

HERBS FOR MEN (continued)

Common Name	Latin Name	Function(s)
Mushrooms (Reishi, Shiitake)	*Ganoderma lucidum; Lentinus edodes*	• adaptogen • stimulates T-helper cells, NK cells, interferons & macrophages • antitumor effect
Saw Palmetto	*Serenoa repens*	• shrinks swollen prostate (BPH) • diuretic • increases sperm count • aids thyroid
Schizandra	*Schisandra chinensis*	• fights fatigue • increases energy • adaptogenic
Yohimbe	*Pausinystalia yohimbe*	• aphrodisiac • dilates blood vessels • aids erections • weight loss

Table 3
HERBS AFFECTING IMMUNITY

Plant	Compound(s)	Type of Compound	Immune Effects
Astragalus *Astragalus membranaceus*	not specified (from dried root)		• interferon induction • natural killer cell enhancement • antiviral
Citrus various species	d-limonene	terpene	• destroys tumors • enhances drug metabolism
Echinacea, Coneflower *Echinacea angustifolia*	echinacosides; unnamed pentadecadiene	caffeic acid glycoside; polysacihandi; hydrocarbon	• antibacterial • nonspecific immune stimulation • antitumor effects
Garlic *Allium sativa*	allicin; methyl allyl trisulphide	allyl sulfide	• antitumor effects • kills *candida* • cycloxygenase & lipoxygenase inhibitor (slows tumor growth)
Goldenseal *Hydrastis canadensis*	berberine; hydrastine; L-canadine	alkaloids	• antibiotic • antiviral
Mathaké *Terminalia catappa*	linoleic acid, palmitic acid & others	fatty acids	• antibacterial (kills *Staphylococcus aureus*) • anti-yeast (kills *Candida albicans*)
Mushrooms A. Reishi *Ganoderma lucidum* B. Shiitake *Lentinus edodes*	arabinoxylo-glucan lentinan; virus-like pachymaran	triterpenes; polysaccharides polysaccharide; double stranded RNA	• adaptogenic • antitumor • immuno stimulant • stimulates T-helper cells • stimulates interferons, NK cells, & macrophages
Oak Bark *Quercus* spp.		tannins	• anti-parasite
Pau D'Arco *Tabebuia impetiginosa*	lapachol; lapa-chone; alpha & beta xyloidone	naphthoquinone; quinoid	• mild antitumor action • Kills *candida*
Seaweeds A. *Laminaria* spp. (brown algae) B. *Chlorella* spp. (micro algae) C. *Lyngbya lagerheimii* & *Phormidium tenue* (blue-green algae)	fucoidan chlorellin containing sulfonic acid	sulfate polysaccharide; fatty acid glycolipid	• antitumor • antifungal • antiviral • immunostimulant • kills AIDS virus
Willow *Salix alba*	Salicin	glycoside	inhibits PG production, enhances immune response, kills cancer cells

Table 4
TYPES OF ANTIBODIES

Antibody	Function
IgG	Most common. Major Ig in defense against microbes. Coats micro-organisms, speeding their destruction by other immune system cells. Confers long-standing immunity.
IgM	Major Ig produced in primary antibody response. Circulates in the blood stream, where it kills bacteria. Increases during acute stage of an infection. Usually forms in star-shaped clusters.
IgA	Concentrates in body fluids (tears; saliva; respiratory, genitourinary, and gastrointestinal secretions) guarding body entrances. First line of defense against invading pathogens and food allergens. Major Ig in defense against viruses.
IgE	Involved in allergic reactions. Attaches to surface of *mast cel,** and on encountering its matching antigen, stimulates the mast cell to pour out its contents. Also fights parasites.
IgD	Major Ig present on surface of B cells; may be involved in differentiation of these cells

* Mast cells are found in connective tissue. They are numerous along blood vessel beds, form the anticoagulant heparin, and *release histamin* in *allergi* and *inflammatory* reactions.

Table 5

HERBS FOR ALLERGY AND INFLAMMATION

Plant	Compound	Type of Compound	Effects
Butcher's Broom *Ruscus aculeatus*	ruscogenin; neo-rusco-genin & flavonoids	steroidal glycosides	• anti-inflammatory • for varicose veins & edema of the legs
Cayenne *Capsicum frutescens*	capsaicin	phenol	• topical anti-inflammatory agent
Ephedra (Ma Huang) *Ephedra* various species	ephedrine; pseudo-ephedrine	alkaloids	• bronchodilation • central nervous system stimulant
Garlic (and onion) *Allium* spp	aliin; allicin thiosulfinate; quercetin	sulfur containing compounds; bioflavonoid	• anti-inflammatory • PAF (platelet activating factor) inhibitor; see *Quercetin*
Ginger *Zingiber officinale*	gingerol; gingerdione	sesquiterpenes	• anti-inflammatory • analgesic (relieves pain) • antipyritic (lowers fever)
Ginkgo *Ginkgo biloba*	ginkgolides; quercetin	diterpene-lactones; bioflavonoid	• anti-allergic • treatment of asthma (PAF inhibitor)
Horse Chestnut *Aesculus hippocastanum*	escin	triterpene glycoside	• for treatment of varicose veins and edema of the legs
Licorice *Glycyrrhiza glabra*	glycyrrizin	triterpene saponin	• like hydrocortisone, inhibits inflammation • soothes mucus membrane • expectorant
Quercetin (a compound)	quercetin	bioflavonoid	• anti-inflammatory (cycloxygenase & lipoxygenase inhibitor) • anti-allergic (blocks histamine release) • anti-oxidant
Turmeric *Curcuma longa*	curcumin	phenol	• anti-inflammatory (cycloxygenase & lipoxygenase inhibitor) • anti-oxidant
White Willow *Salix alba*	salicin	phenolic glycoside	• anti-inflammatory • analgesic (relieves pain) • antipyritic (lowers fevers)

Table 6
HERBS CONTAINING CAFFEINE

Plant Name		Percent Caffeine
Common	Latin	
Arabian coffee	*Coffea arabica*	1-2%
Tea	*Camellia sinensis*	1-4%
Cacao (chocolate)	*Theobroma cacao*	less than 1%
Maté	*Ilex paraguensis*	1-2%
Cola	*Cola acuminata*	about 2.5%
Guaraná	*Paullinia cupana*	2.5-5%

Table 7

SOME HERBS FROM ASIA

Herb	Asian Name	Function(s)
Angelica *Angelica sinensis*	*dong quai,* *tang-kuei*	• balances menstrual irregularities • for many "women's" complaints
Astragalus *Astragalus membraneceus*	*huang qi*	• induces interferons • enhances natural killer cells • antiviral
Bupleurum *Bupleurum falcatum*	*chai hu*	• immune regulation • lowers fevers • elevates brain dopamine levels
Chinese Cucumber *Trichosanthes kirilowii*		• abortifacient • antiviral • antibacterial
Citrus fruits	*chen pi* (& others)	• contains d-limonene • destroys tumors (in animal experiments) • lowers cholesterol
Ephedra *Ephedra sinica*	*Ma huang*	• anti-asthmatic • diminishes allergic rhinitis & hay fever
Fo-Ti *Polygonum multiflorum*	*fo ti* *ho-shou-wu*	• utilized in geriatrics • anti-inflammatory •255 lowers cholesterol • kills viruses • prevents deposition of lipids on inner membrane of arteries • (traditionally said to reverse hair graying)
Garlic *Allium sativum*	*da Suan*	• antiparasitic • immune enhancing • cholesterol-lowering
Ginkgo *Ginkgo biloba*	*yin-hsing* *pai-kuo*	• memory enhancement • impotence alleviated • improves circulation • ginkgolic acid & ginnol inhibit TB bacteria & fungi
Ginseng *Panax ginseng*	*ren shen*	• balances energies • reverses irradiation damage

ASIAN HERBS (continued)

Herb	Asian Name	Function(s)
Gotu Kola *Centella asiatica*	*chi-hsueh-tsao*	• sedative • accelerates wound healing (anti-bacterial)
Licorice, Chinese *Glycyrrhiza uralensis*	*gan cao*	• most commonly utilized Chinese herb--appears as an ingredient in most prescriptions • steroid-like effects • i.e., anti-inflammatory
Mathaké *Terminalia* species	*ho-tzu* (*T. Chebula* is closely related to *T. catappa* from Malaysia & the Pacific Islands)	• kills yeast, staphylo-cocci & typhoid bacteria • weakens influenza virus • inhibits smooth muscle (antispasmodic) • protects mucous membranes against microbial effects
Mushrooms *Ganoderma lucidum, G. japonicum; Lentinus edodes*	*reishi & shiitake*	• adaptogenic; antitumor • immuno stimulant • stimulates T-helper cells, NK cells, interferons & macrophages
Pine *Pinus palustris*	*sheng-sung-chih*	• destroys scabies • traditionally used to dispel rheumatic pain, "discharge pus," "remove toxin," "control pain" (the ground powder was applied externally)
Schizandra *Schisandra chinensis*	*wu wei zei*	• adaptogenic • energy enhancing
Seaweeds Brown Algae *Laminaria* spp.; Micro Algae *Chlorella* spp. Blue-Green Algae *Lyngbya lagerheimii & Phormidium tenue*	*hai zao*	• iodine rich • contains sulfated-polysaccharides which possess antitumor activity • anti-oxidant • anti-biotic & cholesterol lowering • Immune-enhancing
Wormwood *Artemisia* and other species	*ging-hao;* *ching-hao*	• lowers fevers • it may have a mild ability to kill bacteria

Table 8

HERBS FOR WOMEN

Common Name	Latin Name	Function(s)
Angelica Dong Quai	*Angelica sinensis, A. acutiloba*	• antibacterial • antifungal • immunostimulant • antitumor • stimulates uterine muscle
Astragalus	*Astragalus membranaceus*	• stimulates immunity • antibacterial, useful for vaginitis • anti-cancer • anti-fatigue
Bearberry (Uva Ursi)	*Arctostaphylos uva-ursi*	• diuretic • treats inflammations of urinary tract • antiseptic
Blessed Thistle	*Cnicus benedictus*	• promotes menstruation • diuretic • liver & gallbladder disorders
Butcher's Broom	*Ruscus aculeatus*	• treats varicose veins and hemorrhoids
Chasteberry	*Vitex agnus-castus*	• PMS • menstrual problems
Cohosh, Black	*Cimifuga racemosa*	• lowers blood pressure • proven anti-microbial
Crampbark	*Viburnum opulus*	• relieves cramps of painful menstruation • cardiotonic
Cranberry	*Vaccinium macrocarpon*	• urinary tract infections • dissolves kidney & gall stones
Echinacea	*Echinacea angustifolia, E. purpurea, E. pallida*	• antitumor • anti-viral • immunostimulant • effective against herpes
False Unicorn	*Chamaelirium luteum*	• normalizes ovarian function • infertility • menstrual irregularities

HERBS FOR WOMEN (continued)

Common Name	Latin Name	Function(s)
Ginger	*Zingiber officinale*	• brings on menstruation • reduces thromboxane production, thereby reducing risk of heart attacks & stroke • Anti-nausea
Ginseng, Siberian	*Eleutherococcus senticosus*	• anti-stress • anti-inflammatory • improves memory • useful to combat depression, fatigue, or nervous conditions
Horse Chestnut	*Aesculus hippocastanum*	• treats varicose veins and hemorrhoids
Licorice	*Glycyrrhiza glabra*	• stimulates immunity • antiviral activity • soothes irritated urinary tract • anti-depressant • hormonal activity • protects liver
Pau D'Arco (Taheebo Tea)	*Tabebuia impetiginosa* and other species	• anti-cancer • anti-yeast • anti-parasite
Raspberry, Red	*Rubus* spp.	• anti-nausea • drunk during pregnancy to strengthen & tone uterus
Shavegrass (Springtime Horsetail)	*Equisetum hyemale, E. arvense*	• contain silica (important in bone health) • for connective tissue health • diuretic • weight loss • arthritic swelling eased
Squaw Vine (Partridge Berry)	*Mitchella repens*	• diuretic • facilitation of childbirth
Walnut, Black	*Juglans nigra*	• anti-fungal • anti-parasitic • anti-asthmatic

Table 9

VITAMIN/MINERAL SUPPLEMENTATION FOR MENOPAUSE

Supplement	Function
Vitamin A	Supports immune system; promotes growth of skin cells
Beta Carotene	Antioxidant
Vitamin D	Promotes calcium absorption
Vitamin E	Protects against hot flushes; protects against breast lumps; antioxidant protection
Vitamin C	Antioxidant; required for collagen synthesis (to hold cells together)
Vitamin B Complex	For stress management; for protein, carbohydrate and fat metabolism
Calcium	Promotes new bone growth; prevents and treats osteoporosis; lowers high blood pressure; helps prevent colon cancer
Magnesium	For regular heart beats; enhances immune-response; prevents osteoporosis; treats diabetes; treats PMS; enhances physical performance
Phosphorous	Required for bone formation and ATP production; decreases muscular fatigue; helps treat alcoholism
Potassium	Prevents and treats hypertension; prevents stroke
Iron	Enhances immunity and performance
Boron	Helps prevent and treat osteoporosis
Chromium	Prevents and treats diabetes; reduces blood cholesterol, increase HDL's; may regress atherosclerotic plaques
Copper	Helps ameliorate arthritis and inflammatory conditions; enhances immune responses; normalizes blood lipids
Iodine	Treats iodine-deficiency states (helps maintain thyroid hormones)
Manganese	Enhances immune response; balances glucose
Molybdenum	May prevent cancer; may stop sulfite-induced asthma
Selenium	For cancer prevention and treatment; enhances immunity; protects against heavy metal toxicity
Zinc	For cancer prevention and treatment; treats arthritis; alcoholism; helps wound healing; may help treat inflammatory bowel disease

Table 10
SEDATIVES

Herb	Latin	Part(s) Used	Effect
Chamomile, German	*Matricaria chamomilla*	Flowers	• Mild sleep inducer
Cohosh, Black	*Cimicifuga racemosa*	Rhizome & root	• Smooth muscle & nerve relaxant
Gotu Kola	*Centella asiatica (Hydrocotyl asiatica)*	Whole plant	• Reduces hypertension
Hops	*Humulus lupulus*	Strobiles	• Mild sleep inducer
Kava Kava	*Piper methysticum*	Root	• Intoxicant • Anticonvulsant
Lettuce, Wild	*Lactuca elongata*	Latex	• Mild pain killer & calmative
Marigold	*Calendula officinalis*	Flowers	• Lowers blood pressure
Mistletoe	*Viscum album* (European), *Phoradendron flavescens* (American)	Berries, leaves & wood	• Nervine
Motherwort	*Leonurus cardiaca*	Tops & leaves	• Nervine
Passionflower	*Passiflora incarnata*	Plant & flower	• For insomnia, dysmenorrhea, nervous tension & fatigue, hyperactivity
Scullcap	*Scutellaria laterifolia*	Whole plant	• Relaxant
Valerian	*Valerian officinalis*	Root	• Treats insomnia & hyper activity
Yarrow	*Achillea millefolium*	Flowering tops & leaves	• Calming

HERB INDEX

Introduction

No plant is complete by common name alone. Common names often vary according to country, sometimes by region. The correct name for every plant is, by convention, based on a Latin binomial. The first name is the genus to which the plant belongs, the second name the precise species.

In the following lists you will find common English names and their universal Latin equivalents. While Latin names may sometimes vary according to new discoveries by taxonomists or plant hunters, I have chosen those names most frequently found in modern guides to herbs.

ENGLISH/LATIN

LATIN/ENGLISH

INTEGRATED INDEX

A

Abdominal pains, 85, 144, 153, 238

Abortifacient, 109 - 110, 118, 133, 135, 147, 174, 205, 229, 235, 255, 259, 282 - 283, 289, 304, 318, 389, 406

Acacia, 56

Acetic acid, 372

Acne, 319

Acrylic acid, 372

Adaptogen, 71, 98, 151, 168 - 169, 171 - 172, 278, 292, 389, 398, 401 - 402, 407

Adder's Tongue, 57

Adsorbent, 389

Agar-Agar, 295 - 296

Agrimony, 58, 348

Ague, 108

AIDS, *see* HIV

Alfalfa, 59, 348

Alkaloid, 43 - 44, 52, 57, 70, 76, 81 - 82, 88, 90, 93, 96, 121, 130, 140, 145, 147 - 148, 162, 173 - 174, 186, 188, 199, 202, 204, 222, 231, 249, 261 - 262, 268, 282, 330, 336, 389

Allergy, 81, 112, 144 - 145, 163, 166, 252, 272, 275, 278, 284, 292, 302, 403 - 404, 406

Allergy and Inflammation, Herbs for, 404

Aloe Vera, 60, 62, 348, 374, 384

Alterative, 389

Amenorrhea, 61, 110, 113, 192, 218, 239, 282, 324, 389

Amino acid, 80, 161, 273, 389

Anabolic, 390

Analgesic, ix, 60, 71, 81, 96, 108, 134, 140, 202, 210, 234, 245, 249, 270, 390, 398 - 399, 404, 411

Anaphrodisiac, 330

Anemia, 66, 68, 73, 80, 107, 320, 328, 342, 390

Anemone, 62 - 63, 349, 374

Anesthetic, 52, 76, 88, 122, 125, 203, 222, 338, 390

Angelica, 40, 64 - 65, 338, 348, 374, 398, 406, 408

Anise, 49, 66, 279, 300, 338, 349

Anodyne, 82, 189, 204, 222, 226, 269, 336, 390

Antacid, 390

Anthelmintic, 83, 90, 111, 221, 273, 282, 315, 338 - 339, 390

Anthocyanin, 84, 136, 390

Anthraquinone, 62, 97, 105, 157, 168, 279, 300, 342, 390

Anti-inflammatory, 61, 70 - 71, 81, 84, 91, 95 - 96, 101 - 102, 107 - 108, 112, 118, 125, 127 - 128, 131, 139, 145, 150, 152 - 153, 156 - 157, 160, 163, 165, 171, 173, 175, 179, 183, 186 - 187, 191, 196, 205, 213, 226, 242, 245, 263, 275, 298, 300, 306, 312, 320, 322 - 323, 328, 333, 335, 339, 404, 406 - 407, 409

Antibodies, Types of, 403

Antioxidant, 160, 177, 179, 234, 275, 296, 323, 390, 400, 404, 407, 410

Antipyretic, 71, 118, 338, 390

SUPPLIERS

Please contact the following companies for herbal products:

(1) For Nature's Herbs Products:
Nature's Herbs Company
1113 North Industrial Park Drive
Orem, Utah 84057
Telephone: 1-800-437-2257

(2) For Alvita Herbal Teas:
Alvita Tea Company
A Subsidiary of Twinlabs, Inc.
2120 Smithtown Avenue
Ronkonkoma, New York 11779
Telephone: 1-800-645-5626

(3) For Twinlabs Herbal Products:
Twinlabs, Inc.
2120 Smithtown Avenue
Ronkonkoma, New York 11779
Telephone: 1-800-645-5626

(4) For all other herbs inquiries:
Fiji Tea Company
6 Knoll Lane, Suite D
Mill Valley, CA 94941
1-415-388-1006